Everyday Ethics &

Occupational Therapy

Edited by **Brenda Kornblit Kennell, MA, OTR/L, FAOTA, and Brenda S. Howard, DHSc, OTR, FAOTA**

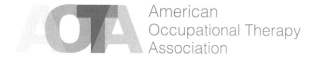

American Occupational Therapy Association

AOTA Vision 2025
As an inclusive profession, occupational therapy maximizes health, well-being, and quality of life for all people, populations, and communities through effective solutions that facilitate participation in everyday living.

Mission Statement
The American Occupational Therapy Association advances occupational therapy practice, education, and research through standard-setting and advocacy on behalf of its members, the profession, and the public.

AOTA Staff
Laura Collins, *Director of Communications and Publications*
Ashley Hofmann, *Acquisitions & Development Manager, AOTA Press*
Amy Ricci, *Product Manager & Business Analyst, AOTA Press*

Rebecca Rutberg, *Director, Marketing*
Amanda Goldman, *Marketing Manager*
Jennifer Folden, *Brand Designer*

American Occupational Therapy Association, Inc.
6116 Executive Boulevard, Suite 200
North Bethesda, MD 20852-4929
www.aota.org
To order: 1-800-729-AOTA (2682) or store.aota.org

Disclaimers
This publication is designed to provide accurate and authoritative information in regard to the subject matter covered. It is sold or distributed with the understanding that the publisher is not engaged in rendering legal, accounting, or other professional service. If legal advice or other expert assistance is required, the services of a competent professional person should be sought.
—*From the Declaration of Principles jointly adopted by the American Bar Association and a Committee of Publishers and Associations*

It is the objective of the American Occupational Therapy Association to be a forum for free expression and interchange of ideas. The opinions expressed by the contributors to this work are their own and not necessarily those of the American Occupational Therapy Association.

ISBN: 978-1-56900-641-2
eBOOK ISBN: 978-1-56900-642-9
Library of Congress Control Number: 2023951796

Cover design by Steve Parrish, AOTA, North Bethesda, MD
Composition by Manila Typesetting Company, Manila, Philippines
Printed by Gasch Printing, Odenton, MD

Suggested citation: Kennell, B. K., & Howard, B. S. (Eds.). (2024). *Everyday ethics & occupational therapy.* AOTA Press.

Contents

Acknowledgments

The editors gratefully acknowledge the following people for serving as readers and providing feedback on the ethics Advisory Opinions, many of whom were also authors.

Arameh Anvarizadeh
Rebecca Argabrite Grove
Jana Cason
Natalie Chang Wright
Aseel Dalton
Brigitte Desport
Melissa Gibson
Shanese Higgins
Megan Huber
Andre' Johnson
Barbara Kornblau
Kirstin Krause
Ed Myers
Rena Purohit
Tammy Richmond
Joyce Rioux
Deborah Yarett Slater
Cristina Reyes Smith
Megan Suman
Melissa Tilton
Michael Urban
Wayne Winistorfer

About the Editors

Brenda Kornblit Kennell, MA, OTR/L, FAOTA, has over 45 years as an occupational therapy practitioner and as an occupational therapist and occupational therapy assistant educator. Her clinical practice experience was with adults and pediatrics in various settings, including driver rehabilitation and hippotherapy. She has served the profession in various state associations, the North Carolina Board of Occupational Therapy, the Roster of Accreditation Evaluators for Accreditation Council for Occupational Therapy, and as the former Education Representative to the American Occupational Therapy Association (AOTA) Ethics Commission (2015–2021). She has published in national journals and presented at local, state, and national conferences, primarily on ethics and education.

Brenda Howard, DHSc, OTR, FAOTA, is an Associate Professor at the University of Indianapolis School of Occupational Therapy. She has been Chairperson (2020–2023) and Interim Chairperson (2019–2020) of the AOTA Ethics Commission and served 4 years as the Ethics Commission Member-at-Large (2015–2019). After more than 30 years of clinical experience in productive aging and rehabilitation/disability, she transitioned to academic education. She has published in national and international journals and has presented at international, national, and regional conferences on ethics, spirituality and occupation, vestibular rehabilitation, and falls prevention.

Figures, Tables, Exhibits, and Case Examples

Case Examples

Introduction and Foundations

Introduction: How to Use This Book

BRENDA S. HOWARD, DHSc, OTR, FAOTA

> "The time is always right to do what is right."
> —Martin Luther King, Jr., Chicago, 1966

Introduction

Occupational therapy practitioners enter the profession with a strong sense of morality and justice and a desire to do good in the world. They are quickly confronted with a health care system in which ethical principles conflict on a daily basis, and they must make decisions regarding what ethical principles and professional values they will prioritize. *Ethical decision making* can include deciding what issue is most important or should be prioritized, such as client autonomy and maintaining a secret, or veracity and beneficence—sharing the secret to benefit the client. A practitioner may want to do the right thing but not always know what that right thing is. Many ethical decisions, small and large, must continually be made in occupational therapy practice, and the practitioner must practice ethically while juggling multiple responsibilities. Often, the practitioner does not know where to find help to resolve the ethical issues they confront.

This book aims to provide help and resources to occupational therapy practitioners managing ethical problems, and provide resources to educators and students to prepare the next generation of practitioners to confront daily ethical challenges. This text takes the approach of *applied ethics,* which focuses less on the philosophical underpinnings of ethics and more on providing tools for working through and solving ethical problems as they emerge in real time. For practitioners, educators, and students, the goal is the same: by having a prepared mind for ethical reasoning and decision making, one can make sound ethical decisions in the moment.

What Are Ethics?

Ethics is defined as the study of morality (Doherty & Purtilo, 2016). *Morality* is made up of societal guidelines for right and wrong, relational factors, judgments made within specific contexts, a sense of duty, and one's own personal values. Morality ideals can vary among people; ethics, however, are what a group, organization, or society has agreed on as the way things ought to be (Doherty & Purtilo, 2016). Ethics provide ways of "examining, understanding, and applying moral principles that guide behavior and actions to address specific problems or dilemmas" (Rogers & Schill, 2021, p. 2). Ethics provide a basis for reasoning, problem solving, and decision making (Rogers & Schill, 2021).

AOTA's Code of Ethics (referred to as the Code) houses AOTA's core values and ethical principles, which comprise the aspirational aspects of the Code; and standards of conduct, which constitute the enforceable aspects of the Code. The most recent version of the Code is available on AOTA's website (https://www.aota.org/practice/practice-essentials/aota-official-documents).[1]

Language and Terminology

In this text, the term *occupational therapy practitioners* indicates both occupational therapists and occupational therapy assistants. *Clients* refers to persons, groups, or populations.

How This Book Is Organized

This book begins with an introduction to the occupational therapy profession's core values and principles and a guide to ethical decision making. Chapters on moral distress, addressing health disparities, ethics related to cognitive ability, and ethics in evaluation discuss aspects of ethical practice that are applicable to all occupational therapy practitioners. Chapters specific to practitioners working in the health care system and schools provide overviews of ethics relevant to those practice areas.

The remainder of this book is divided into seven sections that correlate to the standards sections in the Code. Each section of this book contains adaptations of ethics Advisory Opinions developed by the AOTA Ethics Commission on relevant issues that directly relate to the standards in the respective sections. These Advisory Opinions are intended to increase awareness of ethical issues and provide guidance for ethical decision making. Each Advisory Opinion contains a summary of key points, an introduction with current literature regarding the topic, discussion of the relationship of the topic to the Code, references to AOTA documents and other standards and resources to consider, tips or next steps, and one or more case examples.

The Advisory Opinions do not tell an occupational therapy practitioner what to do; rather, they inform the practitioner about the ethical issues at stake so they can weigh values, prioritize desired outcomes, and reflect on potential consequences of decisions. An appropriate response to one scenario may be inappropriate in a different ethical decision-making situation; there are no absolutely correct answers. The point is for practitioners, students, and educators to work through ethical decision-making scenarios so they can develop the ability to apply ethical reasoning in real-time situations in the clinic, community, classroom, and beyond.

---

[1] Readers who purchased this book from AOTA automatically have the Occupational Therapy Code of Ethics on their AOTA Digital Library bookshelf at https://library.aota.org.

For Practitioners

At the heart of the ethical decision-making process for every occupational therapy practitioner is the goal of collaborating with clients and providing client-centered care while upholding high ethical standards (Erler, 2016). Barriers such as time and resource constraints, reimbursement limitations, employer mandates, client wishes, and other factors may prevent a practitioner from carrying out their desired plan for ethical care, resulting in ethical or moral distress (Doherty & Purtilo, 2016). Practitioners may also face true ethical dilemmas in which they must choose between two equally good (or bad) outcomes of an ethical conflict. Even when they know the right thing to do, practitioners may be prevented from doing the right thing because they do not have the decision-making authority to enact their chosen plan (Doherty & Purtilo, 2016). In all of these circumstances, using an ethical decision-making framework can help practitioners make decisions they can live with, even if the ideal result is not achievable.

The chapters and Advisory Opinions in this book can help occupational therapy practitioners make informed, logical, and ethical decisions regarding specific ethical issues on the basis of current evidence and best practices. These Advisory Opinions, along with the Code, can also serve as references to support and defend a practitioner's position to their employer, supervisor, colleague, or external organizations. Other resources practitioners should consider using are their state, territory, or district practice act; AOTA's most recent *Occupational Therapy Practice Framework: Domain and Process*; and employer or organizational policies that uphold their position. Further, each Advisory Opinion contains references to AOTA resources and external professional resources to learn more about specific issues. Often, managing ethical issues requires a substantial amount of time and energy to investigate and gather resources to assist in the decision-making process.

Occupational therapy practitioners may wish to use this book as a

- reference in the workplace to consult when ethical issues arise,
- part of a book club with other practitioners to practice making ethical decisions,
- springboard for interprofessional discussions on ethical issues that arise frequently in a practice setting, and
- guide to consult when unsure of appropriate ethical conduct.

Although ethics may sometimes make for dry reading, they come to life when cases are considered in context with real-life situations that practitioners confront every day.

For Educators and Students

Occupational therapy educators work to instill a sense of professionalism in their students that calls them to live up to high ethical standards. Educators hope that the conduct of these soon-to-be practitioners positively reflects the values and ethics of the profession. The only way to achieve this goal is through practice of ethical reasoning, first in the classroom and then in clinical education. Students must be actively engaged in learning to develop ethical reasoning. Lectures, papers, and tests have not been as effective in instilling ethical decision making (Howard, Berger, et al., 2023). Active learning strategies such as in-person or online discussions, role playing, debates, clinical simulations, case studies, and mock ethics proceedings have demonstrated greater gains in students' ability to engage in ethical reasoning (Dieruf, 2004; Geddes et al., 2008; Howard, Berger, et al., 2023; Hudon et al., 2014). Researchers have recommended both focused ethics courses (Dieruf, 2004; Geddes et al., 2008) and ethics content integrated throughout the curriculum (Hudon et al., 2014).

Students often encounter real-world ethical problems for the first time on fieldwork. Recommendations for ethics education during fieldwork have included ethics mentorship and ethics rounds that focus on team discussions of ethical issues (Howard et al., 2020). Targeting ethics discussions on the issues most frequently encountered in practice may help prepare students better to make decisions regarding these ethical issues (Howard, Govern, et al., 2023). This book provides literature, cases, and resources for exploring the most pressing current ethical issues in occupational therapy practice.

Educators and students may wish to use this book by

- using the case examples questions to spark discussion among peers on how they would apply the Code to guide their ethical reasoning;
- applying an ethical decision-making framework to a scenario, using resources provided in an Advisory Opinion, to determine a course of action and evaluate its outcome;
- debating two or more possible courses of action regarding an ethical scenario and evaluating which course of action best aligns with occupational therapy's core values and ethical principles as outlined in the Code;
- creating an interprofessional education event where students from a variety of health professions can discuss case scenarios, compare and contrast each profession's ethical guidance on the topic, and work together to determine courses of action;
- role playing and interjecting additional context into the scenarios, to determine how differences in context may influence ethical decision making and evaluate the outcome;
- using a scenario to determine what a poor action and outcome looks like, and acting out a mock ethics proceeding using the Enforcement Procedures to determine if the poor judgment rises to the level of a violation of the Code;
- searching for real-life examples of violations of the ethical principles and standards highlighted in an Advisory Opinion, and discussing the penalties for acting unethically;
- using educator resources to compare and contrast classroom discussions with points discussed by the authors.

AOTA Ethics Process

The AOTA Ethics Commission has two roles: enforcement and education (AOTA, 2023). In the enforcement role, the Ethics Commission only has jurisdiction over AOTA members. If an occupational therapy practitioner is not a member of AOTA, the AOTA Ethics Commission has no jurisdiction over their conduct. Likewise, the AOTA Ethics Commission has no jurisdiction over persons, groups, or organizations who are not occupational therapy practitioners, unless they are members of AOTA. The Ethics Commission closely follows the Enforcement Procedures for the Code to determine whether conduct brought forth in a complaint violates the Code. If the Ethics Commission determines that a member has violated the Code, they may bring sanctions against the AOTA member that pertains to their membership (reprimand, censure, probation, suspension, or revocation). The AOTA Ethics Commission cannot bar a person from practicing occupational therapy; only a state, district, or territory licensure board has the ability to terminate a practitioner's right to practice in that jurisdiction. The Ethics Commission can, however, refer a practitioner who has behaved unethically to a licensing board or to the National Board for Certification in Occupational Therapy for review of ethical misconduct.

The Ethics Commission's educational role is to inform the AOTA membership on the Code and its application. The Code was developed through multiple iterations of membership input and was adopted through voting of the AOTA Representative Assembly, thus ensuring that the Code represents ethical standards that members have agreed truly reflect the ethical standards of the occupational therapy profession in the United States. These standards protect the public, the recipients of occupational therapy services, and the practitioners themselves (Reed & Slater, 2016). In fulfilling its educative role, the AOTA Ethics Commission has written 27 advisories, presented in this book and on the AOTA website (AOTA, 2023). The Ethics Commission members present frequently at the AOTA Annual Conference on current ethics topics. In the past, the Ethics Commission produced several editions of the *Reference Guide to the Occupational Therapy Code of Ethics* (Slater, 2016). This current volume replaces the previous Reference Guide as the educational compilation provided to the occupational therapy profession by the AOTA Ethics Commission. The editors designed this book to serve as a practical, useful guide to navigate the treacherous waters of ethical issues that occur every day in occupational therapy practice.

Summary

Managing ethical issues is never easy. Even seasoned occupational therapy practitioners encounter situations they have never faced before and must use ethical reasoning to confront these issues. However, a practitioner's ability to engage in the process of ethical reasoning does improve with practice. Using tools and resources, such as the chapters and Advisory Opinions in this book and an ethical decision-making framework, will help occupational therapy practitioners and entry-level students develop a prepared mind for ethical decision making.

REFERENCES

American Occupational Therapy Association. (2023). *Practice essentials: Ethics*. https://www.aota .org/practice/practice-essentials/ethics

Dieruf, K. (2004). Ethical decision-making by students in physical and occupational therapy. *Journal of Allied Health, 33*(1), 24–30.

Doherty, R. F., & Purtilo, R. B. (2016). *Ethical dimensions in the health professions* (6th Ed.). Elsevier.

Erler, K. (2016). Shared decision making in occupational therapy practice. In D.Y. Slater (Ed.), *Reference guide to the occupational therapy code of ethics: 2015 edition* (pp. 63–67). AOTA Press.

Geddes, E. L., Salvatori, P., & Eva, K. W. (2008). Does moral judgment improve in occupational therapy and physiotherapy students over the course of their pre-licensure training? *Learning in Health and Social Care, 8*(2), 92–104. https://doi.org/10.1111/j.1473-6861.2008.00205.x

Howard, B., Berger, P., Hendricks, M., Moll, A., Rusconi, E., Shamdin, A., & Swindemann, J. (2023, April 22). *Educational interventions for managing ethical problems in occupational therapy: A survey of practitioners' experiences* (Poster presentation). American Occupational Therapy Association INSPIRE 2023 Conference, Kansas City, MO.

Howard, B., Govern, M., Gambrel, M., Haney, M., Ottinger, H., Rippe, T., & Earls, A. (2023). Encounters with ethical problems during the first five years of practice in occupational therapy: A survey. *Open Journal of Occupational Therapy, 11*(3), 1–14. https://doi.org/10.15453/2168-6408.2078

Howard, B., Kern, C., Milliner, O., Newhart, L., & Burke, S. (2020). Comparing moral reasoning across graduate occupational and physical therapy students and practitioners. *Journal of Occupational Therapy Education, 4*(3), 5. https://doi.org/10.26681/jote.2020.040305

Hudon, A., Laliberte, M., Hunt, M., Sonier, V., Williams-Jones, B., Mazer, B., Badro, V., & Feldman, D. E. (2014). What place for ethics? An overview of ethics teaching in occupational therapy and physiotherapy programs in Canada. *Disability and Rehabilitation, 36*(9), 775–780. https://doi.org/10.3109/09638288.2013.813082

Reed, K. L., & Slater, D. Y. (2016). The function of professional ethics. In D. Y. Slater (Ed.), *Reference guide to the occupational therapy code of ethics: 2015 edition* (pp. 59–62). AOTA Press.

Rogers, B., & Schill, A. L. (2021). Ethics and Total Worker Health®: Constructs for ethical decision-making and competencies for professional practice. *International Journal of Environmental Research and Public Health, 18*(19), 10030. https://doi.org/10.3390/ijerph181910030

Slater, D. Y. (Ed.). (2016). *Reference guide to the occupational therapy code of ethics: 2015 edition*. AOTA Press.

Occupational Therapy Core Values and Principles

Introduction

Occupational therapy practitioners are committed to promoting ethical care, inclusion, participation, safety, and well-being for all recipients of service, and ethical behavior toward current and future colleagues. The AOTA Code of Ethics (the Code), an official document, outlines aspirational core values and ethical principles. These core values and ethical principles, along with enforceable standards of conduct, set expectations for conduct that the public can expect in practitioners. All occupational therapy personnel in all areas of occupational therapy are expected to abide by the Code, including occupational therapist and occupational therapy assistant practitioners and professionals (e.g., direct service, consultation, administration); educators; students in occupational therapy and occupational therapy assistant professional programs; researchers; entrepreneurs; business owners; and those in elected, appointed, or other professional volunteer service. Adherence to the Code is a commitment to benefit others, to the virtuous practice of artistry and science, to genuinely good behaviors, and to noble acts of courage.

Core Values

The occupational therapy profession is grounded in seven long-standing core values: altruism, equality, freedom, justice, dignity, truth, and prudence (American Occupational Therapy Association, 1993). The seven core values provide a foundation to guide occupational therapy personnel in their interactions with others. These core values should be considered when determining the most ethical course of action:

1. *Altruism* indicates demonstration of unselfish concern for the welfare of others. Occupational therapy personnel reflect this concept in actions and attitudes of commitment, caring, dedication, responsiveness, and understanding.
2. *Equality* indicates that all persons have fundamental human rights and the right to the same opportunities. Occupational therapy personnel demonstrate this value by maintaining an attitude of fairness and impartiality and treating all persons in a way that is

free of bias. Personnel should recognize their own biases and respect all persons, keeping in mind that others may have values, beliefs, or lifestyles that differ from their own. Equality applies to the professional arena as well as to recipients of occupational therapy services.

3. *Freedom* indicates valuing each person's right to exercise autonomy and demonstrate independence, initiative, and self-direction. A person's occupations play a major role in their development of self-direction, initiative, interdependence, and ability to adapt and relate to the world. Occupational therapy personnel affirm the autonomy of each individual to pursue goals that have personal and social meaning. Occupational therapy personnel value the service recipient's right and desire to guide interventions.

4. *Justice* indicates that occupational therapy personnel provide occupational therapy services for all persons in need of these services and maintain a goal-directed and objective relationship with recipients of service. Justice places value on upholding moral and legal principles and on having knowledge of and respect for the legal rights of recipients of service. Occupational therapy personnel must understand and abide by local, state, and federal laws governing professional practice. Justice is the pursuit of a state in which diverse communities are inclusive and are organized and structured so that all members can function, flourish, and live a satisfactory life regardless of age, gender identity, sexual orientation, race, religion, origin, socioeconomic status, degree of ability, or any other status or attributes. Occupational therapy personnel, by virtue of the specific nature of the practice of occupational therapy, have a vested interest in *social justice:* addressing unjust inequities that limit opportunities for participation in society (Ashe, 2016; Braveman & Bass-Haugen, 2009). They also exhibit attitudes and actions consistent with *occupational justice:* full inclusion in everyday meaningful occupations for persons, groups, or populations (Scott et al., 2017).

5. *Dignity* indicates the importance of valuing, promoting, and preserving the inherent worth and uniqueness of each person. This value includes respecting the person's social and cultural heritage and life experiences. Exhibiting attitudes and actions of dignity requires occupational therapy personnel to act in ways consistent with cultural sensitivity, humility, and agility.

6. *Truth* indicates that occupational therapy personnel in all situations should be faithful to facts and reality. Truthfulness, or veracity, is demonstrated by being accountable, honest, forthright, accurate, and authentic in attitudes and actions. Occupational therapy personnel have an obligation to be truthful with themselves, recipients of service, colleagues, and society. Truth includes maintaining and upgrading professional competence and being truthful in oral, written, and electronic communications.

7. *Prudence* indicates the ability to govern and discipline oneself through the use of reason. To be prudent is to value judiciousness, discretion, vigilance, moderation, care, and circumspection in the management of one's own affairs and to temper extremes, make judgments, and respond on the basis of intelligent reflection and rational thought. Prudence must be exercised in clinical and ethical reasoning, interactions with colleagues, and volunteer roles.

Principles

Principles guide ethical decision making and inspire occupational therapy personnel to act in accordance with the highest ideals. These principles are not hierarchically organized. At times, conflicts between competing principles must be considered in order to make ethical decisions. These principles may need to be carefully balanced and weighed according to professional values, individual and cultural beliefs, and organizational policies.

PRINCIPLE 1. BENEFICENCE

Occupational therapy personnel shall demonstrate a concern for the well-being and safety of persons

The principle of *beneficence* includes all forms of action intended to benefit other persons. The term *beneficence* has historically indicated acts of mercy, kindness, and charity (Beauchamp & Childress, 2019). Beneficence requires taking action to benefit others—in other words, to promote good, to prevent harm, and to remove harm (Doherty & Purtilo, 2016). Examples of beneficence include protecting and defending the rights of others, preventing harm from occurring to others, removing conditions that will cause harm to others, offering services that benefit persons with disabilities, and acting to protect and remove persons from dangerous situations (Beauchamp & Childress, 2019).

PRINCIPLE 2. NONMALEFICENCE

Occupational therapy personnel shall refrain from actions that cause harm

The principle of *nonmaleficence* indicates that occupational therapy personnel must refrain from causing harm, injury, or wrongdoing to recipients of service. Whereas beneficence requires taking action to incur benefit, nonmaleficence requires avoiding actions that cause harm (Beauchamp & Childress, 2019). The principle of nonmaleficence also includes an obligation not to impose risks of harm even if the potential risk is without malicious or harmful intent. This principle is often examined in the context of *due care*, which requires that the benefits of care outweigh and justify the risks undertaken to achieve the goals of care (Beauchamp & Childress, 2019). For example, an occupational therapy intervention might require the service recipient to invest a great deal of time and, perhaps, even discomfort; however, the time and discomfort are justified by potential long-term, evidence-based benefits of the treatment.

PRINCIPLE 3. AUTONOMY

Occupational therapy personnel shall respect the right of the person to self-determination, privacy, confidentiality, and consent

The principle of *autonomy* expresses the concept that occupational therapy personnel have a duty to treat the client or service recipient according to their desires, within the bounds of accepted standards of care, and to protect their confidential information. Often, respect for autonomy is referred to as the *self-determination principle*. Respecting the autonomy of service recipients acknowledges their agency, including their right to their own views and opinions and their right to make choices in regard to their own care and based on their own values and beliefs (Beauchamp & Childress, 2019). For example, persons have the right to make a determination regarding care decisions that directly affect their lives. In the event that a person lacks decision-making capacity, their autonomy should be respected through the involvement of an authorized agent or surrogate decision maker.

PRINCIPLE 4. JUSTICE

Occupational therapy personnel shall promote equity, inclusion, and objectivity in the provision of occupational therapy services
The principle of *justice* relates to the fair, equitable, and appropriate treatment of persons (Beauchamp & Childress, 2019). Occupational therapy personnel demonstrate attitudes and actions of respect, inclusion, and impartiality toward persons, groups, and populations with whom they interact, regardless of age, gender identity, sexual orientation, race, religion, origin, socioeconomic status, degree of ability, or any other status or attributes. Occupational therapy personnel also respect the applicable laws and standards related to their area of practice. Justice requires the impartial consideration and consistent observance of policies to generate unbiased decisions. For example, occupational therapy personnel work to create and uphold a society in which all persons have equitable opportunity for full inclusion in meaningful occupational engagement as an essential component of their lives.

PRINCIPLE 5. VERACITY

Occupational therapy personnel shall provide comprehensive, accurate, and objective information when representing the profession
The principle of *veracity* refers to comprehensive, accurate, and objective transmission of information and includes fostering understanding of such information. Veracity is based on the virtues of truthfulness, candor, honesty, and respect owed to others (Beauchamp & Childress, 2019). In communicating with others, occupational therapy personnel implicitly promise to be truthful and not deceptive. For example, when entering into a therapeutic or research relationship, the service recipient or research participant has a right to accurate information. In addition, transmission of information must include means to ensure that the recipient or participant understands the information provided.

PRINCIPLE 6. FIDELITY

Occupational therapy personnel shall treat clients (persons, groups, or populations), colleagues, and other professionals with respect, fairness, discretion, and integrity
The principle of *fidelity* refers to the duty one has to keep a commitment once it is made (Veatch et al., 2015). This commitment refers to promises made between a provider and

a client, as well as maintenance of respectful collegial and organizational relationships (Doherty & Purtilo, 2016). Professional relationships are greatly influenced by the complexity of the environment in which occupational therapy personnel work. For example, occupational therapy personnel should consistently balance their duties to service recipients, students, research participants, and other professionals, as well as to organizations that may influence decision making and professional practice.

Summary

The Code is not exhaustive; that is, the core values, principles, and standards of conduct cannot address every possible situation. Therefore, before making complex ethical decisions that require further expertise, occupational therapy personnel should seek out resources to assist with resolving conflicts and ethical issues. Resources can include, but are not limited to, ethics committees, organizational ethics officers or consultants, the AOTA Ethics Commission, and an ethical decision-making framework (see Chapter 3, "An Ethical Decision-Making Framework"). The Code helps guide and define decision-making parameters. However, ethical action goes beyond rote compliance with these core values and principles, and is a manifestation of moral character and mindful reflection.

Note. This chapter is adapted from the AOTA (2020) Code of Ethics.

REFERENCES

American Occupational Therapy Association. (1993). Core values and attitudes of occupational therapy practice. *American Journal of Occupational Therapy, 47,* 1085–1086. https://doi.org/10.5014/ajot.47.12.1085

American Occupational Therapy Association. (2020). AOTA 2020 occupational therapy code of ethics. *American Journal of Occupational Therapy, 74*(Suppl. 3), 7413410005. https://doi.org/10.5014/ajot.2020.74S3006

Ashe, A. (2016). Social justice and meeting the needs of clients. In D. Y. Slater (Ed.), *Reference guide to the Occupational Therapy Code of Ethics (2015 Edition).* AOTA Press.

Beauchamp, T. L., & Childress, J. F. (2019). *Principles of biomedical ethics* (8th ed.). Oxford University Press.

Braveman, B., & Bass-Haugen, J. D. (2009). Social justice and health disparities: An evolving discourse in occupational therapy research and intervention. *American Journal of Occupational Therapy, 63,* 7–12. https://doi.org/10.5014/ajot.63.1.7

Doherty, R., & Purtilo, R. (2016). *Ethical dimensions in the health professions* (6th ed.). Elsevier Saunders.

Scott, J. B., Reitz, S. M., & Harcum, S. (2017). Principle 4: Justice. In J. B. Scott & S. M. Reitz (Eds.), *Practical applications for the Occupational Therapy Code of Ethics (2015)* (pp. 85–95). AOTA Press.

Veatch, R. M., Haddad, A. M., & English, D. C. (2015). *Case studies in biomedical ethics: Decision-making, principles, and cases* (2nd ed.). Oxford University Press.

3

An Ethical Decision-Making Framework

BRENDA S. HOWARD, DHSc, OTR, FAOTA

Introduction

An occupational therapy practitioner's first response to an ethical issue is often one of emotion—a vague feeling that something is not quite right about a decision being made, a situation that is occurring, a thought someone has spoken, or an action someone has taken. Initially, the practitioner may have difficulty putting into words what has troubled them. They may try several ways to process the situation, including avoiding others, talking about it with a peer, or engaging in self-care. In the end, these ways of processing the ethical issue may not achieve the desired result of managing the concern or making an ethical decision. A practitioner may experience *moral distress*, or psychological distress caused by exposure to a moral event (Morley et al., 2022), if they are unable to reach an acceptable conclusion to the moral event. To find a satisfactory outcome to an ethical problem, practitioners must engage in an ethical decision-making process.

An Ethical Decision-Making Framework

An *ethical decision-making framework* is a guide in the analysis of ethical problems that requires an occupational therapy practitioner to use thoughtful reflection and judgment to determine an ethical course of action that produces a caring response (Doherty & Purtilo, 2016). Using an ethical decision-making framework is one of the best tools for taking ethical problems out of the realm of emotion and allowing oneself to examine the issues in a logical way. By rehearsing with an ethical decision-making framework, one can develop a prepared mind for managing ethical problems. Figure 3.1 depicts a composite of several ethical decision-making frameworks, such as Doherty and Purtilo's (2016) Six-Step Guide, Rogers and Schill's (2021) components of ethical decision making, and Juntunen et al.'s (2023) Socially Responsive Model. Although the steps to making ethical decisions vary and may be ordered differently among these frameworks, the elements of the process are essentially the same.

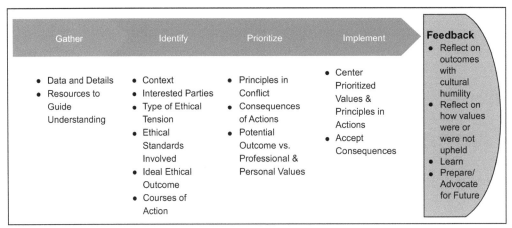

Figure 3.1. Ethical decision-making framework.

Source. Created by Ashley Wagner (Wagner et al., 2023). Used with permission.

UNDERSTAND PRINCIPLES AND CORE VALUES

First, occupational therapy practitioners must prepare to make ethical decisions by possessing a fundamental understanding and skill in applying the core values and aspirational ethical principles of the profession, housed in the AOTA Code of Ethics (the Code). These core values and principles are described in Chapter 2, "Occupational Therapy Core Values and Principles."

GATHER INFORMATION

Next, when confronted with an ethical problem, issue, dilemma, or distress, the occupational therapy practitioner should begin by gathering information. This information gathering should include a detailed understanding of the situation prompting the ethical problem; an articulation of the resources that may be helpful, including organizational policies, state and federal laws, and codes of conduct; and an understanding of who the interested parties and decision makers are in the situation (Doherty & Purtilo, 2016; Rogers & Schill, 2021).

The occupational therapy practitioner should also determine what type of ethical problem the situation exemplifies, what values or ethical principles or standards may be at stake or in conflict, or what ethical theories or approaches (e.g., deontological theories of right and wrong, teleological theories of utilitarianism, narrative approaches) may be useful to analyze the situation (Doherty & Purtilo, 2016). Following the identifying phase of ethical decision making, the practitioner should be able to clearly articulate the ethical conflict to others.

IDENTIFY POSSIBLES COURSES OF ACTION

In the next phase of ethical decision making, the occupational therapy practitioner identifies possible courses of action, considers potential outcomes of each, and applies an ethical ideal (values, theories, principles) to these actions and outcomes. If the practitioner has not already done so, this is a good point at which to involve others in the decision-making process. A trusted mentor, an interprofessional team, an organizational ethics consultant, or a supervisor may be helpful to talk over the options and consider the outcomes of each, both desirable and undesirable. The practitioner, along with other professionals as needed, can then determine which action to employ and carry out that action (Brandt & Slater, 2011; Doherty & Purtilo, 2016).

PRIORITIZE

Next, the occupational therapy practitioner should identify the highest-priority values and ethical principles for the current ethical problem and determine what the ideal ethical outcome would be (Brandt & Slater, 2011). These values and principles can be gleaned from the Code, other codes of conduct, organizational values and principles, and personal values. This prioritization is an important step, especially when personal and professional values conflict. Determining which value or principle is most important to follow in any given situation helps the practitioner decide the course of action most likely to uphold the prioritized value or principle.

IMPLEMENT

After gathering information, identifying possible courses of action, and prioritizing values and principles, it is time to select a course of action and carry it out. It is important that the occupational therapy practitioner be able to articulate their reasoning for the decision they made. The practitioner must be able to demonstrate how they considered all options and chose the one they believed to be the most effective and appropriate, based on the best available information and the priorities, and focused on providing the most caring response for the client and all involved (Brandt & Slater, 2011; Doherty & Purtilo, 2016).

SEEK FEEDBACK

Finally, and perhaps most importantly, the occupational therapy practitioner should seek feedback and reflect on the outcome of the decision made (Doherty & Purtilo, 2016; Rogers & Schill, 2021). The practitioner should consider whether the desired outcome was achieved, if prioritized values and principles were upheld, if the response to the action warrants repeating it in the future, and what preventative measures might be taken to avoid this situation in the future. The practitioner should also consider whether the ethical decision-making process was effective and what changes should be made to the process for future ethics cases (Doherty & Purtilo, 2016).

CONSIDER MULTIPLE PERSPECTIVES

A sense of cultural humility should be infused throughout the entire ethical decision-making process (Juntunen et al., 2023). *Cultural humility* is a "reflective process of understanding one's biases and privileges, managing power imbalances, and maintaining a stance that is open to others in relation to aspects of their cultural identity that are most important to them" (U.S. Department of Health & Human Services, n.d., para. 4). The occupational therapy practitioner should gather information using multiple perspectives. They should engage in self-reflection to determine if bias has any role in how they are viewing the situation. Practitioners should consult with others, perhaps of different personal and professional backgrounds from themselves, to look at the situation from a different perspective. Practitioners should consider multiple pathways toward resolution and how they may be viewed by people from differing cultural backgrounds, and they should reflect on perceptions of the chosen resolution's outcome from the perspectives of those who may hold different values (Juntunen et al., 2023).

Summary

The desired outcome of any ethical decision-making process is to have a caring response (Doherty & Purtilo, 2016). Ideally, this decision should be made with the interprofessional team and not in isolation. The decision should be one that the team may not like or love, but that they can live with and that ultimately meets the needs of the recipient of services and their support system. When an occupational therapy practitioner has prepared their mind to address ethical issues and has collaborated with others to develop a network of support, they can develop a workplace culture that supports ethical conduct.

REFERENCES

Brandt, L. C., & Slater, D. Y. (2011). Ethical dimensions of occupational therapy. In K. Jacobs & G. L. McCormack (Eds.), *The occupational therapy manager* (5th ed., pp. 469–483). AOTA Press.

Doherty, R. F., & Purtilo, R. B. (2016). *Ethical dimensions in the health professions* (6th Ed.). Elsevier.

Juntunen, C., Crepeau-Hobson, F., Riva, M. T., Baker, J., Wan, S., Davis III, C., & Caballero, A. M. (2023). Centering equity, diversity, and inclusion in ethical decision-making. *Professional Psychology: Research and Practice, 54*(1), 17–27. https://doi.org/10.1037/pro0000488

Morley, G., Bradbury-Jones, C., & Ives, J. (2022). The moral distress model: An empirically informed guide for moral distress interventions. *Journal of Clinical Nursing, 31*(9–10), 1–18. https://doi.org/10.1111/jocn.15988

Rogers, B., & Schill, A. L. (2021). Ethics and Total Worker Health®: Constructs for ethical decision making and competencies for professional practice. *International Journal of Environmental Research and Public Health, 18*(19), 10030. https://doi.org/10.3390/ijerph181910030

U.S. Department of Health & Human Services. (n.d.). *Think cultural health: CLAS, cultural competency, and cultural humility.* https://thinkculturalhealth.hhs.gov/assets/pdfs/resource-library/clas-clc-ch.pdf

Wagner, A., Amin-Arsala, T., Ungco, J. C., & Argabrite Grove. (2023). Ethical approaches to occupational justice & inclusion for LGBTQIA+ individuals [Powerpoint slides]. Presented at AOTA INSPIRE Conference, Kansas City, MO.

Moral Distress

KIMBERLY S. ERLER, PhD, OTR/L

Introduction

Health care is an evolving, dynamic environment that is often filled with uncertainties and challenges. For health care professionals, including occupational therapy practitioners who rely on rapport building and therapeutic use of self as integral parts of practice, these complexities can sometimes lead to ethical tensions. *Moral distress* is a type of ethical tension that occurs when a practitioner knows the right course of action but experiences constraints or barriers that prevent them from acting accordingly (Doherty & Purtilo, 2016; Jameton, 1984). Moral distress creates a discomfort that arises from discord between ethical action and practical limitations.

This chapter describes the background of moral distress and the related literature, including factors that contribute to its rise. It also explores the potential negative consequences of unidentified or unaddressed moral distress in occupational therapy. Finally, the chapter outlines evidence-based strategies for preventing moral distress, recognizing it when it occurs, and taking steps to combat it.

Essential Considerations

BACKGROUND

Occupational therapy practitioners commit to providing evidence-based, comprehensive, ethical care to clients. The AOTA Code of Ethics (the Code) outlines principles and standards of conduct to guide ethical practice while acknowledging that ethical action extends beyond rote compliance. It is imperative to understand the ethical principles of *beneficence* (to do or promote good), *nonmaleficence* (to do no harm), *autonomy* (self-determination), *justice* (fairness), *veracity* (honesty), and *fidelity* (faithfulness); yet, judgment and moral character are also essential for ethical decision making (Beauchamp & Childress, 2013).

Because of the complexities of health care and the messy elements of human nature, situations arise that cause ethical tension or conflict. When these ethical concerns surface, health care professionals must recognize their role as a *moral agent*, that is, a person who can differentiate between right and wrong. Although moral agents strive to maintain the highest standards of integrity while providing empathic care, obstacles often appear. The lack of clarity during ethical tensions or conflict in conjunction with the impetus to be a moral agent can result in moral distress.

Jameton (1984) is credited with coining the term *moral distress,* referring to the feeling or experience that occurs when a moral agent knows the right thing to do but encounters constraints that prevent them from acting in such a way. Moral distress was originally identified and has been extensively investigated in the field of nursing. The research has shown that moral distress in nursing has negative consequences on the clinician's well-being, patient care, and the entire health system (Burston & Tuckett, 2013; Henrich et al., 2017). In today's health care climate, the construct of moral distress extends beyond the field of nursing and is recognized as a growing problem for all health care professionals (Ulrich et al., 2010).

Although studies have confirmed that moral distress exists in occupational therapy (Brazil et al., 2010; Mukherjee et al., 2009; Penny et al., 2014; Slater & Brandt, 2009), research on moral distress specific to occupational therapy is in its infancy compared to the field of nursing. Slater and Brandt (2009) suggest that occupational therapy practitioners are at high risk of moral distress, and until further research specific to occupation therapy is completed, the similarities to moral distress in nursing should be considered. Penny et al. (2016) describe the development of a moral distress scale for occupational therapists that has the potential to expand the understanding of moral distress in occupational therapy through further research with a valid and reliable instrument.

CONTRIBUTING FACTORS

Moral distress typically occurs when there are ethical concerns, tensions, or conflicts. In occupational therapy, practitioners experience a broad range of ethical tensions. Some of these are unique to occupational therapy, while others are overarching across health care professions. Bushby et al. (2015) reviewed the current peer review literature on ethical tensions in occupational therapy practice and found seven themes, including

- resource and system issues,
- ethical principles and values,
- safety,
- vulnerable clients,
- interpersonal conflicts,
- professional standards, and
- practice management.

Another study (Mukherjee et al., 2009) explored moral distress among rehabilitation professionals, including occupational therapy practitioners, and found three broad categories of moral distress, including

- institutional ethics (e.g., health care environment, reimbursement pressure),
- professional practice (e.g., codes of conduct or behavior, professionalism), and
- clinical decision making (e.g., goal setting, discharge planning).

Clear overlaps exist between the ethical tensions that occupational therapy practitioners experience and the reported categories of moral distress. Slater and Brandt (2009) found that external factors, which are typically market driven, were major contributors to moral distress in occupational therapy practitioners and suggest that this is related to service delivery models in which occupational therapy services are a source of revenue. Practitioners are being asked to do more in less time and with fewer resources. Although nurses may feel financial or budget constraints indirectly, health professionals like occupational therapists, physical therapists, speech therapists, and physicians are more likely to experience the economic pressure directly from current practice and reimbursement models; this pressure, in turn, contributes to moral distress. Although early research demonstrates that occupational therapy practitioners experience moral distress, there are no indicators that practice setting, degree earned, age, or years of practice increase a practitioner's risk for moral distress (Penny et al., 2014). These findings indicate that no practitioner is immune to moral distress and further research is needed to understand the extent of moral distress in occupational therapy to create effective interventions and, more importantly, prevention strategies.

IMPLICATIONS

Moral distress in occupational therapy can have a negative impact on the emotional and physical well-being of the practitioner, the culture of the workplace, the care of clients, job satisfaction, and staff retention (Burston & Tuckett, 2013; Penny et al., 2014; Whitehead et al., 2015). Moral distress is a type of stress that can lead to burnout. *Burnout* is the state of emotional and physical exhaustion from chronic stress that results in frustration, inability to meet the demands of the job, and disengagement from others (Lydon, 2015).

Research has shown that occupational and physical therapy practitioners experience emotional exhaustion and negative feelings about their work, clients, and personal accomplishments at concerning rates (Balogun et al., 2002). Some research suggests that the lack of professional identity among occupational therapy practitioners is associated with burnout and that practitioners are at risk for all aspects of burnout, including depersonalization (Edwards & Dirette, 2010).

Vision 2025 (American Occupational Therapy Association, 2017) states "Occupational therapy maximizes health, well-being, and quality of life for all people, populations, and communities through effective solutions that facilitate participation in everyday living" (p. 1). To enact this vision, the occupational therapy workforce needs to be healthy, motivated, and satisfied. Addressing moral distress is crucial to the continued excellence and expansion of occupational therapy.

Practical Applications in Occupational Therapy

There are two categories of approaches to combat moral distress in occupational therapy: prevention and intervention. All occupational therapy practitioners, or moral agents, should be empowered to have moral courage and advocate for what they perceive to be right and ethical. *Moral courage* is the courage to overcome the fear of adverse consequences and act in accordance with ethical standards and values (Doherty & Purtilo, 2016).

Occupational therapy managers are uniquely situated to influence a culture of moral courage and ethical action. Occupational managers should implement processes and supports that aim to both prevent and reduce moral distress (Penny et al., 2014). Slater and Brandt (2009) proposed six strategies:

- recognizing moral distress
- implementing educational strategies
- facilitating interdisciplinary research
- improving communication
- creating healthy organizational work environments
- promoting ethical leadership.

RECOGNIZING MORAL DISTRESS

Identifying and naming moral distress in occupational therapy practice is a powerful strategy for mitigating the distress. If an occupational therapy practitioner has the knowledge to recognize and the ability to describe their feelings of powerlessness in an ethical situation, they can seek support or resources, (e.g., societal statements, ethics advisory opinions, ethics committees). By recognizing the ethical tension as moral distress, a practitioner can identify sources or patterns of the distress and create a starting point for intervention.

IMPLEMENTING EDUCATIONAL STRATEGIES

Continuing education on ethical matters related to health care and occupational therapy is a crucial component to combating moral distress. Engaging in or creating opportunities for professional growth strengthens one's professional identity and enhances one's ability to engage in dialogue around ethical tensions. Managers can support both formal and informal forums for education on ethics and moral support.

FACILITATING INTERDISCIPLINARY RESEARCH

Further research is required to understand moral distress in occupational therapy, but because occupational therapy practitioners function as part of a health care team, interdisciplinary moral distress research is also essential. As discussed previously, many members of the interdisciplinary team experience moral distress. Understanding how team dynamics negatively or positively affect moral distress will lead to more effective interventions and elevation of the team effectiveness.

IMPROVING COMMUNICATION

Communication continues to be one of the biggest challenges in health care today. Fostering an environment where all individuals feel comfortable expressing their opinions in a professional manner is central to mitigating moral distress. Managers must create a safe space for open dialogue around difficult topics. Although individuals may have different values and opinions, respectful communication allows for necessary discourse and often leads to actionable solutions.

CREATING A HEALTHY WORK ENVIRONMENT

Many of the strategies already discussed contribute to the creation of a healthy work environment. Communication among health care leaders, managers, and front-line clinicians is crucial. If all occupational therapy practitioners see themselves as moral agents with moral courage, the health of a practice environment will be strengthened. Occupational therapy managers must emphasize respect for all individuals, both clients and staff.

PROMOTING ETHICAL LEADERSHIP

Ethics and leadership are inextricably intertwined. A leader cannot be effective without careful consideration of ethics. Even in challenging situations, an ethical leader will advocate for optimal solutions and processes that adhere to the professional and ethical standards. A strong ethical leader will set the example for all staff members and create an environment that upholds the highest expectations.

OCCUPATIONAL THERAPY ETHICS ROUNDS

Occupational therapy ethics rounds are forums that bring together occupational therapy practitioners and create an opportunity to discuss emerging ethical issues and honestly reflect on practice (Erler, 2017). These rounds allow practitioners to practice communication skills for difficult topics, demonstrate a commitment to education and ethics by leadership, and strengthen the ability to recognize an ethical issue. These rounds may be initiated by managers or practitioners and be held at a specific frequency (e.g., quarterly) or on an as-needed basis when challenging cases arise. Not only do ethics rounds enhance a practitioner's ability to recognize moral distress, the rounds also act as a support system and strategy for preventing and mitigating moral distress.

Summary

Moral distress exists in occupational therapy and can have serious negative consequences to the practitioner, the client, and the health care system (see Case Example 4.1). Understanding the Code and ethical principles provides occupational therapy practitioners with the foundational knowledge and professional standards that must be upheld in challenging ethical scenarios. All practitioners should recognize their role as a moral agent, and managers should strive to facilitate an environment that emphasizes moral courage. An occupational therapy manager can implement strategies such as occupational

CASE EXAMPLE 4.1. MORAL DISTRESS IN INPATIENT ACUTE CARE

Sun is an occupational therapy manager overseeing a department of 15 practitioners in an inpatient acute care setting. Sun overheard an occupational therapist expressing frustration and feelings of powerlessness about a recent situation with a client. Sun decided to meet with the therapist to learn more about the case.

The therapist explained that she first met the client, Jorge, a few days ago on the neurological intensive care unit. Jorge had flown from Mexico, where he lives, to the United States to attend his niece's college graduation. Upon landing, Jorge was noted to have right-side weakness and speech difficulties. He was immediately taken to the closest emergency room and was found to have a left middle cerebral artery stroke. The neurology team treated him with IV tissue plasminogen activator, a clot-busting medication.

During the initial evaluation, which occurred approximately 30 hours after Jorge was admitted, the therapist noted that Jorge had already demonstrated improved motor strength in his right leg but his right arm did not have any active movement, and he continued to have some expressive communication impairments. Over the next few days, Jorge made steady progress but remained below his baseline. Occupational therapy, physical therapy, and speech therapy all recommended that he be transferred to an inpatient acute rehabilitation facility for intense neurorehabilitation.

Despite the entire interprofessional team recognizing that Jorge had excellent rehabilitation potential, the case manager informed everyone during rounds that he was not eligible for transfer to inpatient rehabilitation because he did not have health insurance in the United States or the personal financial resources to cover the cost. Sun identified that the therapist was experiencing moral distress because she knew that the most client-centered, evidence-based, ethical course should include rehabilitation for the client but felt frustrated and powerless because of an external constraint.

Questions
1. What is contributing to moral distress in this case example?
2. What steps could Sun take to combat moral distress in this situation and future situations that may arise?
3. What are the potential consequences of not addressing the moral distress?

therapy ethics rounds and recognition programs that emphasize ethics, communication, culture, processes, and supports aimed at preventing and reducing moral distress.

Learning Activity

Reflect on a time where you felt a sense of frustration and powerlessness.

- What do you think was contributing to your moral distress in this situation?
- How did you proceed?
- Would you do anything differently if a similar situation occurred today?
- What strategies can you implement to prevent moral distress in your current practice setting?

Note. An version of this chapter was previously published in *The Occupational Therapy Manager, 6th Edition,* edited by Karent Jacobs and Guy L. McCormack. Copyright © 2019 by the American Occupational Therapy Association. Reprinted with permission.

REFERENCES

American Occupational Therapy Association. (2017). Vision 2025. *American Journal of Occupational Therapy, 71*(3), 7103420010. https://doi.org/10.5014/ajot.2017.713002

Balogun, J. A., Titiloye, V., Balogun, A., Oyeyemi, A., & Katz, J. (2002). Prevalence and determinants of burnout among physical and occupational therapists. *Journal of Allied Health, 31*(3), 131–139.

Beauchamp, T. L., & Childress, J. F. (2013). *Principles of biomedical ethics* (7th ed.). Oxford University Press.

Brazil, K., Kassalainen, S., Ploeg, J., & Marshall, D. (2010). Moral distress experienced by health care professionals who provide home-based palliative care. *Social Science and Medicine, 71*(9), 1687–1691. https://doi.org/10.1016/j.socscimed.2010.07.032

Burston, A., & Tuckett, A. G. (2013). Moral distress: Contributing factors, outcomes and interventions. *Nursing Ethics, 20*(3), 312–324. https://doi.org/10.1177/0969733012462049

Bushby, K., Chan, J., Druif, S., Ho, K., & Kinsella, E. A. (2015). Ethical tensions in occupational therapy practice: A scoping review. *British Journal of Occupational Therapy, 78*(4), 212–221. https://doi.org/10.1177/0308022614564770

Doherty, R. F., & Purtilo, R. D. (2016). *Ethical dimensions in the health professions* (6th ed.). Elsevier.

Edwards, H., & Dirette, D. (2010). The relationship between professional identity and burnout among occupational therapists. *Occupational Therapy in Health Care, 24*(2), 119–129. https://doi.org/10.3109/07380570903329610

Erler, K. (2017). The role of occupational therapy ethics rounds in practice. *OT Practice, 22*(13), 15–18.

Henrich, N. J., Dodek, P. M., Gladstone, E., Alden, L., Keenan, S. P., Reynolds, S., & Rodney, P. (2017). Consequences of moral distress in the intensive care unit: A qualitative study. *American Journal of Critical Care, 26*(4), e48–e57. https://doi.org/10.4037/ajcc2017786

Jameton, A. (1984). *Nursing practice: The ethical issues.* Englewood Cliffs, NJ: Prentice Hall.

Lydon, A. (2015). *Burnout among health professionals and its effect on patient safety.* https://psnet.ahrq.gov/perspective/burnout-among-health-professionals-and-its-effect-patient-safety

Mukherjee, D., Brashler, R., Savage, T. A., & Kirschner, K. L. (2009). Moral distress in rehabilitation professionals: Results from a hospital ethics survey. *PM&R, 1*(5), 450–458. https://doi.org/10.1016/j.pmrj.2009.03.004

Penny, N. H., Bires, S. J., Bonn, E. A., Dockery, A. N., & Pettit, N. L. (2016). Moral distress scale for occupational therapists: Part 1. Instrument development and content validity. *American Journal of Occupational Therapy, 70*(4), 1–8. https://doi.org/10.5014/ajot.2015.018358

Penny, N. H., Ewing, T. L., Hamid, R. C., Shutt, K. A., & Walter, A. S. (2014). An investigation of moral distress experienced by occupational therapists. *Occupational Therapy in Health Care, 28*(4), 382–393. https://doi.org/10.3109/07380577.2014.933380

Slater, D. Y., & Brandt, L. C. (2009). Combating moral distress. *OT Practice, 14*(2), 13–18.

Ulrich, C. M., Hamric, A. B., & Grady, C. (2010). Moral distress: A growing problem in the health professions? *Hastings Center Report, 40*(1), 20–22. https://doi.org/10.1353/hcr.0.0222

Whitehead, P. B., Herbertson, R. K., Hamric, A. B., Epstein, E. G., & Fisher, J. M. (2015). Moral distress among healthcare professionals: Report of an institution-wide survey. *Journal of Nursing Scholarship, 47*(2), 117–125. https://doi.org/10.1111/jnu.12115

5

Ethics in the Health Care System

SARAH SHIRLEY PULLANI, DOT, MDiv, OTR/L

Introduction

In today's world with complex and ever-changing health, technology, cultural, and demographic considerations, ethics and ethical reasoning have become integral to how occupational therapy practitioners conduct their everyday professional duties. In this chapter, *ethics* is defined as a systemic process of reflection on the language, conventions, methods, and guidelines of moral action (Doherty, 2020). *Morality* is a system of norms to distinguish between right and wrong that can be influenced by culture, geography, religion, and other binding factors and can also transcend these influences as in the case of "common morality" (Varkey, 2021, p. 18).

Ethics

Ethics are a central characteristic of any professional practice. In addition, *codes of ethics,* along with personal ethics, define the range of appropriate relationships and service delivery within a profession. For most practitioners, their profession's code of ethics mediates how they relate to other professionals, clients, and the profession itself. Within the health care system, occupational therapy practitioners work with many health care professionals, each with their own code of ethics. Still, most codes of ethics within health care have unifying themes based on the four principles of biomedical ethics established by Beauchamp and Childress in their 1979 seminal work *Principles of Biomedical Ethics* (most recently updated in 2019). The American Occupational Therapy Association (AOTA) also provides several resources on how to abide by and articulate ethical conduct, which is discussed in more detail in the following sections.

BIOMEDICAL ETHICS

The field of biomedical ethics gained popularity as a subset of the larger field of Bioethics around the 1970s with the seminal book of *Principles of Biomedical Ethics* by Beauchamp and Childress. *Bioethics* is a multidisciplinary field of study, including research, public health, organizational, and clinical ethics (Varkey, 2021). *Biomedical ethics* and *clinical medical ethics* are interchangeable terms referring to the application of ethical reasoning to specific clinical situations (Varkey, 2021).

The four principles of biomedical ethics delineated by Beauchamp and Childress (2019) are common core values in health care professional ethics and guide professional behavior. Most health care professions use these principles, listed here, as a standard approach toward biomedical ethics:

- *Autonomy* refers to informed consent and awareness that patients have the capacity to make their own decisions.
- *Nonmaleficence* refers to doing no harm (e.g., the Hippocratic Oath) through omission or commission. This principle also relates to health care provider competency.
- *Beneficence* refers to promoting good. This principle goes hand in hand with nonmaleficence. Health care providers should act in ways that benefit the patient or prevent the patient from being harmed. Beneficence may have implications for issues regarding patient safety that conflict with patient autonomy.
- *Justice* refers to equality and fairness in access to treatment and allocation of resources.

CLINICAL MEDICAL ETHICS

Clinical medical ethics (CME) is a field that was established in 1972 by physician Mark Siegler when he wrote the first issue of the *Journal of Clinical Ethics* with Edmund Pellegrino and Peter A. Singer. The journal's goal was to focus on the daily ethical decision making of health care practitioners in their routine interactions with patients (Siegler, 2019). Siegler argued that the lived experiences of physicians and other health care practitioners in navigating daily ethical decisions with their patients could not be fully resolved by theoretical rhetoric developed by bioethicists, theologians, or lawyers who were not health care professionals. Therefore, the evolution of shared decision making between doctors and patients was strongly tied to the development of CME and its emphasis on relationships within the daily practice of medicine.

The central role of the relationship between the health care provider and the patient in CME is an example of how this field approaches typical daily routines to shape an ethical viewpoint for health care practitioners. Daily practices may occur between the provider and the patient or among providers focused on specific patient care. For example, *huddles,* or brief, interprofessional, patient-focused gatherings, can be a daily practice among health care practitioners that have been shown to increase communication, problem solving, and medical error prevention (Lin et al., 2022).

Similar to occupational therapy practitioners, nurses describe relationships as central to their experience in navigating ethical concerns (Barlow et al., 2018). A qualitative nursing study identified four significant themes that nurses consider when resolving ethical dilemmas: what is best for the patient, accountability, collaboration, and concern for others (Barlow et al., 2018). Of these four themes, what is best for the patient was identified as the highest value, and the relationship with the patient was the most important within that category. The other three themes involved different relationships, including those with the patient's family and the health care team.

Ethical Approaches

Different ethical approaches offer distinctive perspectives to consider when deciding the most ethical course of action. The most common ethical approaches used in health care include utilitarianism, deontology, and virtue ethics.

UTILITARIANISM

Utilitarianism is a style of discernment that considers the best choice to do the most good for the most people or the least harm to the fewest people (Internet Encyclopedia of Philosophy, n.d.-a). The philosophy is that the ends justify the means. This approach requires careful examination of all actions and potential consequences. An example of utilitarian discernment is using cost-benefit or cost-effectiveness analysis to determine resource allocation. Marseille and Kahn (2019) proposed three applications for utilitarianism in resource allocation for global health:

1. Resource allocation should follow a cost-effectiveness analysis to maximize overall benefit.
2. Every life has equal value, without bias toward identified individuals, such as those who have sought treatment versus people hoping to avoid illness.
3. No preference is given toward actions that seek to mediate inequality, such as poverty, unless they coincide with the first objective of providing maximal benefit according to a cost-effectiveness analysis.

An example of utilitarian resource allocation would be to mail free COVID-19 test kits to every household and to offer federally sponsored community testing to reduce disease transmission by delivering one test to each person regardless of the presence of disease, living situation, or ability to obtain one on their own.

DEONTOLOGY

Deontology, an approach initially developed by the German philosopher Immanuel Kant (Internet Encyclopedia of Philosophy, n.d.-c), is a rule-based approach that focuses on the duty and obligations of an individual (Birchley, 2021). Deontology prioritizes respect for the individual as an autonomous person. According to deontology, duty is guided by human rights and should always be maintained, even when it does not promote the greater good (Internet Encyclopedia of Philosophy, n.d.-b). The emphasis is on human rights and the dignity and worth of individuals rather than on outcomes in which the ends justify the means (Birchley, 2021).

Health care practices that ensure informed consent and adherence to the standards of the Health Insurance Portability and Accountability Act of 1996 (P. L. 104–191) are examples of deontological ethics at work. Each person has a right to autonomy and privacy in choosing health care options with their doctor.

VIRTUE ETHICS

An older approach from Aristotle and Greek philosophy, *virtue ethics,* focuses on the character of the person rather than the outcome or process. In paraphrasing Aristotle, Lyon (2021) described *virtue* as "a disposition or state which both improves the goodness of the person and causes them to succeed in their role" (p. 2). Virtue ethicists claim that rule- and principle-based ethics are too abstract and that clinicians can more easily identify with virtues such as teamwork, honesty, justice, and fairness (Internet Encyclopedia of Philosophy, n.d.-b; Lyon, 2021).

Virtue ethics are related to the nursing concept of the *ethics of care,* which involves routinely listening to patients, understanding their priorities, and responding to their needs accordingly (Falcó-Pegueroles et al., 2021). Nurses who use a standard of doing what they think is the most caring thing for their patients as a basis for ethical action are using virtue ethics.

Occupational therapy gives similar importance to the virtue of care by placing a high value on client-centered practices and therapeutic use of self. Virtue ethics would lead occupational therapy practitioners to reflect on being more caring, empathetic, and compassionate service providers as part of their professional judgment and clinical decision making. Virtue ethics are person or agent centered, because they focus on the judgment of the individual actor (Barlow et al., 2018).

Ethics Within Occupational Therapy

The central values and tenets of occupational therapy are expressed in official documents such as the *Occupational Therapy Practice Framework (OTPF)* and the AOTA Code of Ethics (the Code). These official documents, AOTA position statements, and advisory opinions provide a full scope of professional values through which occupational therapy practitioners can align their expression of ethical values in clinical and academic settings.

In her AOTA presidential address of 2017, Amy Lamb encouraged occupational therapy practitioners to consider their "OT Why," asking, "What led you to occupational therapy? Why did you choose to give your time and service to this profession?" Knowing the answers to these questions can aid practitioners in prioritizing their values and the profession's core values as they grapple with complex ethical tensions—a clear "OT Why" can sustain individual practitioners and the profession through challenging times.

OCCUPATIONAL THERAPY PRACTICE FRAMEWORK

The *OTPF* delineates four cornerstones of occupational therapy: the profession's core values, therapeutic use of occupation, professional behaviors and attitudes, and understanding of the therapeutic use of self. It describes each of these cornerstones along with what contributes to them, including client-centered practice, cultural humility, ethics, and professionalism, among others. The process section of the *OTPF* lays out the expected actions of occupational therapy practitioners, which can be important in determining courses of action that are consistent with professional ethics.

AOTA CODE OF ETHICS

The Code is a public document comprising three sections: core values, principles, and standards of conduct. The core values guide occupational therapy practitioners' relationships with others and reflect the virtues that would ideally be expressed through occupational therapy practice. They include the following:

- *altruism:* unselfish concern for the welfare of others
- *equality:* impartiality, fairness, respect for diversity, and an awareness of the fundamental human rights and opportunities of all people
- *freedom:* self-determination to choose between autonomy and societal membership and affirming the rights of people to pursue goals that have personal and social meaning to them
- *justice:* delivery of professional services to all needing occupational therapy services and abidance of laws governing professional practice
- *dignity:* respecting the uniqueness and inherent worth of all people
- *truth:* veracity, truthfulness, accountability, and authenticity in all professional dealings
- *prudence:* actions governed by rational thought, discretion, moderation, and reflection.

These core values guide decision making involving professional values, individual and cultural beliefs, and organizational policies. The values are not listed here in any particular order, but the first four align with Beauchamp and Childress's (2019) four principles of biomedical ethics: beneficence, nonmaleficence, autonomy, and justice. In addition, the Code includes the principles of *veracity,* which entails providing accurate, objective, and truthful information at all times, and *fidelity,* which refers to having respect, discretion, fairness, and integrity with colleagues, clients, and other professionals. The final section of this code is the standards of conduct, which include specific, enforceable statements of professional expectations in the areas of professional integrity, therapeutic relationships, documentation and reimbursement, service delivery, professional competence, communication, and professional civility.

AOTA ETHICS COMMISSION

The AOTA Ethics Commission is a representative, voluntary body within AOTA responsible for providing educational resources and enforcing the Code of Ethics among AOTA members. In addition to revising the Code of Ethics to be approved by the Representative Assembly, the commission offers ethics education. It provides advisory opinions on its member-only website on specific matters that apply ethical codes to evolving practice issues. It covers topics such as telehealth, ethics during a pandemic, productivity and reimbursement, and professional boundaries.

ETHICS OUTCOMES AND ENFORCEMENT

Three ethical enforcement pathways exist for reporting and sanctioning occupational therapy practitioners: state regulatory boards, AOTA, and the National Board for Certification in Occupational Therapy (NBCOT). Note that state regulatory boards apply only if the complainant is not a member of the latter organizations. First, if the practitioner accused of ethical violations is a member of AOTA at the time of the violation, a complaint can be made to the AOTA Ethics Commission to determine whether the practitioner should be censured or removed from membership. The commission usually initially discusses the issue with the practitioner, recommending corrective steps to be taken, following appropriate protocols within the practitioner's workplace. Complaints or ethical concerns made to AOTA typically are related to acts that violate the seven areas covered in the standards of conduct (described previously). Second, if the practitioner is certified through NBCOT, a complaint may be made to the board, which maintains a published list of disciplinary actions (NBCOT, 2020).

Third, and most significant, complaints made to a state regulatory board typically entail illegal actions and professional acts that can result in a legal conviction, with the potential to remove the license from the practitioner. Complaints to the state regulatory board generally involve violations of the practice act of that state. They may also be made for violations explicitly stated in the standards of conduct. For most states, any person can contact the office of the secretary of state or go to their website for details on how to file a complaint in writing and what documentation may be needed. Finally, ethics violations can be resolved through the criminal or civil justice system if they involve illegal actions or result in harm caused by improper practices or gross negligence.

Ethical Tensions in the Health Care Settings

Settings such as acute care, inpatient rehabilitation, and skilled nursing facilities require occupational therapy practitioners to collaborate with patients and interprofessional teams to create and carry out a plan of care and a discharge plan. Durocher and Kinsella (2021) identified ethical tensions that are likely to surface in a practice context that may have diverse agendas and the potential for competing allegiances. Refer to Exhibit 5.1 for the five types of ethical tensions and examples of each.

Ethical tensions are also commonly related to resource and systemic issues, upholding ethical principles and values, client safety, working with vulnerable clients, interpersonal conflicts, professional standards, and practice management (Bushby et al., 2015). The results of such tensions can have negative consequences such as decreased standard of care and practitioner burnout. However, they can also have positive outcomes, such as an opportunity for change and increased job satisfaction, if resolved in a productive manner (Bushby et al., 2015).

Ethics Typology

In reflecting on ethical behavior, it is helpful to use definitions of ethics-based scenarios that a clinician may encounter. An *ethical dilemma* is a decision that requires a person to

EXHIBIT 5.1.
ETHICAL TENSIONS AND EXAMPLES

Ethical Tensions	Example
Between two different plans or priorities of care for the patient	A patient who is at risk for falling without further rehabilitation but wants to be discharged home, although it is considered unsafe (could be expressed as competing core values of autonomy and nonmaleficence)
Between the values of the patient and the practitioner	A patient who engages in risky behavior, such as drinking and driving, causing an accident, and now requires rehabilitation
Between loyalty to coworkers and an external entity such as a patient or regulatory board	A situation of ethical silence in which a practitioner knows of a colleague's actions that are not within the standard of care set by an accreditation body but is reluctant to call out or report the colleague's behavior
Between the values of the practitioner and supervisory mandates	A practitioner who wants to delay the discharge of a patient because of evidence of ongoing need for therapy but whose employer is reluctant to extend care because of insurance plan limitations or patient's inability to pay
Between loyalty to patients and regulatory boards	A patient who wants to give a gift to a practitioner, as an important cultural practice, but regulatory entities do not allow gift giving

Note. Types of ethical tensions from Durocher & Kinsella (2021).

prioritize one of two or more ethical principles (Drolet et al., 2017). An ethical dilemma could also be characterized as a choice of right action versus right action or as a situation in which each side could be partially right from a particular viewpoint, even though neither is ideal. Erler (2018) described an ethical dilemma of how to proceed when a patient with a history of drinking and driving wanted to go home to continue drinking rather than be admitted to an inpatient rehabilitation center to address functional performance with ADLs. In this case, neither choice was optimal, and the therapist needed to choose between the ethical action of respecting the client's wishes (autonomy) and the ethical action of doing good (beneficence) or preventing harm (nonmaleficence).

In contrast, an *ethical temptation* occurs when organizational or personal agendas challenge a clear ethical value (Drolet et al., 2017). For example, a clinician is asked to spend less time with Patient A, who has the same diagnosis and condition as Patient B, because Patient A's insurance pays at a lower rate. In this situation, the clinician must choose between an ethical action and a questionable action for which they may experience some degree of internal or external pressure toward selecting the questionable choice.

Another concept related to ethics includes *ethical silence,* which is not taking action to report or correct a known unethical situation or behavior of a colleague (Drolet et al., 2017). *Ethical distress* may occur when a practitioner is in a situation involving moral temptation, ethical dilemma, or ethical silence (Drolet et al., 2017), resulting in anxiety or discomfort. *Ethical tension* refers to any combination of ethical distress, moral dilemma or temptation, and ethical uncertainty (Durocher & Kinsella, 2021).

Ethical Reasoning

Ethical reasoning is the process by which a practitioner can follow a logical path to resolve ethical tensions. One path to resolution is based on the scientific method, taking the following common steps (Doherty, 2019):

1. *Define the problem:* Determine whether it is an ethical, legal, or clinical problem and what ethical values are in jeopardy.
2. *Gather initial data:* Ask, Who is involved? What is at stake?
3. *Formulate a hypothesis:* Create a summary of the ethical principles and/or rationales involved in the situation.
4. *Gather evidence:* Problem solve by considering all the options and the ethical components of each action to various stakeholders.
5. *Take action:* After reviewing all of the reasonable options, make a decision and follow through on the clinical plan that seems most prudent.
6. *Reflect:* Think about how the process worked and how it could be improved, the actions taken, and whether the outcomes were beneficial. Document your thoughts for future reference.

ETHICAL REASONING RESOURCES

The Code and AOTA's Standards of Practice for Occupational Therapy (hereafter Standards of Practice) can help practitioners identify the specific ethics involved in an ethical dilemma (Slater, 2016). In addition, the following tools can assist practitioners in evaluating a dilemma and options for resolution:

- *CELIBATE.* CELIBATE (clinical ethics and legal issues bait all therapists equally; Kornblau & Burkhardt, 2012) uses a 10-step process to guide practitioners in consideration of factors contributing to a dilemma, including who is involved and what the motivations and legal concerns are. It encourages practitioners to use the questions to analyze options and choose an action course.
- *Realm–Individual Process–Situation Model.* This model focuses on the analysis of three primary components of an ethical dilemma: determining the realm involved (i.e., individual, organizational, societal), which of four moral processes are in play (i.e., sensitivity, judgment, motivation, ego strength), and the type of situation (i.e., problem, distress, dilemma, temptation, silence) involved (Kirsch, 2009).

- *Decision-making triangle.* This tool helps practitioners organize evidence and theory within ethical principles as well as guide ethical decision making (Tannahill & Douglas, 2014).

The Joint Commission, an accreditation body for hospitals and health care programs, and payers require that facilities establish formal pathways and processes that clinicians can access to select the most ethical course of action (Caulfield, 2007). The first level of assistance is often the clinician's clinical supervisor. If additional assistance is desired, an organizational ethics committee or other oversight body should be available for consultation or investigation.

CREATING ETHICAL ENVIRONMENTS

Because ethical dilemmas and their associated stress are commonly experienced throughout a career in occupational therapy (Bushby et al., 2015), creating a supportive ethical environment can help resolve and decrease the strain of such problems. Rather than avoiding ethical dilemmas, occupational therapy practitioners need to build the skills necessary to navigate them in a way that expresses the authentic value of occupational therapy.

One way to build skills in ethical reasoning is by engaging in ethics rounds (Erler, 2017). *Ethics rounds* are a process, supported by AOTA, in which groups of colleagues discuss real-life or hypothetical ethical situations within a structured framework. The groups can consist of an interprofessional team of work colleagues; an intraprofessional group of local practitioners (Erler, 2017); or an online group, eliminating geographical boundaries, of interested practitioners.

Ethics rounds have a twofold purpose: to build skills in *ethical sensitivity,* which is increased awareness of ethical tensions, and to create a social support structure for practitioners dealing with ethical tensions (Drolet et al., 2017). The outcomes of ethics rounds may increase *ethical resiliency,* the ability to work through an ethical situation without detrimental moral injury or stress, or inspire *ethical advocacy,* which addresses organizational or systemic challenges to ethical practice (Erler, 2017).

PRACTICAL TIPS IN NAVIGATING ETHICAL TENSIONS

Health care providers are expected to base their clinical and ethical decisions on professional values and societal norms (Kornblau & Burkhardt, 2012). Each situation, even when similar to others, is unique and needs to be considered on its own merits. Factors to keep in mind include the practitioner's moral obligations, responsibilities, and consideration of outcomes that will benefit their patients as well as institutional ramifications and potential unintended consequences (Kornblau & Burkhardt, 2012).

The Code encourages occupational therapy practitioners to seek resources when resolving conflicts and reflect on the decision-making process and outcomes. Practical resources include the AOTA Ethics Commission, ethics committees at the state and organization levels, and ethics rounds (Erler, 2017). Continuing education on ethical practice is also helpful and required by some states for licensure renewal.

When faced with a complex ethical choice, occupational therapy practitioners should document both the outcome of their decision and the process by which they came to the decision. For future use or reflection, an email to self is an efficient way to record the ethical discernment process that was followed. It is also helpful in consolidating all the matters that were considered before action was taken.

When ethical reasoning does not resolve ethical tensions, practitioners must consider the need for alternative decision-making tools or ethical advocacy. In this case, it is important for practitioners to work toward more optimal policies for future situations because unresolved ethical tensions can result in stress and moral injury (Erler, 2017).

Summary

Ethical dilemmas and tensions are a common part of professional occupational therapy life that can cause stress without adequate resources and ethical resiliency (Bushby et al., 2015; Erler, 2017). Ethical approaches such as deontology, utilitarianism, and virtue ethics allow occupational therapy practitioners to think through their actions and reflect on possible outcomes. In addition, many health care professions, including occupational therapy, adhere to ethical principles such as autonomy, nonmaleficence, beneficence, and justice. Ethics in occupational therapy can be anchored by practitioners considering their "OT Why," following the tenants of the *OTPF* and adhering to the Code. The Code contains aspirational values, core principles, and enforceable standards of practice.

Ethical tensions can arise in health care settings when organizational principles of cost containment and maximization of service access conflict with patient autonomy and practitioner perceptions of standards of care. Discharge recommendations, resource use, and client safety are common areas of ethical concern. Practitioners, however, can resolve these tensions and concerns by using ethical reasoning, either individually or in groups of inter- or intraprofessional colleagues.

Resolving ethical dilemmas in health care settings is a dynamic process that needs to be addressed through collaboration and cooperation with institutional and professional entities. Occupational therapy practitioners have several resources they can use when resolving ethical dilemmas, including the Code; the AOTA Ethics Commission; state boards of occupational therapy; and professional reasoning using tools, such as the CELIBATE, Realm Individual Process Situation Model, and decision-making triangle. Ethics rounds can also be used in an ongoing way (Erler, 2017) to promote collaboration and strengthen ethical discernment. Finally, once a decision has been reached and acted on, practitioners are encouraged to document and reflect on the process and outcomes to enhance further development of ethical reasoning.

REFERENCES

Barlow, N. A., Hargreaves, J., & Gillibrand, W. P. (2018). Nurses' contributions to the resolution of ethical dilemmas in practice. *Nursing Ethics, 25*, 230–242. https://doi.org/10.1177/0969733017703700

Beauchamp, T. L., & Childress, J. F. (2019). *Principles of biomedical ethics* (8th ed.). Oxford University Press.

Birchley, G. (2021). The theorisation of "best interests" in bioethical accounts of decision-making. *BMC Medical Ethics, 22*, 1–18. https://doi.org/10.1186/s12910-021-00636-0

Bushby, K., Chan, J., Druif, S., Ho, K., & Kinsella, E. A. (2015). Ethical tensions in occupational therapy practice: A scoping review. *British Journal of Occupational Therapy, 78*, 212–221. https://doi.org/10.1177/0308022614564770

Caulfield, S. E. (2007). Health care facility ethics committees: New issues in the age of transparency. *Human Rights Magazine, 34*(4), 10–13. https://www.americanbar.org/groups/crsj/publications/human_rights_magazine_home/human_rights_vol34_2007/fall2007/hr_fall07_caulfi/

Doherty, R. (2019). Ethical practice. In B. A. Boyt Schell & G. Gillen (Eds.), *Willard and Spackman's occupational therapy* (13th ed.; pp. 513–526). Wolters Kluwer.

Doherty, R. F. (2020). *Ethical dimensions in the health professions* (7th ed.). Elsevier.

Drolet, M. J., Gaudet, R., & Pinard, C. (2017). Preparing students for the ethical issues involved in occupational therapy private practice with an ethics typology. *Occupational Therapy Now, 19*(2), 9–10.

Durocher, E., & Kinsella, E. A. (2021). Ethical tensions in occupational therapy practice: Conflicts and competing allegiances. *Canadian Journal of Occupational Therapy, 88*, 244–253. https://doi.org/10.1177/00084174211021707

Erler, K. (2018). Acute care ethics case example: Sam. *OT Practice, 23*(11), 13.

Erler, K. S. (2017). The role of occupational therapy ethics rounds in practice. *OT Practice, 22*(13), 15–18.

Falcó-Pegueroles, A., Rodríguez-Martín, D., Ramos-Pozón, S., & Zuriguel-Pérez, E. (2021). Critical thinking in nursing clinical practice, education and research: From attitudes to virtue. *Nursing Philosophy, 22*(1), e12332. https://doi.org/10.1111/nup.12332

Health Insurance Portability and Accountability Act of 1996, Pub. L. 104-191, 42 U.S.C. § 300gg, 29 U.S.C §§ 1181–1183, and 42 U.S.C. §§ 1320d–1320d9.

Internet Encyclopedia of Philosophy. (n.d.-a). *Act and rule utilitarianism.* https://iep.utm.edu/util-a-r/

Internet Encyclopedia of Philosophy. (n.d.-b). *Health care ethics.* https://iep.utm.edu/h-c-ethi/#SH2c

Internet Encyclopedia of Philosophy. (n.d.-c). *Immanuel Kant.* https://iep.utm.edu/kantview/

Kirsch, N. R. (2009). Ethical decision making: Application of a problem-solving model. *Topics in Geriatric Rehabilitation, 25*, 282–291. https://doi.org/10.1097/TGR.0b013e3181bdd6d8

Kornblau, B. L., & Burkhardt, A. (2012). Ethics in rehabilitation: A clinical perspective. In *Ethics in Rehabilitation: A Clinical Perspective*: Vol. Second ed (220 p.).

Lamb, A. J. (2017). Unlocking the potential of everyday opportunities. *American Journal of Occupational Therapy, 71*, 7106140010. https://doi.org/10.5014/ajot.2017.716001

Lin, S. P., Chang, C. W., Wu, C. Y., Chin, C. S., Lin, C. H., Shiu, S. I., . . . Chen, H. H. (2022). The effectiveness of multidisciplinary team huddles in healthcare hospital-based setting. *Journal of Multidisciplinary Healthcare, 15*, 2241–2247. https://doi.org/10.2147/jmdh.s384554

Lyon, W. (2021). Virtue and medical ethics education. *Philosophy, Ethics, and Humanities in Medicine, 16*, Article 2. https://doi.org/10.1186/s13010-021-00100-2.

Marseille, E., & Kahn, J. G. (2019). Utilitarianism and the ethical foundations of cost-effectiveness analysis in resource allocation for global health. *Philosophy, Ethics and Humanities in Medicine, 14*(1), Article 5. https://doi.org/10.1186/s13010-019-0074-7

National Board for Certification in Occupational Therapy. (2020). *Procedures for the enforcement of the NBCOT candidate/certificate code of conduct.* https://www.nbcot.org/professional-conduct/procedures-for-enforcement

Siegler, M. (2019). Clinical medical ethics: Its history and contributions to American medicine. *Journal of Clinical Ethics, 30,* 17–26. https://doi.org/10.1086/JCE2019301017

Slater, D. Y. (Ed.). (2016). *Reference guide to the Occupational Therapy Code of Ethics* (2015 edition). AOTA Press.

Tannahill, A., & Douglas, M. J. (2014). Ethics-based decision-making and health impact assessment. *Health Promotion International, 29,* 98–108. https://doi.org/10.1093/heapro/das040

Varkey, B. (2021). Principles of clinical ethics and their application to practice. *Medical Principles and Practice, 30*(1), 17–28. https://doi.org/10.1159/000509119

6

Ethical Reasoning for School Occupational Therapy Practitioners

KATHLYN L. REED, PhD, MLIS, OTR, FAOTA, and
JEAN E. POLICHINO, MS, OTR, FAOTA

Introduction

Occupational therapy practitioners who work in schools must adhere to various federal and state education rules and regulations, as well as state licensure rules and regulations. The AOTA Code of Ethics (the Code) provides further guidance.

In *South Kingstown Sch. Dist., 113 LRP 19804* (2013), for example, the occupational therapist's evaluation of a child with autism spectrum disorder (ASD) created concerns for the hearing officer reviewing the therapist's evaluation report. The therapist was found to have spent only an hour with the student. It was unclear whether the therapist had reviewed the student's records before the evaluation. In addition, the therapist was apparently unaware of the parent's concerns regarding the student's sensory functioning.

In his findings, the hearing officer wrote that the occupational therapy evaluation was not sufficiently comprehensive to identify all of the student's occupational therapy needs and, therefore, was not appropriate. The therapist's evaluation was out of compliance with federal regulations supporting the Individuals With Disabilities Education Improvement Act of 2004 (IDEA) at 34 C.F.R. § 300.304(c)(4) and (6), which state that the evaluation must be sufficiently comprehensive to assess the child in all areas related to the suspected disability and must identify all of the child's special needs. From an ethical perspective, it appears that the therapist failed to adhere to the profession's principles of *beneficence* and *justice*. The legal and ethical violations by the therapist compromised the student's welfare (and proved expensive for the school district).

Ethics is the discipline within philosophy that deals with what is good behavior on the basis of moral principles and practice ("Ethics," 2014). *Ethical reasoning* is used "to recognize, analyze, and clarify ethical problems that arise" (Doherty & Purtilo, 2016, p. 76). The focus is not on what could be done but on what should be done. An *ethical dilemma* occurs when there are "two (or more) morally correct courses of action that cannot both be followed" (Doherty & Purtilo, 2016, p. 66). *Ethical behavior* is the "enactment of ethical principles" (Purtilo et al., 2005, p. 14).

Ethical reasoning and practice constantly change in response to policy, political contexts, team structures, family and school demands, and workloads (Gallagher & Tschudin, 2010). The changes produce a complex environment with various challenges, including maintaining quality services with time and money constraints. Creating an ethical climate is critical (Kurfuerst & Yousey, 2012). A positive and acceptable ethical climate increases employee morale, commitment to the school district, and career engagement and encourages staff retention (Shirey, 2005).

The AOTA Code of Ethics is the profession's summary of ethical behavior, conduct, and practice. Its principles and standards are written to apply to all aspects of occupational therapy but must be interpreted in individual situations. This chapter addresses how the Code applies to practitioners providing occupational therapy services in schools.

Essential Considerations

Essential considerations for ethical reasoning include understanding AOTA's ethics principles, categories of conflicts, and the barriers and supports present in school settings.

AOTA CODE OF ETHICS

The Code asserts six ethics concepts organized into six principles. These principles are delineated in the Code. Four of the principles are considered moral principles:

- beneficence
- nonmaleficence
- autonomy
- justice.

Two principles are viewed as standards of conduct that service providers should follow:

- veracity
- fidelity.

These moral principles and standards that occupational therapy practitioners in schools should follow are summarized in Table 6.1. The primary role of school occupational therapy practitioners with students in special education is to facilitate access to and participation in their individualized education program (IEP). The school occupational therapy practitioner also plays a role in increasing students' engagement and participation by assisting districts in preventing unnecessary referrals to special education. Occupational therapy services must be consistent with and support the educational mission. Thus, for example, the ethics principle of *beneficence* is best illustrated in school practice when occupational therapy services enable students to better perform their educational tasks and roles.

TABLE 6.1. Principles From the AOTA Code of Ethics and School Practice

Principle	Examples	School Practice Applications
Beneficence	Requires taking action to help others by promoting good, by preventing harm, and by removing harm. The term *beneficence* connotes acts of mercy, kindness, and charity (Beauchamp & Childress, 2013); thus, actions that promote participation in educational activities should be the primary focus.	Instructional personnel implemented sensory strategies for students with ASD, including the use of weighted vests and blankets, without consulting the research literature for evidence of effectiveness or benefit to students with ASD or obtaining any formal training. On learning of this situation, the occupational therapist approached the campus principal to alert her to the research evidence, reviewed the precautions and inappropriate use, and offered to provide the needed training.
Nonmaleficence	"Obligates us to abstain from causing harm to others" (Beauchamp & Childress, 2013, p. 3). The obligation includes not imposing risks of harm, even when the potential risk is without malicious or harmful intent. Harm in educational settings may occur when students are denied participation in educational activities in which other students are engaged.	A student with behavioral challenges was having difficulty remaining in his seat. The occupational therapist discovered that the teacher was using another student's positioning chair and seat belt to restrict the student's mobility during instruction. The occupational therapist shared her concerns with the teacher regarding the physical, social, and emotional risks of harm to the student, as well as the legal prohibition of using positioning equipment for restraint.
Autonomy	Acknowledges a person's right to hold views, to make choices, and to take actions based on personal values and beliefs (Beauchamp & Childress, 2013). It also requires obtaining consent before initiation of occupational therapy services and protection of a student's confidential information and records.	An 18-year-old high school student no longer wanted occupational therapy services as part of his transition IEP. His parents insisted the school continue to provide occupational therapy "in case something comes up." The occupational therapy practitioner reminded the IEP team that the student is of age for making his own (self-) determinations and reassured the team that occupational therapy was available should the IEP team, including the student, want assistance in the future.

(Continued)

TABLE 6.1. Principles From the AOTA Code of Ethics and School Practice *(Cont.)*

Principle	Examples	School Practice Applications
Justice	Relates to the fair, equitable, and appropriate treatment of persons (Beauchamp & Childress, 2013). Occupational therapy practitioners should respect all applicable laws, policies, rules, regulations, and standards related to their area of practice. The focus is on upholding the idea that all individuals have an equitable opportunity to achieve occupational engagement as an essential component of the life.	A student was referred to occupational therapy because of concerns that his sensory processing may be the source of his behavioral difficulties. The occupational therapist performed an evaluation, using interviews with the teacher and parents; observations in the classroom, cafeteria, and playground; and standardized testing, including data from school and home. She provided a fair, objective report of her findings, indicating that although the student processes sensory input differently from others in some areas, the responses did not present as affecting his participation in learning, self-help, and social activities, nor did they serve as a trigger for the unexpected behaviors.
Veracity	This refers to comprehensive, accurate, and objective transmission of information and includes fostering the client's understanding of such information. The recipient of care or participant in research enters into a contract that includes a right to truthful information (Beauchamp & Childress, 2013). Parents and caregivers remain informed, and records should be complete and accurate.	The occupational therapy practitioner noticed that student documentation submitted by an occupational therapy colleague did not completely and accurately represent the time or activities provided by a colleague. She was concerned that the report should be comprehensive and accurate when it is submitted for Medicaid billing. She shared her concerns with her supervisor so that an investigation could be initiated.
Fidelity	This refers to being faithful, which includes obligations of loyalty and of keeping promises and commitments (Veatch et al., 2010). This principle specifically addresses the need for practitioners to consistently balance their duties to service recipients and other interested parties, who may influence ethical reasoning and professional practice.	As part of the early intervening team at her school, the occupational therapist recommended simple accommodations for students to enhance their participation and performance in curriculum activities. Teachers had not been implementing the recommendations in a matter that demonstrated integrity to student learning objectives. The therapist reached out to the teachers to seek understanding of their reticence to use the strategies and to determine whether she needed to provide training or model their use.

Note. ASD = autism spectrum disorder; IEP = individualized education program.

In school practice, adherence to these basic ethical principles encourages occupational therapy practitioners to ensure that their conduct is beyond reproach. Practitioners should avoid actions that would compromise or prevent student participation in education activities and should actively support student self-determination. They should ensure that students and their parents or guardians understand their rights regarding consent for services and assure them of the confidentiality of provider interactions and documentation. Practitioners should make the effort to limit how health disparities and social inequality affect student outcomes.

Occupational therapy practitioners have an ethical obligation to know and follow all laws, rules, regulations, and policies that apply to school practice and should be sure that state or district policies, practice guidelines, and procedures ensure the protection of the recipients of occupational therapy. Respect should be demonstrated through truthfulness and accuracy in all actions, deeds, and communications.

CATEGORIES OF CONFLICT

In educational settings, conflicts may arise around administrative directives, supervision, Medicaid billing, staffing, and resource allocation decisions. Clear lines of administrative supervision need to be established. Job descriptions will clarify the line of supervisory authority, as well as the specific duties and responsibilities of occupational therapy practitioners.

Job descriptions need to be reviewed annually and updated as needed to ensure that they are an accurate and current reflection of the job. A convenient time for supervisors and their employees to review job descriptions is during the annual employee performance evaluation. *Veracity*, a principle of the Code, states that occupational therapy practitioners must accurately describe the type and duration of occupational therapy services in professional contracts, including the duties and responsibilities of all involved parties.

Conflicts with administrative supervision and directives may also occur when rules and policies are written without adequate input from the people who have to carry them out. School administrators may not be familiar with occupational therapy and may have little understanding of what occupational therapy practitioners know and do. Practitioners need to take responsibility for ensuring that employers are aware of occupational therapy's ethical obligations as set forth in the Code and of the implications of those obligations for occupational therapy practice, policy, education, and research.

Third-party billing for services may also be a source of conflict for occupational therapy practitioners in schools. School systems often seek reimbursement for services, depending on how the student's services are classified. For example, when providing services for students who have disabilities, districts may seek cost recovery under the state's Medicaid program for schools. In some instances, they may bill private insurance or seek reimbursement from a state agency. Different sources of funding have different rules for documentation and submission of claims. Practitioners may find it frustrating to comply with the requirements, but it is an ethical responsibility under the fourth principle of *justice*.

Occupational therapy practitioners must ensure that documentation for reimbursement purposes is done according to applicable laws, guidelines, and regulations.

In addition, the Code states that fees are to be collected legally and justly in a manner that is fair, reasonable, and commensurate with services delivered. Occupational therapy practitioners whose schools bill third parties are also cautioned not to let the need for third-party funds drive the recommendations they make for student services (Royeen et al., 2000). The standard to determine whether occupational therapy should be part of the student's educational program is driven by educational need. Through the team process, consideration is given to the occupational therapy evaluation data, as well as the student's academic, behavioral, self-help, and social goals for the IEP period. Together, the team members determine whether occupational therapy is needed for the student to benefit from special education, not whether third-party funds can be accessed.

If occupational therapy services for a student are desired by others to garner reimbursement, or if they appear unnecessary, then the occupational therapy practitioner uses the principle of *fidelity*, using conflict resolution to resolve disputes and interpersonal conflicts, as well as perceived institutional ethics violations. Conversely, in accordance with the principle of *justice*, if the practitioner feels that services are needed but that others do not want them provided so as not to incur associated costs, then the practitioner will make efforts to advocate for changes to systems and policies that are discriminatory or unfairly limit or prevent access to occupational therapy services.

Desired allocation of limited occupational therapy resources by stakeholders may be another source of conflict in school practice. Doherty and Purtilo (2016) define a *stakeholder* as "a person, group, or other entity that has a deep and compelling interest in a situation that it wants to protect" (p. 187). Stakeholders have a vested interest in the outcome of a situation or issue of concern and may include family members, school administrators, educators, school staff, providers of related services, private therapists, advocates, and the community as a whole. Stakeholders can be allies in ethical reasoning and decision making, or they may complicate the situation because of the interests that they want to promote or protect. Understanding the perspective and interests of stakeholders can assist in determining options and choices. The provision of occupational therapy requires professional time, supplies and materials, space, and equipment. All may be in short supply. Determining how to allocate the available resources requires consideration of the ethical principle of *justice*.

CONFLICTS RESULTING FROM THE SUPERVISORY RELATIONSHIP

Occupational therapists and occupational therapy assistants in schools will both experience ethical conflicts, but their views of the conflicts may differ on the basis of their unique professional perspectives. For example, supervision and the supervisory relationship will look different depending on each practitioner's role in the partnership. However, AOTA's official document, Guidelines for Supervision, Roles, and Responsibilities During the Delivery of Occupational Therapy Services, notes that both supervisors and practitioners have a responsibility for ensuring the success of the professional relationship. As stated in this document, professional standards specify that, to provide occupational therapy services, occupational therapy assistants should receive supervision from an occupational therapist. Together, they are responsible for collaboratively developing a plan for supervision.

Although state requirements vary regarding the specifics for supervision of occupational therapy assistants, the occupational therapist is, in all cases, responsible for all aspects of occupational therapy and is accountable for the safety and effectiveness of services. State occupational therapy licensure laws and regulations, as well as state and local educational agency administrative directives, should be consulted.

In states in which supervision is specified, the ethical and legal responsibility is to follow the regulations. Where regulations are not spelled out, occupational therapy practitioners should collaboratively develop a working plan for supervisory relationships and review the plan at least annually. Whether one occupational therapist supervises one occupational therapy assistant or one occupational therapy assistant has multiple occupational therapist supervisors, a well-developed working plan is important. Considerations should include factors such as

- the amount of experience and competency level of the assistant;
- any expertise or specialized training the assistant may have acquired, such as knowledge of assistive technology or feeding techniques;
- the complexity of students' disabling conditions and needs and of the intervention process; and
- the needs and requirements of each school setting.

The AOTA official document on supervision provides the following guidance relevant to school practice:

- The occupational therapist is responsible for all aspects of occupational therapy service delivery and is accountable for the safety and effectiveness of the occupational therapy service delivery process.
- The occupational therapist must be directly involved in the delivery of services during the initial evaluation and regularly throughout the course of intervention, intervention review, and outcomes evaluation.
- The occupational therapy assistant delivers occupational therapy services under the supervision of and in partnership with the occupational therapist.
- It is the responsibility of the occupational therapist to determine when to delegate responsibilities to an occupational therapy assistant.

BARRIERS AND SUPPORTS WITHIN SCHOOL SETTINGS

Ethical conflicts and dilemmas can seem overwhelming. Providing support to staff dealing with ethical issues is essential. When the occupational therapist is the only therapist in the district or the only one assigned to a school or set of schools, a system of support is especially necessary. Taking steps in advance can reduce the barriers and increase the support system. Resources such as state occupational therapy rules and regulations (typically accessible on the Internet), the Code, and samples of effectively written documents may provide guidance. Activities that enhance support include the following:

- developing a network of other school occupational therapy practitioners (e.g., district, state, national), which may provide support when the need arises
- establishing working relationships with occupational therapy practitioners working in nearby districts and with other related services practitioners in the same district, such as physical therapists and speech-language pathologists
- building relationships with local administrative leaders and human resources personnel, and involve them when necessary in resolving ethical dilemmas
- joining AOTA and accessing resources, including the pediatric coordinator, the members of the Children and Youth Special Interest Section, and official AOTA guidelines and documents.

EMOTIONAL DISTRESS AND ETHICAL DILEMMAS

It is common to experience emotional distress when dealing with ethical dilemmas. The practitioner may feel that something was done incorrectly, may experience self-doubt about their professional role, may be overwhelmed with decisions that need to be made, may feel that an individual is incompetent or not up to performing the job, or may experience anger directed at administrators and coworkers for allowing a situation to occur. To process emotional distress constructively, consider the following steps:

- acknowledge the emotions, and attempt to clarify the problem and determine possible solutions
- identify whether the problem at hand is a legal problem (e.g., conflict with federal or state law), an employment problem (e.g., conflict with employment policies, procedures, and practices of your employer), or an ethical problem (e.g., violation of the code of conduct), keeping in mind that all three areas may be applicable in some cases
- when there is an ethical element to the issue, follow the suggested guidelines for ethical reasoning outlined in the next section.

Best Practices

Best practices for using the ethical reasoning process include developing partnerships with team members and documenting communication and actions related to occupational therapy services and any conflict that may have transpired. The following section presents strategies for dealing with ethical issues, an ethical reasoning process for resolving ethical dilemmas, and guidance on what actions to take when the Code appears to be violated. Finally, occupational therapy practitioners are encouraged to gather additional resources on ethical reasoning and practice.

DEVELOP PARTNERSHIPS WITH TEAM MEMBERS

Decisions about occupational therapy services in special education are made in teams. It is important to collaborate with other team members and document those discussions. Doing so ensures that different professional perspectives are considered when issues arise, and that multiple perspectives factor into decision making when a course of action must be determined. For example, practitioners may encounter a parent who refuses to release medical information and restricts medical provider access regarding their child's health. Despite the child's unknown medical history, the occupational therapy practitioner might identify critical health concerns (e.g., gagging or choking during snack or lunch). This information must be immediately reported to the student's team, including the administrator, case manager, and school nurse. The team must determine steps to ensure a safe mealtime program for the student. In these instances, a team effort is often likely to produce successful outcomes for obtaining needed information.

For a student in regular education whose cognitive processing is slower than that of others or who is depressed and withdrawn, occupational therapy practitioners may find themselves advocating along with the parent in an early intervening effort to address the student's issues with simple accommodations or modifications. Clarifying the existence and impact of the student's "hidden" difficulties for other members of the team may provide insight that will assist instructional personnel with more effective delivery of curriculum content and may help prevent social isolation.

DOCUMENT COMMUNICATION AND ACTIONS

Conflicts may arise at any time. Documentation of therapy services as well as phone calls and occupational therapy practitioner actions, may be key in resolving conflicts. Documentation should occur immediately after the occurrence and should succinctly articulate what transpired. Keep in mind that if no record of a phone call, service, or action exists, then there is no proof that it ever occurred. Such proof could become important when attempts are made to resolve a conflict.

USE ETHICAL REASONING PROCESS TO RESOLVE ETHICAL DILEMMAS

One method of resolving ethical dilemmas is to use a systematic method of ethical reasoning that is outlined in Table 6.2, which illustrates the ethical reasoning process used in the following scenario:

> A 6-year-old student has a congenital disorder that typically results in death before puberty. The student has been evaluated by the occupational therapist, who recommends occupational therapy services to modify the classroom environment and curriculum activities to ensure continued participation in school. School personnel indicate in a written report that they think occupational therapy for this student is a waste of time and money. They ask the therapist not to recommend services. The therapist respectfully disagrees with her colleagues, explaining specifically how her services will help the student participate with peers (reflecting the ethical principle of *justice*) and restates her recommendations. She moves forward with presenting these recommendations at the IEP meeting.

TABLE 6.2. Applying Doherty and Purtilo's (2016) Ethical Reasoning Process for Resolving Ethical Dilemmas

Steps	Information
1. **Gather relevant information.** Identify the major issue or essential problems using facts (data) that help to organize the thinking process.	Can occupational therapy services be withheld because of the beliefs or preferences of school personnel? Should occupational therapy services be provided to a student with a degenerative condition, particularly if resources are scarce?
2. **Identify the type of ethical problem.** Usually one of the concepts described in Table 6.1 is the primary ethical concern, but there may also be secondary issues.	The principles of *justice* (fair treatment and an impartial share of the benefits of society) and Beneficence (protecting and defending the rights of others) are involved.
3. **Use ethical theories or approaches to analyze the problem.** • If the ethical issue is based on a duty, there is usually an actual or implied law, rule, regulation, policy, or procedure to be followed. • If the issue is based on a consequence, then the consequences can be identified and evaluated. Often, both occur together and can be evaluated together.	Here, the occupational therapy practitioner has a duty to treat the client with equality, fairness, and justice. The consequences should be based on need and not on factors such as age, race, ethnicity, economic status, or disability.
4. **Explore the practical alternatives.** Exploring practical alternatives allows for a discussion about options and choices. If one approach cannot be followed, perhaps another approach can be substituted. Occasionally, discussion of options allows a better choice to be made.	To meet the student's needs, consider strategically scheduling sessions such as a 1-hour session the first 2 weeks of service for making initial modifications, then a 30-minute session each grading period thereafter to make any needed adjustments as the student's condition progresses. This pattern ensures student participation in school activities. Work with the teacher to adapt new tasks related to curriculum content.
5. **Complete the action.** Implement the best choice of action.	Provide the service, problem solving continuously with the student and teacher.
6. **Evaluate the process and outcomes.** Evaluate the choice of action to determine whether the desired outcome was obtained.	Together with the teacher and student, collect data at predetermined intervals (such as every Tuesday), to monitor progress. Analyze the data, and adjust the intervention plan on the basis of the results.

If the aforementioned steps are followed, then the desired outcome should occur. Sometimes the steps need to be repeated to obtain a satisfactory resolution to the ethical dilemma.

TAKE ACTION WHEN ETHICAL VIOLATIONS ARE SUSPECTED

If occupational therapy practitioners suspect that an ethical violation has occurred, then what course of action should be taken? First, as the ethical reasoning process previously discussed suggests, clarify the problem, and identify the ethical principle that may have been violated. Next, consider what steps can be taken to correct the violation. Often, the best approach is to talk with the person directly. Is the person aware that his or her actions appear to violate an ethical principle? If the person does not know or realize that a violation has occurred, educating the person may solve the problem. If the person knows the violation is occurring but chooses not to correct their behavior, then the approach depends on administrative policies, which may include written notice to a supervisor or administrator.

Again, if the violation can be corrected within the institutional guidelines, that course of action should be pursued first. However, if the violation cannot be corrected within the facility or organization, then the next step is to contact the state regulatory board (SRB). Forms for filing complaints are usually available online or by calling the SRB. The online address or phone number may be on the license itself. The person making the complaint is often asked to identify what rule or regulation appears to be violated, so it is useful to have a copy of the regulations available to consult.

If the ethical violation is covered by the Code and the occupational therapy practitioner is an AOTA member, then the AOTA Ethics Commission should be notified. The enforcement procedures for the Code outline the process and include the form needed to file a complaint. A written statement should be attached that summarizes the facts and circumstances, including dates and events. If the person has maintained their certification with the National Board for Certification in Occupational Therapy (NBCOT), then NBCOT should also be notified. Information on how to file a complaint and related forms are available online at NBCOT's website (https://www.nbcot.org).

GATHER RESOURCES TO GUIDE ETHICAL REASONING AND PRACTICE

Occupational therapy practitioners should have access to documents (e.g., federal, state, local) that guide ethical reasoning and practice. These resources may be used to resolve ethical dilemmas. Most documents are available online. Practitioners should be knowledgeable about the federal, state, and district education laws and procedures. State regulations for billing Medicaid or other funding sources should be accessed by practitioners. All practitioners must follow their state credentialing regulations (e.g., licensure, practice act, and rules).

Summary

Ethical behavior is based on moral judgment. To facilitate ethical reasoning and help with decision making, professions organize moral judgment into codes of ethics. Although issues in school practice may appear to be unique, the ethics concepts and the ethical reasoning process are the same for all areas of practice, policy, education, and research.

Note. A version of this chapter was previously published in *Best Practices for Occupational Therapy in Schools, 2nd Edition,* edited by Gloria Frolek Clark and Joyce Rioux. Copyright © 2019 by the American Occupational Therapy Association. Reprinted with permission.

REFERENCES

Beauchamp, T. L., & Childress, J. F. (2013). *Principles of biomedical ethics* (7th ed.). Oxford University Press.

Doherty, R. F., & Purtilo, R. B. (2016). *Ethical dimensions in the health professions* (6th ed.). Elsevier/Saunders.

Ethics. (2014). In *Merriam-Webster dictionary and thesaurus.* Author.

Gallagher, A., & Tschudin, V. (2010). Educating for ethical leadership. *Nurse Education Today, 30,* 224–227. https://doi.org/10.1016/j.nedt.2009.11.003

Individuals With Disabilities Education Improvement Act of 2004, Pub. L. 108–446, 20 U.S.C. §§ 1400–1482.

Kurfuerst, S., & Yousey, J. R. (2012). Leading with ethics: Creating an ethical climate in your occupational therapy department. *OT Practice, 17*(13), CE1–CE7.

Purtilo, R. B., Jenson, G. M., & Royee, C. G. (2005). *Educating for moral action: A source book in health and rehabilitation ethics.* Philadelphia: F. A. Davis.

Royeen, C. B., Duncan, M., Crabtree, J., Richards, J., & Frolek Clark, G. (2000). Effects of billing Medicaid for occupational therapy services in schools: A pilot study. *American Journal of Occupational Therapy, 54,* 429–433. https://doi.org/10.5014/ajot.54.4.429

Shirey, M. (2005). Ethical climate in nursing practice: The leader's role. *JONA's Healthcare Law, Ethics, and Regulation, 7*(2), 59–67.

South Kingstown Sch. Dist., 113 LRP 19804 (R.I. SEA Jan. 12, 2013)

Veatch, R. M., Haddad, A. M., & English, D. C. (2010). *Case studies in allied health ethics.* Oxford University Press.

Ethical Considerations in Cognition

KATHLEEN M. GOLISZ, OTD, OTR/L, FAOTA, and
DEBORAH YARETT SLATER, MS, OT/L, FAOTA

Introduction

Occupational therapy practitioners are expected to abide by the principles and standards detailed in the AOTA Code of Ethics (the Code) as they work to promote inclusion, participation, safety, and well-being for clients in various stages of life, health, and illness. Working with individuals who have cognitive impairments resulting from brain injury or disease can pose ethical challenges for occupational therapy practitioners in research and clinical contexts. The nature of the cognitive impairments, whether temporary, stable, or progressive in nature, can impede the individual's awareness of his or her capabilities and limitations. Balancing the principles of *autonomy*, *beneficence*, and *nonmaleficence* can be challenging when cognitive impairments affect a client's judgment and decision making. Impairments in areas such as attention, memory, executive functions, or emotional regulation can cause individuals to face restrictions on their freedoms. This increases the risk of becoming socially and economically marginalized. Determining *capacity,* an individual's ability to make an informed decision, will ultimately determine how much autonomy and freedom the individual retains. Capacity may differ based on the functional task or domain. For example, an individual with cognitive impairments may function autonomously enough to live alone but not to drive a car or handle his or her finances.

Cognitive impairments can be caused by various conditions, including autism spectrum disorder, Alzheimer's disease (AD), and other forms of dementia, stroke, traumatic brain injuries, Parkinson's disease, developmental disabilities, or mental health conditions such as schizophrenia or depression. More than 15 million individuals were estimated to be living with cognitive impairments in the United States in 2015 (Erickson et al., 2016), and this number is expected to grow as the Baby Boomer generation ages, thus experiencing increased risk for illnesses that may have associated cognitive impairments.

This chapter presents an overview of ethical challenges related to working with individuals with cognitive impairments and provide guidance in addressing these challenges.

Essential Components of Ethical Practice

Regardless of practice setting or diagnostic group, core concepts of ethical practice form a foundation for appropriate professional conduct and the provision of occupational therapy services. The current health care environment can present numerous and diverse ethical challenges related to patient care and interprofessional relationships among colleagues. However, one consistent and perhaps classic example of ethical tension can arise between the principle of *autonomy* (the patient's right to self-determination in making health care decisions) and the principle of *beneficence* (well-being/"doing good"). This can be an issue when a patient's cognitive capacity to understand health-related information and to make rational decisions based on that information is questionable.

A further challenge is defining the line between patient decisions that run counter to health care professionals' recommendations but may be appropriate for that patient. In these situations, decisions may unknowingly cause harm because the patient did not possess cognitive capacity or competence to understand fully the implications of his or her decision.

The trend in health care has moved away from a more paternalistic relationship between providers and their patients (Capron, 2015) toward more transparency and collaboration with patients, with overarching respect for autonomy in the patient's decision-making process within the limits of medical norms. However, individuals in these situations can benefit from guidance (not coercion), and we have an ethical obligation to promote patient welfare and, above all, prevent harm (Huddle, 2016). Therefore, accurately assessing cognitive *competency* (a global assessment of capabilities made within the legal system by a judge in court) or capacity can be of great importance to providing care that meets professional and ethical standards, thereby promoting respectful and valid health care decisions. An additional challenge is accurately assessing the dynamic concept of competency that fluctuates and is open to influence. These factors must be considered as part of the analysis of an ethical issue or dilemma to make a defensible decision or recommendation.

Principles of the AOTA Code of Ethics

An understanding of relevant ethical principles in the Code is a good first step in providing guidance to address ethical issues or dilemmas. An *ethical dilemma* is when a "moral agent is faced with two or more conflicting courses of action but only one can be chosen" (Doherty & Purtilo, 2016, p. 68). However, ethical issues of varying seriousness can arise throughout the process of providing health care services in all settings and with all patient populations across the lifespan.

The principles of *beneficence, nonmaleficence, autonomy,* and *justice* form a foundation to guide ethical decision making and professional practice. In addition to knowledge about the application of these principles to clinical practice, an organized framework for ethical decision making can provide a systematic method of reasoning through ethical dilemmas to reach a resolution that is best suited to the situation (even when not perfect) and is defensible. Many such models exist, but most have common elements.

BENEFICENCE AND NONMALEFICENCE

Of primary importance is *beneficence*, a principle found in the codes of ethics of most health care professions. It means that care should benefit patients and do good. It also includes preventing or removing harm to provide benefit, good, or well-being and aligns with altruism—a value typically shared by health care providers.

The principle of *nonmaleficence*, according to the Code, means to "refrain from actions that cause harm" and to reinforce the ethical obligation of providers to "not impose risks of harm even if the potential risk is without malicious or harmful intent." Both beneficence and nonmaleficence underscore the importance of recommendations by practitioners related to safety in daily activities. Impaired cognition is clearly a critical factor in the practitioner's clinical reasoning when making these recommendations and guiding outcomes.

AUTONOMY

Autonomy is the "self-governing right of an individual to make his or her own informed choices free from coercion; self-determination" (Slater, 2016, p. 291). Risk and ethical responsibility to mitigate damage extends to awareness of potential for abuse of patients with cognitive impairment. Abuse can occur in institutions as well as in the home environment at the hands of caregivers. Practitioners must be alert to health care decisions made by the patient with impaired cognition or by another individual in the legal role of surrogate that may result in personal harm, as this is a vulnerable population. The challenge for clinicians is to respect autonomy while promoting good and preventing undue risk or harm. Accurate assessment of competency and capacity is important to allow self-determination to the extent feasible. Patients deemed adequately competent to understand and make health care decisions may still make decisions that compromise safety and defy provider recommendations. This is difficult for practitioners to accept, but *paternalism,* "the act of a person or group in a position of authority that limits the freedom of another person with the intent to protect or benefit that person" (Slater, 2016, p. 292), is no longer acceptable in the patient–health care provider relationship.

JUSTICE

The principle of *justice* reinforces the role of laws and regulations related to safeguarding the rights of patients. It also supports the need to provide services that are objective, unbiased, and fair. This principle includes an ethical obligation to advocate for patients to access needed services, even when barriers exist.

The framework for ethical decision making in Exhibit 7.1 provides an approach to analyzing an ethically challenging situation.

Analysis of Ethical Dilemmas

Ethical issues can be complex and require a thoughtful and comprehensive approach to resolve them in the best way possible. There is at least one model of ethical decision making that relies on consensus among all involved parties to move forward with an action (Slater,

EXHIBIT 7.1.
FRAMEWORK FOR ETHICAL DECISION MAKING

- What is the nature of the perceived problem (ethical distress, ethical dilemma), and what is the specific problem (similar to clinical reasoning, "name and frame" the problem)?
- Who are the players—not only those immediately involved, but also others who may be influenced by the situation or any decision that is made?
- What information is known, and what additional information is needed to thoroughly evaluate the situation and formulate options?
- What resources are available to assist?
- What are the options and likely consequences of each option?
- How are values prioritized (e.g., prioritize moral values, despite potential negative personal repercussions, to act on best decision)?
- What action is being taken, and is it defensible?
- Was the outcome expected? Would one make a different decision if confronted with a similar situation in the future?

Source. From "Ethical Dimensions of Occupational Therapy," by L. C. Brandt & D. Y. Slater, 2011, *The Occupational Therapy Manager* (5th ed., p. 478), AOTA Press. Copyright © 2011 by the American Occupational Therapy Association. Used with permission.

2016). However, this requires repeating the decision analysis process until consensus is reached and may also be unrealistic in many situations. Exhibit 7.1 represents a systematic consideration of relevant factors that should support an ethical decision when an ethical issue or dilemma is identified.

The first step in addressing an ethical "problem" is to decide whether the situation is, in fact, an ethical dilemma, *ethical distress* (i.e., the practitioner knows what to do, but a barrier prevents her or him from doing it), or just a disagreement of opinion. It is difficult to solve a problem when it is not clearly defined. If, in fact, a true ethical issue or dilemma exists, then the players who are involved must be identified. The players may be broader than the patient, clinician, and family group and can extend to other individuals or groups that may be affected by any decision made. Likewise, it is important to think broadly when gathering information that may be relevant to the decision-making process. There may be a need for significant, additional information to understand the issues fully and to formulate options to address them.

Because ethical issues typically are not "black and white," and may include factors that add to complexity, occupational therapy practitioners should avail themselves of all potential resources. This helps to ensure that options are not limited by the individual clinician's values, opinions, or biases. Multiple perspectives can be enlightening and helpful. Practitioners can take advantage of ethics committees in the workplace if they exist and are highly competent. Other resources can include, but are not limited to, the ethics staffs and committees of professional associations, the Code, and the highly regarded ethics texts.

The result of this deliberative process should be one or more options that will, it is hoped, resolve the ethical dilemma or issue. Each option needs to be weighed in terms of potential consequences to make a reasoned decision about which is most appropriate, keeping in mind benefiting the patient, preventing harm, respecting patient autonomy to the extent feasible, and considering any applicable laws, regulations, or obstacles to promoting access to services. Prioritizing values may be an important component as options are weighed. Some potential decisions may result in negative personal repercussions that not every occupational therapy practitioner is willing to withstand. This reinforces the difficulty that ethically challenging situations may pose.

Finally, the occupational therapy practitioner or health care team must act. Without action, the process is an intellectual exercise, but one that does not resolve the ethical dilemma, the goal of which is to end up in a better or at least more acceptable place than the initial one. Equally important is reflection on the outcome as a final step. Was the outcome as expected or did the situation turn out totally different? This is an important learning experience because the same or similar dilemma could arise in the future, and the practitioner must decide whether to handle it the same way, depending on perceived effectiveness and the result.

Health care can present numerous, often significant, ethical challenges. Understanding and accessing relevant resources and tools can assist the occupational therapy practitioner and the health care team in making ethically sound recommendations and decisions that respect and benefit the patients they treat. Case Example 7.1 describes a client with cognitive impairments that may affect his health, safety, and autonomy. This case includes some common ethical issues that practitioners encounter when working with individuals with cognitive impairments. Application of the framework for ethical decision making can assist practitioners' analysis of the ethical dilemma.

CASE EXAMPLE 7.1. MR. WILSON: AN ETHICAL DILEMMA

Mr. Wilson was recently admitted to an acute care hospital after breaking his hip from a fall. Following surgery, Mr. Wilson was referred to occupational therapy for assessment of his ADLs in preparation for his discharge home alone (Mr. Wilson's expressed desire). The occupational therapist who completed the initial evaluation was concerned that Mr. Wilson may have cognitive impairments. He had difficulty recalling the therapist's name, the day of the week, and following instructions during treatment sessions. The physician speculated that the observed impairments were likely to be related to the surgical anesthesia. Mr. Wilson's neighbor visited during one of the occupational therapy treatment sessions and expressed concern with the plans for Mr. Wilson to return home alone. The neighbor reported that Mr. Wilson had been seen walking in the neighborhood in his pajama bottoms with a jacket in cold weather. He ran over his mailbox when backing his car out of the garage, and neighbors were concerned that Mr. Wilson wasn't safe in his home alone.

Mr. Wilson presented ethical challenges to the occupational therapist. Physically, he was recovering well and appeared to have the strength and stamina to return home. During performance-based assessment of simple IADL tasks, Mr. Wilson appeared confused when asked to make a can of soup and cold sandwich. He required cues to read the soup can instructions and forgot to turn off the stove

(Continued)

CASE EXAMPLE 7.1. MR. WILSON: AN ETHICAL DILEMMA *(Cont.)*

when he removed the pot. The therapist followed up with a comprehensive cognitive evaluation, which indicated impairments in memory, executive functioning, and attention. The therapist was concerned about Mr. Wilson's ability to be safely discharged home and to return to driving.

At the family conference, Mr. Wilson's daughter and son, who both lived nearby, did not agree about their father's ability to live independently and to return to driving. The daughter thought her father should return to his own home, while the son thought his father should go to live with his sister (Mr. Wilson's daughter). Neither believed their father would be willing to stop driving and stated he'd rather "die than give up his keys."

What is the nature of the perceived problem (ethical distress, ethical dilemma), and what is the specific problem (similar to clinical reasoning, "name and frame" the problem)?
This case presents a clear ethical dilemma—two or more ethical courses of action where doing one will preclude doing the other, although both are correct. Mr. Wilson wishes to go home and is physically able to do so. Respecting the ethical principle of *autonomy*, the right of individuals to make decisions about their care, would support this decision. However, there is significant objective and observational information from multiple sources that contradicts this option in terms of patient safety (and potentially public safety if Mr. Wilson continues to drive). The children are also not in agreement about the appropriate discharge plan, further complicating the decision-making process.

Who are the players—not only those immediately involved but also others who may be influenced by the situation or any decision that is made?
In this case, the individuals who must be considered in any decision are Mr. Wilson, his son and daughter, the treating occupational therapist, Mr. Wilson's physician, and potentially his neighbors, given the safety concerns. Another consideration may be public safety implications if Mr. Wilson continues to drive.

What information is known, and what additional information is needed to thoroughly evaluate the situation and formulate options?
We know that, although physical recovery for Mr. Wilson has been adequate to make a home discharge potentially realistic, there is objective information from the occupational therapist's initial evaluation, subsequent cognitive assessment, and observations during treatment sessions that functional cognition is impaired. There is cognitive dysfunction in multiple areas that affect his ability to perform IADLs safely as well as other daily living activities, including driving. The physician also recognized cognitive impairment, and at least one of Mr. Wilson's children understands that discharge to live alone may not be an appropriate plan. Further, neighbors have recognized and shared several incidents that indicate likely cognitive impairment with safety implications. Another consideration is that Mr. Wilson fell and broke his hip. Although he has physically recovered, is he at further risk for falls (either from a home safety hazard, a musculoskeletal problem, or inattention because of cognition impairment)? It may be helpful to get additional information about what supports would be available in the home (e.g., family, friends, paid help) and the community to help Mr. Wilson and ensure safety if that ends up being the discharge plan, despite recommendations to the contrary. What alternative living options that offer more protection and services are potentially available in Mr. Wilson's community? What are the state laws regarding reporting an individual with a medical condition that may negatively affect his or her ability to drive safety?

(Continued)

CASE EXAMPLE 7.1. MR. WILSON: AN ETHICAL DILEMMA *(Cont.)*

What resources are available to assist?
The hospital ethics committee, if one exists, can be consulted to assist with discussion and options, although committee members will not make the decision. Case management services may also be helpful to identify options. A family/team meeting would seem appropriate to discuss the patient's wishes, but the team must reach some consensus on recommendations, with a rationale to support them. The team members must balance patient autonomy or self-determination with their ethical obligations to safeguard the patient's well-being and to protect him from harm (beneficence and nonmaleficence).

What are the options and likely consequences of each option?
Option 1: Mr. Wilson goes home alone despite recommendations to the contrary. Consequences will depend on what, if any, supports are put in place to assist with ADLs and IADLs to ensure safety (e.g., the stove may be disconnected; an aide may come in to prep meals, assist with ADLs, and drive Mr. Wilson as needed; his children or sister may assist as they are able). If there are no supports or inadequate support, it is likely that Mr. Wilson will be unable to safely, independently, and competently complete ADLs and IADLs to manage daily activities. If he drives despite warnings, there is potential for personal or public harm, or for him to get disoriented, lost, and unable to get back home. Occupational therapy practitioners have an ethical, and possibly a legal, responsibility (principles of *beneficence* and *nonmaleficence*, of the Code), as do physicians, to warn patients and families, and potentially state agencies, when they have objective evidence that an individual may have a medical impairment that affects the ability to drive safely.

   Even if Mr. Wilson goes home, the children will need to (it is hoped in collaboration and discussion with their father) address his inability to continue to drive safely. This may entail taking away the keys, disabling the car, and looking at alternative community mobility options in conjunction with the occupational therapist. This option respects Mr. Wilson's desire to return to his home, but with parameters that minimize risk. However, there may be a challenge if the children do not have the will, ability, or tenacity to go against their father's wish to continue driving and take action.

Option 2: Mr. Wilson goes home with his daughter, who is able to provide assistance or hire additional help (if financially feasible) to facilitate his daily activities. The car is taken away, even if Mr. Wilson protests, as his safety and that of the public supersede his wish to drive independently based on ethical and professional obligations of the health care providers. The rationale for no longer driving is reinforced, even though Mr. Wilson's cognitive limitations may preclude him from understanding the risk and may provoke significant anger or another negative response. If he continues to drive, safety concerns will persist.

Option 3: Mr. Wilson's family and case manager explore alternative housing, such as assisted living, if there is the financial ability to pay for additional help through the day. Housing is close to his sister or at least one of the children, so they can check on him as well. The stove in the assisted living apartment is disabled, and any other potential safety hazards in the apartment are mitigated to the extent feasible. Again, the car is no longer available, so driving is not an option. If he is able to continue driving, safety concerns and potential danger will still exist.

(Continued)

CASE EXAMPLE 7.1. MR. WILSON: AN ETHICAL DILEMMA *(Cont.)*

How are values prioritized (e.g. prioritize moral values, despite potential negative personal repercussions, to act on best decision)?
Ideally, the physician, occupational therapist, and any other team members have reached consensus on the best plan to recommend to the patient and his family. Regardless, the therapist has an ethical obligation to be honest and direct in conveying clinical data and recommendations, to provide supporting rationale for his or her professional judgment, and to warn about potential consequences of a decision that does not consider these facts. This may result in a negative response from the patient or his family. In addition, if the providers are not in agreement about the best option and approach, there may be a backlash from colleagues.

What action is being taken, and is it defensible?
Make a recommendation that is objective and data driven (as noted earlier) and offers alternative options that are more appropriate to the patient's status and abilities.

Was the outcome expected? Would one make a different decision if confronted with a similar situation in the future?
What strategies worked and what, if any, did not. If they did not work, what could be done differently to bring about a better outcome?

Competence vs. Capacity for Treatment Consent or Research Participation

Competence and *decisional capacity* are central concepts in health care law and ethics. Although often used interchangeably, the concepts differ. *Competency* is a global assessment of capabilities made within the legal system by a judge in court, and *capacity* is a determination of functional abilities within a clinical setting (Dastidar & Odden, 2011). Because both concepts affect autonomous decision making, when "clinicians determine that a patient lacks decision-making capacity, the practical consequences may be the same as those attending a legal determination of incompetence" (Grisso & Appelbaum, 1998, p. 11).

Individuals may make decisions or choices that, although risky or "ill advised," do not necessarily imply they lack decisional capacity. Neurotypicality and neurodiversity fall along a continuum with murky boundaries. Individuals displaying eccentric cognitive, behavioral, or affective presentations may still retain decision-making capacity (Banja & Fins, 2013).

The ability to provide informed consent is dynamic in nature and dependent on multiple factors, including the individual's diagnosis; decision-making capacity, which lies along a continuum from complete capacity to a complete lack of capacity; complexity of the treatment choice; level of risk; and individual values and beliefs (see Figure 7.1).

INFORMED CONSENT

Providing *informed consent* requires that an individual display at least four abilities: understanding, appreciation, reason, and choice (Appelbaum, 2007; Grisso & Appelbaum, 1998). All

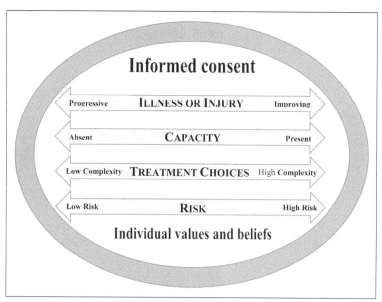

Figure 7.1. Dynamic nature of determining capacity.

these components of capacity require cognitive capabilities, including memory and executive functioning (EF). The individual must have a basic understanding of the facts involved in his or her decision to consent or refuse treatment or involvement in research. The simple requirement of "understanding" can be complex based on how it is defined and the behaviors required to demonstrate "understanding." In a medical setting, understanding is a complex cognitive experience potentially affected by many cognitive impairments. Gurreraet et al. (2014) suggest that "understanding may be the most cognitively mediated consent task" (p. 7).

The ability to appreciate the significance of the decision to be made requires not only the understanding of basic facts of the treatment or research but also the potential alternatives, along with their risks and benefits and how each relates to his or her personal values and priorities. The individual should be able to provide a rational reason for his or her choice, explaining the consequences of the choice on daily activities. This component of capacity to consent requires higher cognitive functions such as mental manipulation of information. Weighing the risks and benefits and potential consequences of a decision requires awareness of one's current health status and generation of possible outcomes based on one's choices. Making a choice that goes against medical advice is not an indication of a lack of decision-making capacity and reason for medical paternalism (Capron, 2015; Dastidar & Odden, 2011).

Finally, individuals should be able to choose an option from those presented and to make the choice known. Consider physical and communicative impairments that may accompany injuries and conditions (e.g., stroke) that may impair cognition. A patient may be able to meet the first three conditions for capacity but be unable to express a choice because of the inability to consent verbally or through gestures (e.g., nodding, blinking, hand gesture). Individuals with language deficits may benefit from the involvement of a speech–language pathologist during the capacity appraisal (Brady Wagner, 2003). Frequent changes in the choice initially made may be seen in individuals with psychiatric or neurological conditions, and indicate a lack of capacity (Appelbaum, 2007). In situations where individuals are deemed to lack capacity to consent to treatment or research participation, surrogates or proxies for decision making may be used.

SURROGATE DECISION MAKERS

Obtaining consent from a *surrogate decision maker* or proxy raises issues related to the ethical principle of *autonomy*, especially if the surrogate is court appointed rather than self-selected by the individual prior to the loss of decisional capacity. How well does the proxy represent the individual's beliefs and values? Is the surrogate struggling to find a balance between respect for the autonomy of the individual and performing his or her caring duties? Is the proxy's decision clouded by emotions related to the relationship with the individual or financial implications of treatment? Surrogates may consider both patient-centered factors and surrogate-centered factors, including their own wishes and interests, as well as those of the family; religious beliefs; and feelings of obligation and guilt (Fritsch et al., 2013).

There is a rising need for surrogate decision makers because of the growing number of adults with dementia or other cognitive impairments who do not have the capacity to engage in medical decision making. Torke et al. (2013) report that surrogates were involved with nearly half of hospitalized older adults, yet approximately only 26% of Americans have an *advance directive, not advanced* (Rao et al., 2014) or a durable power of attorney for health care. Forty-four states in the United States have established hierarchy surrogate consent laws that allow a family member or the closest relative to the patient who did not prepare an advance directive prior to becoming incapacitated to become the designated surrogate for that individual and make medical decisions. However, formal court appointment of a guardian or surrogate occurs less often than a more informal arrangement of a family member who assumes the role of surrogate decision maker (Banja & Fins, 2013).

Without an advance directive, a surrogate uses knowledge of the person's lifestyle, preferences, behaviors, and decisions made prior to being incapacitated to respect and protect the individual's values, beliefs, preferences, and autonomy. The surrogate attempts to make the decision based on *substitute judgment* most resembling what the incapacitated individual would have made. In situations where the individual has not shared his or her values and beliefs with the surrogate, the *best interest standard* may apply. This requires the surrogate to decide based on the principle of what would be good for the individual who lacks the capacity to decide for him or herself. This approach is based on the moral principle of *beneficence*.

Practitioners may encounter cognitively impaired patients who are considered "unbefriended" individuals. This population includes individuals who do not have the capacity to give informed consent, have no advance directive nor the current capacity to execute an advance directive, and have no appointed guardian, family, or friends. Only 14 states in the United States have provisions for unbefriended patients in their surrogate consent laws. These provisions typically permit the attending physician to make medical decisions with consultation of the institution's ethics committee to provide a safeguard and form of consensus decision making (Wynn, 2014).

Individuals with brain injuries or neurological or psychiatric disorders may present with anosognosia, where the individual appears unaware (underlying neurological dysfunction) or denies (underlying psychological etiology) the existence of physical, cognitive, or behavioral impairments. This condition affects engaging the individual in treatment. An occupational therapy practitioner who treats a patient who does not see the necessity for the intervention and refuses treatment violates the individual's autonomy and could be charged with assault or battery (Cherney, 2006; Egbert, 2017). However, the practitioner may view providing the intervention as honoring the ethical principles of *beneficence* and *nonmaleficence*. The rehabilitation team may need to engage a surrogate decision maker while attempting to restore decisional capacity through interventions aimed at increasing self-awareness (Toglia & Kirk, 2000).

In situations where the patient's capacity to consent is questioned, occupational therapy practitioners should first inquire about the existence of an advance directive. If one exists, the practitioner should discuss with the surrogate any medical decisions, providing clear information on the recommended intervention and alternatives available. In addition, when possible, the practitioner should include the patient in these conversations. Depending on the complexity of the information discussed, the individual may be able to contribute information on his or her values and wishes. Over time, with improvements in cognitive capabilities, the individual's autonomy may return in part or wholly, shifting decision making from the surrogate back to the individual (Banja & Fins, 2013).

ASSESSING CAPACITY FOR CONSENT

Capacity to consent to treatment is a component of personal autonomy in which an individual demonstrates the cognitive and emotional capabilities to select a course of treatment among options or to refuse treatment. Capacity to consent may improve over time in some diagnoses (e.g., psychiatric illnesses [Dornan et al., 2015], traumatic brain injury [Steward et al., 2016]), fluctuate (e.g., Lewy body dementia [Dornan et al., 2015]), or decline as with dementia (Trachsel et al., 2015). Factors such as infection, medication, time of day, and therapeutic rapport with the evaluator may affect a patient's performance on a capacity assessment (Dastidar & Odden, 2011).

Assessing individuals with cognitive impairments to determine their capacity to consent to treatment or research participation should combine clinical judgment with standardized assessments of capacity. There are a variety of capacity assessments (see Table 7.1) that typically assess the four components of capacity (i.e., understanding, appreciation of situation, reasoning, ability to express a choice) through interactive interviews in which the components are discussed between the health care provider and the patient. Hypothetical situations are presented to the patient that are either from the first-person perspective (Capacity to Consent to Treatment Intervention [CCTI; Marson et al., 1995] and MacArthur Competence Assessment Tool for Treatment [MacCAT–T; Grisso & Appelbaum, 1998]) or a third-person perspective (Hopemont Capacity Assessment Interview [HCAI; Edelstein, 1999]).

Physicians and psychiatrists typically perform capacity assessments, especially if there are legal proceedings to establish conservatorship. However, all health care professionals

TABLE 7.1. Examples of Capacity Assessments

Assessment	Description
Aid to Capacity Evaluation (ACE) Etchells et al. (1999)	Semistructured interview tailored to individual's diagnosis and treatment. Designed for use with medical inpatients. Assesses capacity components of • Understanding, • Appreciation, and • Reasoning. The tool takes 10–20 minutes to administer. Developers recommend users attend a standardized ACE training session prior to use.
Assessment of Capacity to Consent to Treatment Moye & Marson (2007)	Interview of values and preferences related to medical decisions using 1 of 3 vignettes (i.e., acute, chronic, advanced illness). The clinician selects the vignette closest to the level of complexity of the patient's decisional situation. The interview addresses the patient's perspective on the following: • Effect of treatment choices on valued activities and relationships, • Decision-making style (autonomous, shared, deferred), and • Value of quality versus length of life. Developed for research applications but can be adapted for clinical use. This tool has been used with patients with dementia and schizophrenia, as well as cognitively healthy populations.
CCTI Marson, Ingram, Cody, & Harrell (1995)	Two clinical vignettes of hypothetical medical problems (i.e., neoplasm, cardiac disease), symptoms, and risks/benefits of two alternative treatment options. Presented in oral and written formats using a structured interview. Standardized scoring of patient's oral responses to the following: • Understanding of treatment situation, • Expressing a treatment choice, • Providing a rational for treatment choice, and • Appreciation of personal consequences. The tool takes approximately 20–25 minutes to administer. It has been used with patients with Alzheimer's disease, dementia, and Parkinson's disease.
HCAI Edelstein (1999)	Semistructured interview using hypothetical vignettes on eye infection and cardiopulmonary resuscitation to assess • Understanding, • Appreciation, and • Expressing a choice. The tool takes 30–60 minutes to administer. It has been used with nursing home residents as well as adults with and without dementia. It can be administered by nonclinicians.

(Continued)

TABLE 7.1. Examples of Capacity Assessments *(Cont.)*

Assessment	Description
MacCAT–T Grisso & Appelbaum (1998)	Semistructured interview using information from each patient's medical chart to explore the elements of decision making: • Understanding, • Reasoning, • Appreciation, and • Choice. The tool does not specify a passing score. It takes approximately 15–20 minutes to administer. The tool requires formal training to administer (manual and training video available) and has been used with individuals with schizophrenia, psychosis, dementia, and depression.
MacCAT–CR Appelbaum & Grisso (2001)	Semistructured interview to assess capacity for consent to participate in research. Provides a format for disclosure of study-specific information: • Understanding basic elements of research as required by U.S. Federal Common Rule, • Appreciating that the research may not provide individual benefit and that they are free to decline participation without penalty, • Reasoning that involves comparing the consequences of the alternatives presented, and • Expressing a choice or selecting a desired option. The tool takes approximately 15–20 minutes to administer. Requires training for valid administration and interpretation. Includes structured aggregated scores on scales for each of the four abilities. A composite score is not generated, as poor performance on any scale may indicate impaired capacity. It can be sold to any researcher doing research on human subjects.

should have a basic understanding of the components of capacity. Occupational therapy practitioners may encounter patients and clinical situations where the question of capacity arises and a basic assessment of capacity should be performed. Capacity assessments vary in the training and education required of the rater (see Table 7.1). Some assessments (e.g., HCAI, MacCAT–T) provide detailed training manuals to guide administration, scoring, and interpretation (Lamont et al., 2013), with a training video available for the MacCAT–T. Occupational therapy practitioners should abide by the Code and only perform assessments within their level of competence and scope of practice.

Individuals may have difficulty with specific components of capacity on the assessments based on the nature of their diagnosis and cognitive impairments. The assessment tool used may result in varying decisions on the individual's capacity as the tools differ in how they assess the components. For example, in the assessment of the capacity component of understanding, two assessments (CCTI and HCAI) require the individual to recall information presented, while the MacCAT–T requires the individual to paraphrase information. These skills may be particularly difficult for individuals with dementia (Moye et al., 2004).

The component of appreciation may show less impairment in individuals with dementia unless the CCTI is used to determine capacity because this assessment requires foresight—an abstract concept for individuals with cognitive impairment. Individuals with psychiatric illness may struggle more on assessment of the appreciation component because of delusional symptoms and executive dysfunction (Owen et al., 2013). The capacity component of reasoning is typically impaired in individuals with dementia when tested using the CCTI and MacCAT–T as reasoning requires comprehension, encoding, and retrieval of alternating treatment options.

Specific cognitive impairments appear to affect different components of capacity. As defined, capacity requires appreciation and reasoning of alternatives that rely on intact executive skills. Performance on neuropsychological assessments more strongly predicts individuals' understanding and reasoning abilities than the appreciation and expression of choice components of capacity (Gurrera et al., 2014). Variability in an individual's neuropsychological test performance is associated with reduced consent capacity in community-dwelling adults, independent of overall neuropsychological performance. This suggests that decisional capacity may be related to undefined interactions between a variety of cognitive functional domains (Gurrera et al., 2014).

Cognitive assessments alone may not directly translate to understanding an individual's decision-making capacity (Owen et al., 2017). The Mini-Mental State Examination (MMSE; Folstein et al., 1975) was not developed for assessing decision-making capacity; however, high and low scores on the MMSE have been found to correlate with clinical judgments of incapacity and capacity assessment scores (Raymont et al., 2004). Midrange scores of 17–23 do not correlate well with capacity, requiring additional assessments as necessary (Dastidar & Odden, 2011). Individuals with Parkinson's disease and cognitive concerns may have a wide range of decisional capacity capabilities.

Lower scores on the Montreal Cognitive Assessment (MoCA) and MMSE have been found to predict impaired MacCAT–T subscores (Abu Snineh et al., 2017). Cognitive assessments of attention (i.e., Digit Span subtest from the Wechsler Adult Intelligence Scale), phonemic and semantic verbal fluency, verbal memory (i.e., Hopkins Verbal Learning Test—Revised), and processing speed (i.e., Digit Symbol subtest and Trail Making Test Parts A and B) have been associated with the understanding component of capacity in the CCTI in patients newly diagnosed with brain metastases (Gerstenecker et al., 2015).

Parkinson's disease

Individuals with Parkinson's disease perform below neurotypical controls on all four capacity components when tested with the CCTI (Dymek et al., 2001). In particular, difficulties were seen in the reasoning and comprehension abilities. Simple measures of executive function (i.e., the Executive Interview—EXIT–25) and to a lesser extent measures of memory and orientation (i.e., Memory subscale of the Dementia Rating Scale) were predictors of capacity. Moelter et al. (2016) similarly found research consent capacity, as measured on the MacArthur Competence Assessment Tool for Clinical Research (MacCAT–CR), to be associated with executive functions and delayed recall. Scores on the visuospatial/executive subscale of the MoCA predicted experts' ratings of capacity. The progressive nature of Parkinson's disease suggests decision-making capacity should be assessed throughout the course of patients' illness.

Acquired brain injuries

Individuals with acquired brain injuries and executive dysfunction may have limitations in decision-making capacity because of the limited ability to appreciate or use the knowledge of their cognitive impairments in weighing their decisions (Owen et al., 2017). Individuals may show evidence of awareness of their impairments and metacognitions (i.e., ability to think about one's thinking) during conversations; however, they may not demonstrate "online" awareness to use this information to engage in decision making in real or hypothetical scenarios (Owen et al., 2017). Owen et al. (2013) found the appreciation component of the MacCAT–T was a better "test" of capacity to consent to treatment in individuals with psychiatric illness, whereas individuals with cognitive impairments in medical facilities who had poorer reasoning showed a lack of capacity.

Alzheimer's disease

Research on biomarkers and diagnostic and treatment studies for memory loss in AD may seek to enroll individuals with mild cognitive impairments (MCI), as approximately half of individuals with MCI are diagnosed as having AD within a 4-year period (Jefferson et al., 2012). Individuals with MCI may have limitations to their decisional capacity. Individuals with MCI assessed risk differently than cognitively neurotypical peers when completing a risk assessment task. This task involved ranking four hypothetical vignettes for memory loss research (i.e., brain autopsy, blood draw, oral medication, neurosurgery) on a scale from least to most risk. Participants with MCI often overestimated the risk of brain autopsy and overestimated the benefit of oral medication (Jefferson et al., 2012).

Dementia

The progressive nature of dementia poses specific challenges in determining capacity. Neuropsychological factors such as conceptualization and confrontation naming predict performance on the understanding concept of capacity (Moye & Marson, 2007), but not other aspects of capacity. Currently, there is no simple method to predict when decisional capacity has deteriorated to the point that a surrogate decision maker should be involved. Okonkwo et al. (2008) found declining trajectories in the understanding component of decision-making capacity of individuals who converted from MCI to dementia. Other capacity components assessed by the CCTI in a longitudinal study of people with MCI were not affected. Clinicians and researchers may need to reassess capacity to consent over time when engaging in longitudinal studies or longer-term intervention with clients with cognitive impairments. As dementia progresses, so does the impairment in capacity to consent.

As with any assessment, clinicians must consider the numerous factors that may interfere with performance, including lack of motivation, inattention, mistrust, or misunderstanding of expectations (Sturman, 2005). The measures presented in Table 7.1 are not intended to replace clinical judgment of capacity but to support a determination (Triebel et al., 2012). Capacity assessments need continued validity testing. A review of studies focusing on reliability between capacity-assessment tools (Moye & Marson, 2007) found limited agreement between evaluators, multiple tools, or clinician and an assessment measure. Agreement is highest for the construct of understanding and lowest for appreciation (Moye & Marson, 2007).

Research With Individuals With Cognitive Impairment

Research with human participants is guided by ethical principles related to respect for people, autonomy, human dignity, beneficence, and justice (Dunn et al., 2015). Researchers are ethically bound to ensure their research includes a comprehensive consent process that provides the potential participant with adequate information to make an informed decision on whether to volunteer. Individuals with cognitive impairments may find it challenging to understand abstract or hypothetical concepts related to randomization, risks, and benefits required to make an informed decision. Occupational therapy researchers may question if it is acceptable to enroll individuals who cannot consent in research that poses risks exceeding those considered part of ordinary, daily life.

The Office for Human Research Protections, under the auspices of the U.S. Department of Health and Human Services, provides guidance on ethical and regulatory issues in biomedical and social-behavioral research (Office for Human Research Protections; 45 CFR part 46). Federal regulations provide specific guidance on enrolling adults who may lack the capacity to consent as a result of trauma, intellectual or developmental disability, some forms of mental illness, or dementia, whether the impairment is temporary, progressive, or permanent. Unless informed consent is waived by an institutional review board for research, only a legally authorized representative for the adult can give consent for participation in research.

As part of their advance health care directive documents (i.e., advance directives), individuals may have designated someone, by the *durable power of attorney* (DPA) legal document, with special moral and legal authority to make decisions on the individual's behalf (Kim & Appelbaum, 2006). This DPA may have the authority to enroll the individual in a research study if there is sufficient reason to believe that participation in the study is consistent with the individual's values. The individual's advance directives may also state that the DPA has authority to enroll the individual in research that might be detrimental to his or her health. There is evidence that many individuals with cognitive impairments (e.g., early-stage AD) retain the ability to appoint a surrogate for making decisions concerning research (Kim et al., 2011). Participants with progressive diseases affecting cognition and capacity should be asked to designate a family member or friend to serve as their surrogate should the participant's ability to assess his or her willingness to continue in the research be later compromised. Court-appointed guardians, such as those appointed for individuals with intellectual or developmental disabilities, are often permitted to make research decisions even though they were not appointed by the individual for these specific responsibilities. In situations where surrogate consent is obtained, assent should still be sought from the individual in a simple, understandable form.

Ethical Issues of Technology Supporting Individuals With Cognitive Impairments

Over the past several years, there has been a growing interest and market for Internet-based, brain-training games that promise to increase intelligence and cognitive capabilities. Clients with intact cognitive function or MCI may seek the advice of occupational therapy practitioners about the benefits of purchasing a "brain-training" program. These companies may provide published data on their program's effectiveness, but it is often self-published company data. There is limited, if any, evidence on a connection between observed improvements of the games' and tasks' results and performance of everyday functions (Purcell & Rommelfanger, 2015). Using a citizen scientist approach, these companies partner with researchers, sometimes without oversight by a research ethics board. In exchange for free access to their products, researchers permit inclusion of their participants' performance on the product in the company's large data pool collected on users. Occupational therapy practitioners should consider ethical issues related to privacy of clients' neurodata and cost benefits of products with limited supporting evidence. These issues should be discussed with clients prior to recommending these products.

Current everyday technology, such as electronic devices and health-smart homes, has health care applications that offer potential to improve the lives and levels of independence for individuals with cognitive impairments. Although technology may provide increased independence, peace of mind for family members, and a greater sense of security, there are ethical issues related to dignity, privacy, and choice for the individual that need consideration (Birchley et al., 2017; Landau & Werner, 2012; Yang & Kels, 2017). Both physical privacy and data privacy should be considered when deciding on whether to track or safety monitor an individual with cognitive impairments. Finding an acceptable balance between some loss of privacy, safety of the individual, and greater autonomy should be discussed with patients and caregivers.

Reimbursement and Ethics

Delivering occupational therapy services without a patient's consent violates the Code. There may be a higher risk of ethical conflict in therapeutic situations when patients with cognitive impairments do not have the capacity to consent to care, participate in financial decisions about their care, or advocate for their health care rights under insurance.

Occupational therapy practitioners are expected to exercise professional and ethical judgment when providing services in the current complex health care system, where business practices may appear to drive service delivery. The business of health care can result in a conflict of interest, ethical dilemma, or moral distress for practitioners. Employers or administrators may pressure practitioners to provide specific (e.g., higher reimbursement level services) or excessive services to individuals. These services may not be medically necessary or beneficial, or based on evidence supporting achievement of patient outcomes and the practitioner's clinical judgment. In other clinical situations, based on the reimbursement structure, practitioners may be mandated to limit services provided to individuals with cognitive impairments to maximize profits for the parent company. This can result in conflicts between honoring the ethical principles of *beneficence, justice,* and *veracity*.

Individuals with cognitive impairments may have a lengthy recovery, potentially exhausting traditional reimbursement sources prior to reaching their recovery. Occupational therapy practitioners may be challenged by their duty to advocate for services patients need and to identify funding options and access to services (Winistorfer et al., 2016).

Summary

Although it is not typically in the scope of practice of an occupational therapy practitioner to determine a patient's decision-making capacity, practitioners working with individuals with cognitive impairments may be able to contribute a valuable perspective of their patients' cognitive abilities related to consent capacity. Practitioners should monitor therapeutic encounters to ensure that a consult with a surrogate decision maker occurs when needed. Jensen et al. (2012) state the concept of ethical mindfulness is an extension of reflective practice. Ethical mindfulness allows the practitioner to seek understanding of the meaning and lived experience of the patient, family, and caregivers, recognizing personal bias and judgment rather than relying solely on ethical principles for clinical reasoning and decision making.

Autonomy and individual freedom are highly valued in the United States and other liberal democracies, yet not all cultures place as strong a value on this concept. Many cultures hold a value system that places the family or community above the individual and use a collective or family-centered, decision-making process (Wells, 2017). Occupational therapy practitioners should provide culturally sensitive care, seek knowledge of the mores and beliefs of their clients, and ask clients or their surrogates how they wish to receive information and make decisions. Practitioners should provide services that reflect cultural humility and knowledge of the mores and beliefs of their clients (Tervalon & Murray-García, 1998). This involves acknowledging one's own limited knowledge of other cultures as well as the potential influence of one's own assumptions and prejudices. This approach to working with individuals from different cultures helps practitioners to keep an open mind and remain respectful.

Occupational therapy practitioners working with clients with cognitive impairments in awareness, memory, and EF may face some unique ethical challenges. Issues of autonomy, decision-making capacity, involvement of surrogate decision makers, and ethical principles of *beneficence* and *nonmaleficence* may all need to be considered during the intervention process. Guidance from the Code, reflection on the structured questions proposed in the framework for ethical decision making, and consultation with experts or an institutional ethics committee should support practitioners' ethical practice with this population.

Key Points

- Providing ethical care to patients with cognitive impairments, whether fluctuating or progressive, requires a balance between respecting patient autonomy (or surrogate decisions) and providing guidance within the limits of medical norms to promote well-being and to prevent harm.
- Occupational therapy practitioners should use relevant principles and related standards of practice, along with a framework for ethical decision making and other ethical resources to make decisions that are reasoned and defensible in ethically challenging situations.
- Capacity to consent to treatment or research participation may vary along a continuum based on the complexity of the decision and context.
- Providing informed consent requires at least four abilities: understanding, appreciation, reason, and choice.
- Determining capacity to consent to treatment or research participation should combine clinical judgment with standardized assessments of capacity.
- Cognitive assessments alone may not predict an individual's decision-making capacity.
- Emerging technology can be beneficial to patients with varied levels of cognitive impairment, but can also pose ethical challenges related to limited research and privacy concerns.
- Administrative directives designed to increase revenue, sometimes at the expense of clinical judgment and appropriate patient care, can lead to unethical or illegal practice.

Note. An earlier version of this chapter was previously published in *Cognition, Occupation, and Participation Across the Lifespan: Neuroscience, Neurorehabilitation, and Models of Intervention in Occupational Therapy, 4th Edition*, edited by Noomi Katz and Joan Toglia. Copyright © 2018 by the American Occupational Therapy Association. Reprinted with permission.

REFERENCES

Abu Snineh, M., Camicioli, R., & Miyasaki, J. M. (2017). Decisional capacity for advanced care directives in Parkinson's disease with cognitive concerns. *Parkinsonism & Related Disorders, 39*, 77–79. https://doi.org/10.1016/j.parkreldis.2017.03.006

Appelbaum, P. S. (2007). Assessment of patients' competence to consent to treatment. *New England Journal of Medicine, 357*, 1834–1840. https://doi.org/10.1056/nejmcp074045

Appelbaum, P. S., & Grisso, T. (2001). *MacArthur Competence Assessment Tool for Clinical Research (MacCAT–CR)*. Sarasota, FL: Professional Resource Press/Professional Resource Exchange.

Banja, J., & Fins, J. (2013). Ethics in brain injury medicine. In N. Zasler, D. Katz, & R. Zafonte (Eds.), *Brain injury medicine* (pp. 1374–1390). Demos Medical Publishing.

Birchley, G., Huxtable, R., Murtagh, M., Ter Meulen, R., Flach, P., & Gooberman-Hill, R. (2017). Smart homes, private homes? An empirical study of technology researchers' perceptions of ethical issues in developing smart-home health technologies. *BMC Medical Ethics, 18*(1), 23. https://doi.org/10.1186/s12910-017-0183-z

Brandt, L. C., & Slater, D. Y. (2011). Ethical dimensions of occupational therapy. In K. Jacobs & G. L. McCormack (Eds.), *The occupational therapy manager* (5th ed., pp. 469–483). AOTA Press.

Brady Wagner, L. C. (2003). Clinical ethics in the context of language and cognitive impairment: Rights and protections. *Seminars in Speech and Language, 24*(4), 275–284. https://doi.org/10.1055/s-2004-815581

Capron, A. M. (2015). Not taking "yes" for an answer. *Journal of Clinical Ethics, 26*(2), 104–107.

Cherney, L. R. (2006). Ethical issues involving the right hemisphere stroke patient: To treat or not to treat? *Topics in Stroke Rehabilitation, 13*(4), 47–53. https://doi.org/10.1310/tsr1304-47

Dastidar, J., & Odden, A. (2011, August). How do I determine if my patient has decision-making capacity? *The Hospitalist.* https://www.the-hospitalist.org/hospitalist/article/124731/how-do-i-determine-if-my-patient-has-decision-making-capacity

Doherty, R. F., & Purtilo, R. B. (2016). *Ethical dimensions in the health professions.* St. Louis, MO: Elsevier.

Dornan, J., Kennedy, M., Garland, J., Rutledge, E., & Kennedy, H. G. (2015). Functional mental capacity, treatment as usual and time: Magnitude of change in secure hospital patients with major mental illness. *BMC Research Notes, 8,* 566. https://doi.org/10.1186/s13104-015-1547-4

Dunn, L. B., Alici, Y., & Roberts, L. W. (2015). Ethical challenges in the treatment of cognitive impairment in aging. *Current Behavioral Neuroscience Reports, 2*(4), 226–233. https://doi.org/10.1007/s40473-015-0055-0

Dymek, M. P., Atchison, P., Harrell, L., & Marson, D. C. (2001). Competency to consent to medical treatment in cognitively impaired patients with Parkinson's disease. *Neurology, 56*(1), 17–24. https://doi.org/10.1212/WNL.56.1.17

Edelstein, B. (1999). *Hopemont Capacity Assessment Interview manual and scoring guide.* West Virginia University.

Egbert, A. R. (2017). A framework for ethical decision making in the rehabilitation of patients with anosognosia. *Journal of Clinical Ethics, 28*(1), 57–66. https://doi.org/10.1086/JCE2017281057

Erickson, W., Lee, C., & von Schrader, S. (2016). *2015 disability status report: United States.* Cornell University Yang Tan Institute on Employment and Disability.

Etchells, E., Darzins, P., Silberfeld, M., Singer, P. A., McKenny, J., Naglie, G., . . . Strang, D. (1999). Assessment of patient capacity to consent to treatment. *Journal of General Internal Medicine, 14*(1), 27–34. https://doi.org/10.1046/j.1525-1497.1999.00277.x

Folstein, M. F., Folstein, S. E., & McHugh, P. R. (1975). Mini-mental state: A practical method for grading the cognitive state of patients for the clinician. *Journal of Psychiatric Research, 12,* 189–198. https://doi.org/10.1016/0022-3956(75)90026-6

Fritsch, J., Petronio, S., Helft, P. R., & Torke, A. M. (2013). Making decisions for hospitalized older adults: Ethical factors considered by family surrogates. *Journal of Clinical Ethics, 24*(2), 125–134.

Gerstenecker, A., Meneses, K., Duff, K., Fiveash, J. B., Marson, D. C., & Triebel, K. L. (2015). Cognitive predictors of understanding treatment decisions in patients with newly diagnosed brain metastasis. *Cancer, 121*(12), 2013–2019. https://doi.org/10.1002/cncr.29326

Grisso, T., & Appelbaum, P. S. (1998). *Assessing competence to consent to treatment: A guide for physicians and other health professionsals.* Oxford University Press.

Gurrera, R. J., Karel, M. J., Azar, A. R., & Moye, J. (2014). Neuropsychological performance within-person variability is associated with reduced treatment consent capacity. *American Journal of Geriatric Psychiatry, 22*(11), 1200–1209. https://doi.org/10.1016/j.jagp.2013.03.010

Huddle, T. (2016). Putting patient autonomy in its proper place: Professional norm-guided medical decision-making. *Kennedy Institute of Ethics Journal, 26*(4), 457–482. https://doi.org/10.1353/ken.2016.0038

Jefferson, A. L., Carmona, H., Gifford, K. A., Lambe, S., Byerly, L. K., Cantwell, N. G., . . . Tripodis, Y. (2012). Clinical research risk assessment among individuals with mild cognitive impairment. *American Journal of Geriatric Psychiatry, 20*(10), 878–886. https://doi.org/10.1097/JGP.0b013e318252e5cb

Jensen, G. M., Randall, A. D., & Wharton, M. A. (2012). Cognitive impairment in older adults: The role of ethical mindfulness. *Topics in Geriatric Rehabilitation, 28,* 163–170. https://doi.org/10.1097/TGR.0b013e31825932d0

Kim, S. Y. H., & Appelbaum, P. S. (2006). The capacity to appoint a proxy and the possibility of concurrent proxy directives. *Behavioral Sciences & the Law, 24*(4), 469–478. https://doi.org/10.1002/bsl.702

Kim, S. Y. H., Karlawish, J. H., Kim, H. M., Wall, I. F., Bozoki, A. C., & Appelbaum, P. S. (2011). Preservation of the capacity to appoint a proxy decision maker: Implications for dementia research. *Archives of General Psychiatry, 68*(2), 214–220. https://doi.org/10.1001/archgenpsychiatry.2010.191

Lamont, S., Jeon, Y. H., & Chiarella, M. (2013). Assessing patient capacity to consent to treatment: An integrative review of instruments and tools. *Journal of Clinical Nursing, 22*(17–18), 2387–2403. https://doi.org/10.1111/jocn.12215

Landau, R., & Werner, S. (2012). Ethical aspects of using GPS for tracking people with dementia: Recommendations for practice. *International Psychogeriatrics, 24*(3), 358–366. https://doi.org/10.1017/S1041610211001888

Marson, D. C., Ingram, K. K., Cody, H. A., & Harrell, L. E. (1995). Assessing the competency of patients with Alzheimer's disease under different legal standards. A prototype instrument. *Archives of Neurology, 52*(10), 949–954. https://doi.org/10.1001/archneur.1995.00540340029010

Moelter, S. T., Weintraub, D., Mace, L., Cary, M., Sullo, E., Xie, S. X., & Karlawish, J. (2016). Research consent capacity varies with executive function and memory in Parkinson's disease. *Movement Disorders, 31*(3), 414–417. https://doi.org/10.1002/mds.26469

Moye, J., Karel, M. J., Azar, A. R., & Gurrera, R. J. (2004). Capacity to consent to treatment: Empirical comparison of three instruments in older adults with and without dementia. *Gerontologist, 44*(2), 166–175. https://doi.org/10.1093/geront/44.2.166

Moye, J., & Marson, D. C. (2007). Assessment of decision-making capacity in older adults: An emerging area of practice and research. *Journals of Gerontology, Series B: Psychological Sciences, 62*(1), P3–P11. https://doi.org/10.1093/geronb/62.1.P3

Office for Human Research Protections. (2010). Code of Federal Regulations, Title 45, Part 46, Protection of Human Subjects. www.hhs.gov/ohrp/regulations-and-policy/regulations/45-cfr-46/index.html

Okonkwo, O. C., Griffith, H. R., Copeland, J. N., Belue, K., Lanza, S., Zamrini, E. Y., . . . Marson, D. C. (2008). Medical decision-making capacity in mild cognitive impairment: A 3-year longitudinal study. *Neurology, 71*(19), 1474–1480. https://doi.org/10.1212/01.wnl.0000334301.32358.48

Owen, G. S., Freyenhagen, F., Martin, W., & David, A. S. (2017). Clinical assessment of decision-making capacity in acquired brain injury with personality change. *Neuropsychological Rehabilitation, 27*(1), 133–148. https://doi.org/10.1080/09602011.2015.1053948

Owen, G. S., Szmukler, G., Richardson, G., David, A. S., Raymont, V., Freyenhagen, F., . . ., Hotopf, M. (2013). Decision-making capacity for treatment in psychiatric and medical in-patients: Cross-sectional, comparative study. *British Journal of Psychiatry, 203*(6), 461–467. https://doi .org/10.1192/bjp.bp.112.123976

Purcell, R. H., & Rommelfanger, K. S. (2015). Internet-based brain training games, citizen scientists, and big data: Ethical issues in unprecedented virtual territories. *Neuron, 86*(2), 356–359. https:// doi.org/10.1016/j.neuron.2015.03.044

Rao, J. K., Anderson, L. A., Lin, F. C., & Laux, J. P. (2014). Completion of advance directives among U.S. consumers. *American Journal of Preventive Medicine, 46*(1), 65–70. https://doi.org/10.1016/ j.amepre.2013.09.008

Raymont, V., Bingley, W., Buchanan, A., David, A. S., Hayward, P., Wessely, S., & Hotopf, M. (2004). Prevalence of mental incapacity in medical inpatients and associated risk factors: Cross-sectional study. *Lancet, 364*(9443), 1421–1427. https://doi.org/10.1016/S0140-6736(04)17224-3

Slater, D. Y. (Ed.). (2016). *Reference guide to the Occupational Therapy Code of Ethics* (2015 ed.). AOTA Press.

Steward, K. A., Gerstenecker, A., Triebel, K. L., Kennedy, R., Novack, T. A., Dreer, L. E., & Marson, D. C. (2016). Twelve-month recovery of medical decision-making capacity following traumatic brain injury. *Neurology, 87*, 1052–2059. https://doi.org/10.1212/WNL.0000000000003079

Sturman, E. D. (2005). The capacity to consent to treatment and research: A review of standardized assessment tools. *Clinical Psychology Review, 25*(7), 954–974. https://doi.org/10.1016/ j.cpr.2005.04.010

Tervalon, M., & Murray-García, J. (1998). Cultural humility versus cultural competence: A critical distinction in defining physician training outcomes in multicultural education. *Journal of Health Care for the Poor and Underserved, 9*(2), 117–125. https://doi.org/10.1353/hpu.2010.0233

Toglia, J., & Kirk, U. (2000). Understanding awareness deficits following brain injury. *NeuroRehabilitation, 15*(1), 57–70.

Trachsel, M., Hermann, H., & Biller-Andorno, N. (2015). Cognitive fluctuations as a challenge for the assessment of decision-making capacity in patients with dementia. *American Journal of Alzheimer's Disease and Other Dementias, 30*(4), 360–363. https://doi.org/10.1177/1533317514539377

Triebel, K. L., Gerstenecker, A., & Marson, D. (2012). Neuropsychological assessment of decisional capacity in an aging society. *Bulletin, 28*(2), 13–15.

Wells, S. A. (2017). In J. B. Scott & S. M. Reitz (Eds.), *Practical applications for the Occupational Therapy Code of Ethics (2015)* (pp. 255–266). AOTA Press.

Winistorfer, W. L., Scheirton, L. S., & Slater, D. Y. (2016). *Ethical considerations for productivity, billing, and reimbursement.* https://www.aota.org/~/media/Corporate/Files/Practice/Ethics/Advisory/ reimbursement-productivity.pdf

Wynn, S. (2014). Decisions by surrogates: An overview of surrogate consent laws in the United States. *Bifocal, 36*(1), 1–6.

Yang, Y. T., & Kels, C. G. (2017). Ethical considerations in electronic monitoring of the cognitively impaired. *Journal of the American Board of Family Medicine, 30*(2), 258–263. https://doi.org/10.3122/ jabfm.2017.02.160219

8

Ethics of Evaluation

WAYNE L. WINISTORFER, MPA, OTR, FAOTA

Introduction

Occupational therapy evaluation and ethics may not appear to have a natural connection, but occupational therapy practitioners recognize its importance. When patients or clients are seen for an occupational therapy evaluation, the process is likely well established within the setting, and practitioners proceed on the basis of their knowledge, experience, and habits. Practitioners are expected to follow the practice standards of the profession and the setting as they apply to the person, group, or population. They must also adhere to the applicable regulations and any specific requirements relative to the source of reimbursement for services. This is considered good practice.

However, whenever an occupational therapy evaluation process is undertaken, it reflects decisions and patterns established by and consistent with values and ethics. Applying ethical principles may not occur at the level of conscious awareness or as the result of deliberate, objective discernment. Using the term *discernment* is common in the realm of ethics; the equivalent term in occupational therapy is *professional judgment*. The application of ethical principles is an essential foundational element for how assessments are actually selected, presented to the client, and interpreted, and how an occupational therapy evaluation process is delivered in practice. In addition, the results of an evaluation, how and with whom they are shared, and how they lead to appropriate intervention plans are certainly affected by general ethical principles and specific professional ethics codes and standards.

All health care professions define, adopt, and attempt to enforce profession-specific codes of ethical conduct. These codes are meant to ensure that, when entering into relationships with health care professionals, members of the public can expect to be treated safely, fairly, and competently. Professional codes of ethics typically address the profession's higher calling and virtues in the form of principles. Honoring these principles is the ethical ideal of the profession and is considered to be aspirational in nature. Problems of professional ethics usually arise from conflicts of values (Beauchamp & Childress, 2013).

This chapter reviews ethics and ethical principles and analyzes how the principles relate to broad areas of occupational therapy evaluation. Applicable standards and ethical dilemmas that may arise with occupational therapy assessment and the occupational therapy evaluation process are discussed. Case examples and guidance for critical analysis, recommended behaviors, and application to evaluation as a component of ethical occupational therapy practice are presented.

What Are Ethics?

When people says they are being ethical, they are referring to beliefs, behaviors, or actions that they have judged as the right thing to do. Although people may have no conscious awareness of why an action is correct, they arrive at a proper personal conclusion as a product of the influences and experiences that have occurred throughout their lifetime. Learning and life experience results in the development of personal values: people's own *moral code.* The influences and values developed from personal experiences, as well as from shared cultural, societal, and organizational expectations, result in shared *moral norms* (Beauchamp & Childress, 2013).

DEFINING *ETHICS*

In the case of occupational therapy or other health care practitioners, biomedical ethics and professional ethics also influence the underlying foundational values and moral norms that guide ethical behavior in professional practice. Beauchamp and Childress (2013), in their classic book *Principles of Biomedical Ethics,* defined *ethics* as a generic term covering several "different ways of understanding and examining the moral life" (Beauchamp & Childress, 2013, p. 7). These well-respected authors have devoted efforts over many years to advancing the features of and challenges unique to biomedical ethics. AOTA has consistently relied on the work of ethicists, as well as the ethical codes of other professions, when regularly updating the AOTA Code of Ethics (the Code) and the numerous resources and Advisory Opinions in this text.

CODES OF CONDUCT

A profession's embrace of ethical principles does not represent professional obligations, nor do the principles form the basis for disciplinary action of members of the profession who violate them (American Psychological Association, 2016). A *code of conduct* has detailed descriptions of requirements and prohibitions intended to minimize vagueness and define clear boundaries for professional behavior. Although a profession's foundational values likely remain constant, the specific expected behaviors and prohibitions may be revised over time. Revisions are typically made in response to emerging issues, cultural or societal evolution, and emerging practice areas and challenges.

At times, specific abhorrent or egregious behavior of a member of a profession reaches a critical level of public awareness. When public notoriety rises to the level of scandal, the unethical behavior may reveal a gap in the breadth or scope of a professional code of conduct. Although the scandal may be blatantly incongruous with the core values of the profession, the violation may not be adequately addressed within the expected or prohibited behavioral standards of the ethics code or code of conduct. The "this has never happened before" response may prompt a professional association to examine its ethics code or code of conduct and adopt new prohibitions designed to address the specific concern, objectionable behavior, or notorious event. The motivation for the association is to ensure that similar offenses do not occur and to preserve the profession's integrity (Beauchamp & Childress, 2013).

OCCUPATIONAL THERAPY CODE OF ETHICS

Professional ethics for the occupational therapy profession did not just begin in 1975 when the AOTA Representative Assembly passed Resolution 461-75 to establish the Commission on Ethics. The genesis of concern for the ethical practice of occupational therapy certainly began before the adoption of the first Code (Slater, 2016). Yet, not until that time could occupational therapy professionals point to a guiding document that addressed ethical behavior and delineated the mechanisms intended "to serve Association members and the public through development, review, interpretation, and education . . . the process whereby they are enforced" (Slater, 2016, p. 3). The purpose of the Code has remained constant since its adoption: "to promote quality care and professional conduct" (Slater, 2016, p. 3).

The intention of professional principles is to guide practitioners' interactions and behavior. As the occupational therapy professional *Code of Ethics* was established, a set of *core values* was codified as the foundation that led to the ethical principles on which the current Code is structured (Table 8.1).

The core values of the occupational therapy profession lay the foundation for how practitioners come to know that an action is ethical or unethical. They do not provide an

TABLE 8.1. AOTA Code of Ethics Core Values

Core Value	Applicability to Occupational Therapy
Altruism	Demonstrate concern for the welfare of others
Equality	Treat all people impartially and free of bias
Freedom	Honor personal choice
	Values and desires of the client guide practice
Justice	A state in which diverse communities are inclusive
	Organize and structure communities such that all members can function, flourish, and live a satisfactory life
Dignity	Promote and preserve individuality by treating the client with respect in all interactions
Truth	Provide accurate information in all forms of oral, written, and electronic communication
Prudence	Use clinical and ethical reasoning skills, use sound judgment and reflection to make decisions in professional roles

authoritative framework or description of specific behaviors that dictate the professional, ethical practice of occupational therapy. The Code is the document that brings the profession's core values into the realm of application. It uses six ethical principles that, along with the associated *related standards of conduct* (RSCs), bring clarity to an array of activities and situations that present ethical dimensions and ethical dilemmas. RSCs prescribe expected, virtuous behaviors and an assortment of prohibitions that are relevant to the contemporary, ethical practice of occupational therapy.

AOTA CODE OF ETHICS AND EVALUATION

The Code directly relates to occupational therapy evaluation. While performing assessments and evaluations, occupational therapy practitioners who violate or do not conform to accepted, recognized standards could be subject to complaints and adverse action by their state or territorial jurisdiction, in addition to sanctions that could be imposed by the national professional association, AOTA. Ethical practice requires that the occupational therapy evaluation process honor general ethical principles enumerated within the Code. More specifically, several RSCs provide authoritative statements of professional expectations and behavioral directives, as well as some prohibitions, that apply to assessments and the process of occupational therapy evaluation. The Code serves as a framework with which to explore issues in occupational therapy assessment and evaluation. Each ethical principle offers specific opportunities to practice ethically and also introduces potential challenges and ethical dilemmas related to practice. Table 8.2 describes how the six ethical principles relate to evaluation.

Throughout the remainder of this chapter, the Code and relevant RSCs are used as the structure for definitions, illustrations, case examples, and analysis.

Beneficence

The principle of *beneficence* includes all forms of action intended to benefit other persons. The term *beneficence* connotes acts of mercy, kindness, and charity (Beauchamp & Childress, 2013). Beneficence requires taking action to help others, promote good, prevent harm, and remove the potential for harm. Examples of beneficence include protecting and defending the rights of others, preventing harm from occurring to others, removing conditions that will cause harm to others, helping persons with disabilities, and rescuing persons in danger (Beauchamp & Childress, 2013).

BENEFICENCE AND RELATED STANDARDS OF CONDUCT

The Code RSCs that are consistent with the principle of *beneficence*, highlighting only those areas that pertain to evaluation, are as follows:

- Provide appropriate evaluation and a plan of intervention for recipients of occupational therapy services specific to their needs.

TABLE 8.2. Ethical Principles for Occupational Therapy Evaluation

Ethical Principle	Code of Behavior	Relevance to Evaluation
Beneficence	All forms of action intended for the well-being and safety of clients	Appropriate evaluation, intervention, reassessment, and reevaluation are provided in a client-centered and evidence-based manner within the scope of occupational therapy practice.
Nonmaleficence	Abstain from causing harm to others	Undue internal and external influences on evaluation that may compromise the occupational therapy process should be avoided.
Autonomy	Respect clients' rights to self-determination, privacy, confidentiality, and consent	Always seek consent before evaluation, and maintain privacy and confidentiality of the reports and results.
Justice	Promote fairness and objectivity	Provide timely response to referral as determined by law, regulation, or policy and promote nondiscriminatory behavior.
Veracity	Truthfulness when representing occupational therapy	Refrain from making false claims on the basis of the evaluation.
Fidelity	Commitment to treat clients and others with respect, fairness, discretion, and integrity	Treat clients and others with respect, and establish collaborative communication.

Note. Ethical principles from the AOTA Code of Ethics.

- Reevaluate and reassess recipients of service in a timely manner to determine whether goals are being achieved and whether intervention plans should be revised.
- Use, to the extent possible, evaluation, planning, intervention techniques, assessments, and therapeutic equipment that are evidence based, current, and within the recognized scope of occupational therapy practice.

The first RSC applicable to the ethical principle of *beneficence* directs occupational therapy personnel to provide appropriate evaluation for recipients specific to their needs, which leads to the question, "What is an appropriate evaluation?" The second RSC relates to the timely reevaluation and reassessment. The third RSC describes the use of evaluations that are evidence based, current, and within the recognized scope of occupational therapy practice. Law and MacDermid (2008) described *evidence-based practice* as "integrating clinical experience with the best available external clinical evidence from systematic research" (p. 5). Their focus on the balance between clinical experience and systematic research relates to the clinical decision-making process to choose appropriate evaluation tools which will lead to evidence-based interventions. Decisions "should be made on the basis of judicious clinical reasoning, sound judgment, insight, experience, and available research" (Slater, 2016, p. 181).

BENEFICENCE: PRACTICAL APPLICATION TO EVALUATION

When selecting ethically beneficent occupational therapy assessments and evaluation processes, occupational therapy practitioners must consider several questions.

Is this assessment current?

When examining the age and current applicability of an assessment, occupational therapy practitioners should consider

- the original development date of the assessment,
- when the assessment was last updated, and
- whether the most current edition of the assessment is available and in their possession.

Using the most current version of an assessment is always indicated as the best and most ethical approach. Many assessments are updated on a regular basis. Keeping current requires research and awareness of developments in the profession and specific areas of practice. The expense of purchasing updated versions is a concern, but best practice requires having the most recent assessments, recording forms, and tools. Occupational therapy practitioners are responsible for using the most recent version of any assessment.

Determine whether an assessment developed during an earlier time period is still relevant to the current situation. For example, the first edition of the Bay Area Functional Performance Evaluation (Bloomer & Williams, 1979) used a paper bank deposit slip, which was later revised because of concerns related to cultural experience and relevance. With the emergence of digital financial transactions, paper bank deposit slips may be foreign to any number of patients referred to occupational therapy. Likewise, a patient who is indigent, has no bank account, and exclusively uses cash for purchases may have little or no exposure to banking in either paper or electronic formats (Houston et al., 1989).

In another example, the original Kohlman Evaluation of Living Skills (KELS; McGourty, 1978) used a bound, paper telephone directory and a desk phone to assess cognition and functional performance. Today, these tools may be unknown to a generation with touch-screen personal cellphones that have contacts features and search functions to access websites and links to contact local businesses. The most current KELS added online banking and bill-pay simulations (Thomson & Robnett, 2016).

Is this assessment evidence based?

To determine whether an assessment is evidence based, occupational therapists should ask,

- What is the assessment's validity and reliability?
- Am I accessing and referencing the most recent data on research applications of the tool?
- Has research been published within the past 5 years that validates the use of this tool?

Many widely used assessments are the subject of research. Occupational therapists have an ethical duty to access research findings and determine their applicability to practice. Research data that verify test validity and performance norms can affect the contemporary interpretation of results and skew a comparison of a person's performance to the results expected of a cohort population.

Affirmative findings pertaining to these questions may bring occupational therapists peace of mind. However, when the currency, applicability, and evidence of an assessment's currency are compromised, practitioners need to consider using other tools or procuring the most recent edition of a tool. Less-than-perfect assessment tools require therapists to be judicious when reporting evaluation results, which are likely compromised in some way. Clinical experience and expertise can supplement the validity of evaluation results, but therapists must also be aware and recognize the shortcomings of the situation and acknowledge them in any reports. Most importantly, the therapist has an ethical responsibility to choose the best assessment based on the needs of the client, which is the essence of beneficence.

Is this evaluation within the scope of the profession or appropriately used by occupational therapists?

It is incumbent on occupational therapists to know whether the assessments they are using, or want to begin using, are appropriately used within the domain of occupational therapy. An easy indicator is that the evaluation tool was designed, developed, and researched by occupational therapy practitioners for populations they see frequently. Some tools are available for purchase or use only by members of specific professions or by occupational therapists with specialized skills or certification.

For example, only certified speech-language pathologists may use the American Speech-Language-Hearing Association's (2019) Functional Communication Measures to submit data to the National Outcomes Measurement System. Similarly, an occupational therapist with a bachelor's-level education must hold certification and have additional training in assessment to purchase and use the Sensory Integration and Praxis Tests (Ayres, 1989).

ARE YOU HONORING THE PRINCIPLE OF BENEFICENCE?

What are occupational therapy practitioners to do when they are presented with a patient in need of occupational therapy evaluation and the available assessments are not current or not quite appropriate?

A decision-making strategy from the field of administration and management can serve as a method for resolving the challenges of the less-than-perfect solution. *Satisficing* entails exploring the available alternatives until an acceptable threshold is met. This mash-up of the words *satisfy* and *suffice,* first introduced by Herbert A. Simon (1956), was popularized by John Rawls (1971) in *A Theory of Justice.* Satisficing explains decision making in circumstances in which an optimal resolution cannot be determined or achieved.

For example, an immediate request to evaluate a patient when optimal tools are not available does not release the occupational therapist from completing the assigned task, but the therapist must choose the most appropriate assessment to meet the needs of the client. Satisficing allows the therapist to do what is requested in ways that are satisfactory for the situation and within the constraints of the environment and available resources. Using a previous version of a standardized assessment may be necessary when there is no other option. Eliminating one component of an assessment tool when the tools or equipment are outdated or broken can fulfill the basics of the questions to be answered by the evaluation process. These variations must be clearly noted when reporting or documenting assessment results. In addition, any limitations or compromises must be considered while identifying priorities for the development of an intervention plan.

However, satisficing is not an acceptable response when an evaluation request is outside the scope of the occupational therapy domain of practice. In the face of this practice dilemma, ethical responses could include offering alternative assessment tools or strategies, suggesting that other professionals or professions perform the evaluation, or simply declining the referral and declining to provide the service (Fleming & Rucas, 2015; see Case Example 8.1).

CASE EXAMPLE 8.1. KANDI: BENEFICENCE AND EVALUATION

Kandi, a new graduate, just started her first job as an occupational therapist providing services to inpatients in an acute care hospital. Kandi is assigned to **Marquis,** a seasoned occupational therapist and long-term employee, for orientation to the setting and to the varied caseload. In the Rehabilitation Services department, Marquis is known as a clinical expert who always connects with patients and their families. A physical therapist in the department told Kandi that Marquis is the best in the department for bringing focus to the critical issues for safe transition to home, home health, or other care settings. While orienting Kandi to her new job, Marquis stated strongly that "there is no evaluation tool that captures the functional deficits and rehab needs of our caseload. I've been doing this for years. I can tell when someone is or isn't going to be safe at home." Kandi finds this odd because during her occupational therapy education program, she learned of several assessments that she understood could be appropriately used in this setting. Kandi knows she has an understanding of assessment tools to effectively identify occupational deficits and characterize the contexts applicable to the person being served, yet Kandi is unsure how to respond to Marquis' comments.

Into the second week of working alongside one another, Marquis regularly checks in with Kandi regarding her day. Kandi's assigned schedule includes a medical staff–ordered occupational therapy evaluation of and treatment for an elderly man admitted to the hospital on observation status from the Emergency Department the prior evening. The man had a serious fall at home, resulting in multiple contusions to his face and suspected concussion and rib fractures. Kandi completed a records review and learned that the man lives alone. It was unclear from the available documentation whether the man's recent fall was a first or repeat occurrence. The documentation from the staff in the Emergency Department reflects that the man was unsure whether, or when, he had fallen in the past, but he reported that he "gets tipsy" at home. The early morning case management notes say, "Because no fractures were found on X-ray, plan to transition home in early afternoon, as soon as cleared by therapies."

Kandi told Marquis about the case and that she brought with her the equipment to administer the Allen Cognitive Level Screen (ACLS–5; Allen et al., 2007), which she intended to use with this elderly man. Marquis questioned why Kandi was using the ACLS–5. Kandi shared what she knew about repeat falls and the level of risk for those with cognitive impairments and that men are less likely to report fall occurrences than women (Bergen et al., 2016).

(Continued)

CASE EXAMPLE 8.1. KANDI: BENEFICENCE AND EVALUATION *(Cont.)*

Marquis scoffed, "I know about that Allen thing. I went to a workshop back in the 1990s, and I know it works for psych patients. I haven't been to any workshops in a long time, but I've been an OT for decades. How is leather lacing going to prevent this old guy from falling again? Just recommend a home health visit. He's going home today, and he'll be just fine!"

Foundational ethics question:
* How does the ethical principle of *beneficence* apply to this scenario?

Considerations:
* How might Kandi approach this conflict with Marquis?
* What standards are applicable, and what resources might Kandi use to advance ethical practice?
* How can a cognitive assessment contribute to an ethical occupational therapy evaluation when there are only one or two occupational therapy encounters before discharge from an acute care setting?
* How does using appropriate assessment tools address individual needs and the development of an ethical intervention plan?
* Why is it important to use, to the extent possible, evaluations that are evidence based, current, and within the recognized scope of occupational therapy practice?
* Is it reasonable to believe that an assessment by occupational therapy could influence the development of a comprehensive and safe transition plan?
* Are there any ethical concerns about Marquis' participation in continuing professional development activities?
* How might Kandi address these ethical concerns?

Nonmaleficence

The principle of *nonmaleficence* "obligates us to abstain from causing harm to others" (Beauchamp & Childress, 2013, p. 150). It also includes an obligation to not impose risk of harm even if the potential risk is without malicious or harmful intent. The standard of *due care* "requires that the goals pursued justify the risks that must be imposed to achieve those goals" (Beauchamp & Childress, 2013, p. 154). The concept of *harm* in health care often means that a health care practitioner injured or wronged a patient. However, a patient could be harmed by "thwarting, defeating or setting back of some party's interests" (Beauchamp & Childress, 2013, p. 153).

Health care practitioners perform services that may cause pain to a client, but their direct intention is not to harm. Actions that cause harm may sometimes be inadvertent. At other times, it may be difficult to identify the specific harm that resulted from a health care practitioner's action or lack of action. When harm is the direct intent of an action, the principle of nonmaleficence is certainly violated. However, clear malevolent intent and proven harm by a health care professional could also result in disciplinary action or even criminal liability.

NONMALEFICENCE AND RELATED STANDARDS OF CONDUCT

The Code RSCs illustrate several scenarios in which an occupational therapist might violate the principle of *nonmaleficence* while engaging in the evaluation process. The RSCs that are consistent with the principle of nonmaleficence are as follows:

- Recognize and take appropriate action to remedy personal problems and limitations that might cause harm to recipients of service, colleagues, students, research participants, or others.
- Avoid compromising the rights or well-being of others on the basis of arbitrary directives (e.g., unrealistic productivity expectations, falsification of documentation, inaccurate coding) by exercising professional judgment and critical analysis.
- Avoid exploiting any relationship established as an occupational therapy clinician, educator, or researcher to further one's own physical, emotional, financial, political, or business interests at the expense of recipients of services, students, research participants, employees, or colleagues.

ARE YOU HONORING THE PRINCIPLE OF NONMALEFICENCE?

In honoring the principle of *nonmaleficence*, occupational therapists have a duty to take action when their personal limitations have the potential to result in insufficient service, as illustrated in Case Example 8.2. Applying the principle of nonmaleficence requires practitioners to address any harm that may result from engaging in relationships and delivery of service that could be considered exploitative or result in lack of due care. For example, devoting an atypical and unnecessary amount of time and charging extended service time for the evaluation of a patient reflects a violation of nonmaleficence if the therapist's motivation is to ensure a desired number of work hours and the size of the next paycheck. When this occurs, the patient and the therapist's employer are both victims of maleficent intent and unethical behavior.

CASE EXAMPLE 8.2. SHEILA: NONMALEFICENCE AND EVALUATION

Sheila works as an outpatient occupational therapist specializing in neurological conditions. Sheila is also a sexual assault survivor, but she has not made this known to her coworkers. Sheila is fully aware of situations that might trigger her anxiety and the overwhelming symptoms of posttraumatic stress disorder that she sometimes experiences.

Today, Sheila had a new, middle-aged male patient on her schedule for an initial evaluation after a mild cerebrovascular accident with residual upper-extremity impairments and related limitations in activities of daily living. Sheila was surprised to discover that the patient was accompanied by a staff member from a local Community Corrections Transitional Living Center. Sheila introduced herself to the patient and opened the patient's electronic medical record. She immediately discovered personal red flags indicating that the patient was listed on the state's Sex Offender Registry. After a

(Continued)

CASE EXAMPLE 8.2. SHEILA: NONMALEFICENCE AND EVALUATION *(Cont.)*

deep breath, Sheila excused herself from the patient and his attendant. She quickly checked with her Outpatient Department's registration and scheduling staff to see whether another therapist might be available to complete this initial evaluation. Discovering that no one else had an opening in their schedule, Sheila returned to the patient, feeling her heart racing and her breathing become shallow and labored. Sheila asked the patient to describe some of his functional limitations and to demonstrate upper-extremity functional movements. The patient reported having difficulty controlling the movement of his right hand and, without prompting, stood up in front of Sheila and demonstrated his challenges with unzipping his pants and tightening his belt. Sheila startled and moved away from the patient as she recognized her skyrocketing anxiety.

After having spent less than 6 minutes with this patient, Sheila informed him and the attendant that the evaluation was completed. Sheila informed the patient, "There is nothing I can do for you" and directed him and his attendant to leave the building. At the same time, she left the treatment area. Sheila immediately documented a brief evaluation report and included a discharge notation: "No therapy indicated at this time." As Sheila left the building, she abruptly announced to the registration staff that she was ill and asked them to cancel her patients for the rest of the day.

Foundational ethics question:

- How does the ethical principle of *nonmaleficence* apply to this scenario?

Considerations and discussion:

The patient has a diagnosis of stroke and functional impairments resulting from that stroke. His condition would typically be considered eligible for occupational therapy evaluation and intervention.

- Does a personal challenge experienced by a therapist justify early termination of an evaluation session?
- Does the reason a therapist experiences distress make a difference in supporting the early termination of an evaluation session?
- Is a therapist acting ethically when discharging a patient for personal reasons when the patient could reasonably have benefited from occupational therapy services?

Did the occupational therapist harm this patient?

What other options might Sheila have explored or used? Abandoning a patient or providing a service that does not meet the expected standard is a violation of the principle of *nonmaleficence*. Intention is always a factor in evaluating nonmaleficence, and justification of the harmful action is obligatory. Sheila terminated the evaluation session without gathering sufficient information about the patient's status. Compelling personal challenges prevented her from fulfilling her professional role at the level of the expected standard of performance. A severe emotional crisis could serve as a rational justification for prematurely terminating an evaluation session. Alternatively, the recommendations for no intervention and immediately discharging the patient appear to be violations of the principle of nonmaleficence. Although no other therapist was immediately available to perform the evaluation, Sheila could have ended the session and directed the patient to reschedule with another therapist at a future date.

(Continued)

CASE EXAMPLE 8.2. SHEILA: NONMALEFICENCE AND EVALUATION *(Cont.)*

Some factors can be considered legitimate when there is a serious barrier to the establishment of a therapeutic relationship. A therapist can take steps to prevent being assigned a new patient for evaluation when there is a risk that the patient's personal characteristics or history will generate a serious adverse emotional reaction and moral distress. Self-disclosure of one's life story is optional, but refusing to serve a patient in need of occupational therapy requires an explanation and request for accommodations. A more egregious violation of the principle of nonmaleficence is a therapist refusing to serve a patient for reasons that most would label as bigoted or racist in some way.

Other violations of the principle of nonmaleficence include exploitation of the therapist–patient relationship. Nonmaleficence can also be violated with the blurring of professional boundaries when personal relationships between the therapist and the patient encroach on professional objectivity.

Conversely, occupational therapists who devote too little time to the completion of a thorough evaluation of a patient, as a result of an organization's unachievable productivity demands, are also acting in a manner contrary to the patient's best interests. Therapists have a duty to focus on the benefit to the patient and not harm the patient by engaging in behaviors and actions that violate the principle of nonmaleficence.

Autonomy

Autonomy is often referred to as the "self-determination" principle. Occupational therapy's core value of freedom honors personal choice and acknowledges that the wishes and values of the client guide the ethical practice of the profession. The right to self-determination also recognizes the patient's right "to hold views, to make choices, and to take actions based on [their] values and beliefs" (Beauchamp & Childress, 2013, p. 106). This principle means that the client should have the occupational therapy evaluation fully explained to them, an opportunity to express their views about the evaluation process, and the choice of whether to engage in it.

AUTONOMY AND RELATED STANDARDS OF CONDUCT

The Code RSCs that are consistent with the principle of *autonomy* are as follows:

- Respect and honor the expressed wishes of recipients of service.
- Fully disclose the benefits, risks, and potential outcomes of any intervention; the personnel who will be providing the intervention; and any reasonable alternatives to the proposed intervention.
- Obtain consent after disclosing appropriate information and answering any questions posed by the recipient of service or research participant to ensure voluntariness.
- Establish a collaborative relationship with recipients of service and relevant stakeholders to promote shared decision making.

- Respect the client's right to refuse occupational therapy services temporarily or permanently, even when that refusal has potential to result in poor outcomes.
- Maintain the confidentiality of all verbal, written, electronic, augmentative, and nonverbal communications, in compliance with applicable laws, including all aspects of privacy laws, and exceptions thereto (e.g., Health Insurance Portability and Accountability Act of 1996 [P. L. 104-191], Family Educational Rights and Privacy Act of 1974 [P. L. 93-380]).
- Facilitate comprehension and address barriers to communication (e.g., aphasia; differences in language, literacy, or culture) with the recipient of service (or responsible party), student, or research participant.

ARE YOU HONORING THE PRINCIPLE OF AUTONOMY?

Patients have the right to be fully informed of the process of occupational therapy evaluation and to consent or refuse to participate in all or any portion of an assessment (see Case Example 8.3). When a patient has been legally declared incompetent or two physicians have examined the patient and determined a temporary or permanent lack of capacity to make decisions about medical care or treatment, an authorized agent must be relied on to engage in decision making. A patient who is in a coma or too ill to make their own decisions may have someone who holds a health proxy to make decisions for them. Additionally, parents have a right to make health decisions for their children who are under the age of majority (generally age 18 years).

CASE EXAMPLE 8.3. SETH: AUTONOMY AND EVALUATION

An 18-year-old high school senior, **Seth,** has been treated for severe symptoms of attention deficit hyperactivity disorder since he was a young child. Seth's wealthy grandfather decided it was time for Seth to be more independent and gifted Seth with a new sport utility vehicle as an 18th birthday present. Seth's parents have refused to allow Seth to test for or obtain his driver's license because they are concerned that Seth will not be sufficiently attentive to drive safely.

Seth's father heard about the Safe Driver Program at the local rehabilitation center, which serves drivers of all ages. Seth's father scheduled an appointment for Seth to have a comprehensive occupational therapy evaluation focused on driving skills. Seth complained to his father about having to take a special test when his friends already have their license. Seth decided to go to the session because his father told him, "You're going to take this test since I'm paying for it. And if you don't I'm selling your car!"

On arrival for his appointment, Seth was asked to sign a Consent to Evaluation and Treatment form. Seth read it carefully, signed the form, and informed his father that he would refuse to take the driving evaluation if his father did not leave the building. Seth's father decided to "let Seth win one" and informed Seth he would return in about 90 minutes. **Peggy,** the occupational therapist, engaged Seth in the standard protocol of assessments of the driving skills evaluation. Peggy identified several deficits, including Seth's environmental scanning, impulse control, and inappropriate attention

(Continued)

CASE EXAMPLE 8.3. SETH: AUTONOMY AND EVALUATION *(Cont.)*

to distracting stimuli presented within the assessment tool. On completion of the evaluation, Peggy summarized the identified deficits and formulated an intervention plan intended to help Seth be successful in his pursuit of the IADL of driving. Peggy finished sharing her findings and recommendations with Seth just as Seth's father returned. As Peggy began to share the evaluation findings with Seth's father, Seth yelled, "I know my rights! You can't tell him how I did unless I say so!" Seth's father admonished Seth, saying, "I paid for this so I have a right to know what Peggy thinks." Seth stormed out of the building. Seth's father told Peggy, "I'll call you!" as he quickly followed Seth out the door.

Foundational ethics question:

- How does the ethical principle of *autonomy* apply to this scenario?

Considerations and discussion:

Seth exercised his newly acquired right to consent to an occupational therapy evaluation and also to have his right to privacy honored. Adults who have the capacity to make their own medical decisions have the right to choose whether and with whom their personal information can be shared. Seth's father is demonstrating his recent former role of parent of a child by exercising his paternalistic impulses. Seth's father is struggling with the fact that the parent of an adult child who has reached the age of consent and who has capacity to make his or her own decisions has no right to that child's health care information (Berg et al., 2001). The fact that Seth's father paid for the evaluation may be relevant but is legally inconsequential to his request to learn about what is now Seth's protected health information.

When Seth's father contacts Peggy to learn about the occupational therapy evaluation and her recommendations, Peggy is bound by federal law, as well as the ethical principle of *autonomy*, to observe Seth's wishes and refuse to provide any information to Seth's father (HIPAA, 1996). If and when Seth consents to having his evaluation results shared with his father, Peggy can reveal the outcome and recommendations. Seth could also decide to personally share the evaluation results with anyone of his choice. If Seth never consents to a release of information, he alone is the client with whom Peggy can confer regarding next steps.

Justice

The ethical principle of *justice* refers to the fair, equitable, and impartial treatment of persons (Beauchamp & Childress, 2013). When occupational therapy practitioners use the principle of justice, they consistently follow established rules and demonstrate a concern for fairness. It is important to emphasize that fair and equitable is not the equivalent of equal. *Equal* denotes the same, whereas equitable refers to even-handed treatment or fair distribution of benefits or resources according to individual or group need (Beauchamp & Childress, 2013).

The process of occupational therapy evaluation emphasizes the unique nature of each person's occupations, contexts, and preferences. When two distinct individuals are treated equally, the perception, the outcome, and the impacts may have disparate results. Providing an equal amount of time or fair amount of services is a matter of subjective judgment. For example, two male patients, both with newly diagnosed rheumatoid arthritis, may be scheduled for the same length of time for their initial occupational therapy evaluation, yet their unique client factors, performance deficits, occupational choices, and priorities could result in one evaluation requiring a second session for completion, and the findings of both evaluations will result in two substantially different occupational therapy intervention plans.

JUSTICE AND RELATED STANDARDS OF CONDUCT

The Code RSCs that are consistent with the principle of *justice* are as follows:

- Respond to requests for occupational therapy services (e.g., a referral) in a timely manner as determined by law, regulation, or policy.
- Maintain awareness of current laws and AOTA policies and official documents that apply to the profession of occupational therapy.
- Hold requisite credentials for the occupational therapy services they provide in academic, research, physical, or virtual work settings.
- Bill and collect fees legally and justly in a manner that is fair, reasonable, and commensurate with services delivered.
- Ensure that documentation for reimbursement purposes is done in accordance with applicable laws, guidelines, and regulations.

ARE YOU HONORING THE PRINCIPLE OF JUSTICE?

It is the responsibility of all occupational therapy practitioners to honor the principle of *justice* in evaluation (see Case Example 8.4). They must follow state laws, hold the requisite state license, and bill according to their work site and the services that have been provided to the patient. Most importantly, practitioners must provide evaluations equitably to all patients on the basis of patients' individual needs. This does not mean providing the same amount of time or the same assessment tool to each patient; rather, practitioners must determine what each individual needs and provide the evaluation that is appropriate for that person.

CASE EXAMPLE 8.4. VERONICA: JUSTICE AND EVALUATION

Veronica, an occupational therapist working in a community mental health center, received a referral for occupational therapy evaluation of **Mildred,** a 49-year-old woman with a long history of depression and bipolar affective disorder. Mildred is experiencing some troubling symptoms that are resulting in significant difficulties with organizing and performing IADLs, so much so that she has recently been tardy to or absent from her job cleaning offices.

At the time of registration for the occupational therapy evaluation, Mildred presented her insurance card from her employer-sponsored health insurance. On first meeting Veronica, Mildred informed her that her insurance requires a $25 per-visit copay, which she had paid in cash. Mildred went

(Continued)

CASE EXAMPLE 8.4. VERONICA: JUSTICE AND EVALUATION *(Cont.)*

on to share that she also has a separate deductible of $2,000. Mildred told Veronica that coming up with $25 was difficult, but she knows it is worth it because an occupational therapist was a big help to her a few years ago. Mildred also explained that she does not know where she will get the money to pay her sizable insurance deductible.

Veronica reassured Mildred that the financial advocate at the center could help with her financial concerns. Veronica knows that in her setting, when patients are not able to pay for services, grant funding and government programs allow for "writing off" their bill. However, when patients have insurance, their insurance benefits are accessed, and patients are responsible for their portion of the fees. Veronica takes her job in community mental health seriously. She is proud of her role and passionate about promoting social justice by providing her services to people who are economically and socially disadvantaged (Braveman & Bass-Haugen, 2009).

As Veronica engaged Mildred in gathering an occupational profile and analyzed Mildred's occupational performance skills and patterns, she identified several co-morbid upper-extremity neuromuscular dysfunctions that likely impede Mildred's independent performance of activities of daily living. The evaluation took much more time than Veronica had estimated, and she had to consider more assessment components than anticipated. When Veronica documented the evaluation results, she realized that she had completed an occupational therapy evaluation of high complexity and CPT® (Current Procedural Terminology) code 97167 should be charged (American Medical Association, 2019). Veronica is well informed about the charge categories and that her employer has established a higher charge for each progressive level of complexity of occupational therapy evaluation. Veronica feels that she really connected with Mildred, and she empathizes with Mildred's financial concerns. Veronica entered the charge for Mildred's occupational therapy evaluation as the low-complexity CPT 97165, knowing that Mildred's total bill for occupational therapy services would be a challenge for Mildred, no matter the final cost.

Foundational ethics question:
- How does the ethical principle of *justice* apply to this scenario?

Considerations and discussion:
Veronica is demonstrating concern for her client and is making accommodations that Mildred might appreciate. However, Veronica is not acting justly for Mildred's best interests or for the best interests of her employer. Reporting that Mildred's occupational therapy evaluation was less complex than it really was may result in Mildred being ineligible for the intensity of occupational therapy services that may be warranted by her current limitations. The insurance reviewer, whose job it is to authorize occupational therapy services, may raise questions about the service provided when comparing the clinical documentation with the billed charge. On the basis of a charge for a low-complexity evaluation, the insurance reviewer could legitimately limit Mildred's number of authorized occupational therapy visits. Limited authorization for a low frequency and duration of approved services could well result in insufficient progress for Mildred's independence.

Veronica's intentional undercharging violates the principle of *justice* in terms of being untruthful and undervaluing her services. Veronica is also not being just to her employer because the organization

(Continued)

CASE EXAMPLE 8.4. VERONICA: JUSTICE AND EVALUATION *(Cont.)*

will be reimbursed for less time and service than Veronica devoted to Mildred's occupational therapy evaluation. Veronica's social justice mindset is clearly violating the broader application of the principle of justice.

The occupational therapy profession identifies *justice* as one of the profession's core values; it is also one of the six ethical principles that frame the Code. The core value of justice highlights inclusion and the development of communities where people can, according to the Code, "function, flourish and live a satisfactory life." The Code directs occupational therapy practitioners to relate in a respectful, fair, and impartial manner and respect laws and standards. Honoring the core value of justice and abiding by the ethical principle of justice are imperatives for all practitioners.

Veracity

The principle of *veracity* refers to comprehensive, accurate, and objective transmission of information and includes fostering an understanding of that information (Beauchamp & Childress, 2013). Truthfulness and honesty are the hallmarks of the principle of veracity. When occupational therapists evaluate a patient, that patient has the right to a full and accurate accounting of the findings and recommendations. Sharing the documentation produced at the end of an evaluation, with abbreviations, medical terminology, and documentation formats that are foreign or beyond the patient's reading comprehension level, is contrary to honoring the principle of veracity. Occupational therapy practitioners have the duty to inform patients and make every effort to ensure that patients understand what is being shared and receive the assistance they need to comprehend the importance of that information to the development of their individualized intervention plan.

VERACITY AND RELATED STANDARDS OF CONDUCT

The Code RSCs that are consistent with the principle of *veracity* are as follows:

- Represent credentials, qualifications, education, experience, training, roles, duties, competence, contributions, and findings accurately in all forms of communication.
- Refrain from using or participating in the use of any form of communication that contains false, fraudulent, deceptive, misleading, or unfair statements or claims.
- Record and report in an accurate and timely manner and in accordance with applicable regulations all information related to professional or academic documentation and activities.

ARE YOU HONORING THE PRINCIPLE OF VERACITY?

Occupational therapy practitioners must accurately and truthfully represent their professional competence, experience, and conformance to professional standards (see Case Example 8.5). An occupational therapist who claims expertise in the evaluation of populations or skill with specific assessments without proper training and experience is clearly violating the principle of veracity.

If an occupational therapist is called on to perform an evaluation for a patient diagnosed with a rare condition with which the therapist has no experience, the principle of *veracity* requires that the therapist make the patient aware of the limits of their competence or refer the patient to a more experienced therapist. That does not mean the patient must be turned away. In some settings and in underserved geographic regions, the less experienced occupational therapist may be the only practitioner available to provide any level of service. In these situations, the therapist must honor the principle of veracity by informing

CASE EXAMPLE 8.5. ELLEN: VERACITY AND EVALUATION

Great Life Senior Care, Inc. (GLSC) is a continuing care community funded by resident funds, local government block grant funding, or, when residents' personal funds are depleted, by state and federal Medicaid. The GLSC brochures and website describe a wide array of services, including professional occupational therapy services. **Amelia,** the daughter of Enid, a soon-to-be new resident, is eager to have a comprehensive evaluation of her mother's functional status. The GLSC transition specialist promptly scheduled Enid for time with **Ellen,** their "very skilled OT" for a comprehensive independent living and community skills evaluation. The transition specialist stated that "the goal of time with the OT is to learn about Enid's challenges and to develop a 'living well plan'" for Enid's residence at GLSC.

When Amelia brought her mother to the scheduled appointment, they were welcomed by Ellen, who is an occupational therapy assistant (OTA). Amelia, an educated health care consumer, questioned Ellen: "You're an OTA; where is the occupational therapist?" Ellen chuckled and replied, "Oh, don't worry. I know what I'm doing. Since we're a community program, I take care of all occupational therapy evaluations. I've been doing these evaluations for over 15 years! There isn't an OTR at GLSC and we really don't need one."

Foundational ethics question:
- How does the ethical principle of *veracity* apply to this scenario?

Considerations and discussion:
Clearly, the occupational therapy assistant in this scenario is not conforming to the AOTA Standards of Practice or the AOTA Guidelines for Supervision, Roles, and Responsibilities During the Delivery of Occupational Therapy Services. This occupational therapy assistant is almost certainly violating the state's licensure statute or administrative code by both claiming to provide and providing what she is representing as an occupational therapy evaluation. Speaking with authority and denigrating the organization's need for a properly trained and credentialed occupational therapist violates the principle of veracity. The organization is not providing what it purports to offer, and consumers are not getting what they expect. The client is bound to suffer from receiving an inadequate evaluation and appropriate intervention plan. The occupational therapy assistant is demeaning the profession and likely damaging the otherwise good reputation of this assisted living facility.

Questions to consider:
- What might Amelia, Enid's daughter, do to address this situation?
- What other options might these consumers pursue?

the patient of the resources and skills offered and rely on the patient to exercise autonomy and accept or refuse the less-than-ideal occupational therapy service. This could mean the patient makes the choice to go without services.

Occupational therapy assistants work under the supervision of occupational therapists. They may perform specific evaluations independently with supervision but require supervision to use evaluative data for setting goals and intervention planning. Once the occupation therapy assistant performs an evaluation, they are required to review the evaluation data with the supervising occupational therapist. Together they can decide on the areas of strength and limitations for the patient. Following this the occupational therapist and the occupational therapy assistant can, as a team, develop the goals for the client and the course of intervention.

Fidelity

The ethical principle of *fidelity* is derived from the Latin root *fidelis,* meaning loyal. *Fidelity* refers to the duty one has to keep a commitment once it is made (Veatch et al., 2010). Health professions make a commitment to fidelity when vowing to be loyal to their clients, consistent, attentive, and acting in the best interests of the person being served. Occupational therapy practitioners would rarely inform patients that they will be loyal to them, but in the interest of establishing a therapeutic relationship, therapists often tell their patients, "I'm here to help you accomplish your goals" and "We're in this together!" The therapist who most embodies the ethical principle of fidelity is the one who is always willing to take on the difficult patient.

FIDELITY AND RELATED STANDARDS OF CONDUCT

The Code RSCs that are consistent with the principle of *fidelity* are as follows:

- Promote collaborative actions and communication as a member of interprofessional teams to facilitate quality care and safety for clients.
- Respect the practices, competencies, roles, and responsibilities of their own and other professions to promote a collaborative environment reflective of interprofessional teams.
- Use conflict resolution and internal and alternative dispute resolution resources as needed to resolve organizational and interpersonal conflicts, as well as perceived institutional ethics violations.
- Self-identify when personal, cultural, or religious values preclude, or are anticipated to negatively affect, the professional relationship or provision of services, while adhering to organizational policies when requesting an exemption from service to an individual or group on the basis of conflict of conscience.

ARE YOU HONORING THE PRINCIPLE OF FIDELITY?

Fidelity also applies to developing respect for and acting respectful toward other occupational therapy practitioners and all other professionals encountered in the practice environment. Behaviors that demonstrate disrespect or that discount the value or contributions of others violate fidelity both within an interdisciplinary team and within organizations and systems (Purtilo & Doherty, 2011).

Adherence to the principle of *fidelity* also requires occupational therapists to share information in ways that promote the patient's understanding of the information and, with the patient's consent, engagement of those invited to participate in the occupational therapy evaluation. Fidelity is violated when therapists opt out of sharing objective assessment findings with patients in the interest of not upsetting or demoralizing them and their hopes and goals for improvement (Veatch et al., 2010). See Case Example 8.6.

CASE EXAMPLE 8.6. HECTOR: FIDELITY AND EVALUATION

Hector Garcia, a middle-aged man, is referred to a comprehensive outpatient postconcussion rehabilitation program to aid his recovery from a serious concussion that occurred during a scaffold collapse at his construction job. Mr. Garcia emigrated from Central America as a teenager, and his primary language is Spanish. Although Mr. Garcia is known to be fluent in English, since the accident he has almost exclusively spoken Spanish and reportedly has had difficulty comprehending spoken English.

The protocol for the postconcussion rehabilitation program includes comprehensive evaluations, which are completed on Day 1. The first team member to evaluate Mr. Garcia was **Carmen,** an occupational therapist trained in Puerto Rico. Carmen is new to the postconcussion program. Mr. Garcia was then evaluated by other members of the team, including Jim, a physical therapist, and **Erin,** a speech-language pathologist.

On Day 2 of the program, the interdisciplinary treatment team typically meets with the patient, so Mr. Garcia and his Workers' Compensation case manager were invited to attend a team meeting to hear the evaluation findings, review recommendations, and arrive at an interdisciplinary intervention plan specific to Mr. Garcia's needs. Because of illness, Carmen is absent from work on Mr. Garcia's Day 2 meeting. Juana, another occupational therapist at the rehabilitation center, volunteered to review the occupational therapy evaluation report before the team meeting and participate in the interdisciplinary team conference in Carmen's place.

As the team conference began, Erin expressed concern about Mr. Garcia's comprehension of the information to be discussed. Erin shared that she had asked Leona, a physical therapy assistant at the clinic who is fluent in Spanish, to join the meeting to provide English-to-Spanish interpretation for Mr. Garcia. On hearing this, Juana scoffed and blurted out, "He's been in this country for over 30 years. He understands English! My ex-husband was from Mexico, and when I'd ask him to do something he didn't want to do, he'd act like he didn't understand English. What a waste of Leona's time!" Despite Juana's objection, Leona joined the meeting and greeted Mr. Garcia, who nodded and smiled in response to Leona's greeting, "Buenos dias."

As Erin shared results of the speech therapy cognitive assessments she had performed with Mr. Garcia, Juana interrupted and questioned why Erin used one of the assessments and why she thought it was appropriate for a postconcussion assessment. Erin calmly explained her rationale and proceeded to deliver the remainder of her report.

(Continued)

CASE EXAMPLE 8.6. HECTOR: FIDELITY AND EVALUATION *(Cont.)*

When Juana's turn came to report the occupational therapy evaluation results, she stated, "I hate to say this, but Carmen didn't know what she was doing! She really doesn't have the skill or experience to evaluate anyone with this level of head injury. I'm not going to share the garbage that she documented! I need to see this *cholo* after our meeting today to start over and use the right occupational therapy evals!" Jim, Erin, and the case manager were so stunned by Juana's statements that they did not speak for a full 20 seconds. Leona observed that Mr. Garcia appeared confused, and she interpreted this to mean that Mr. Garcia did not understand what was going on. Leona invited Mr. Garcia to join her in leaving the meeting, and they both exited the room. The Workers' Compensation case manager followed behind. Juana also left the room, exclaiming to Erin and Jim, "I've had it! Carmen is on her way out of this department!"

Foundational ethics question:
- How does the ethical principle of *fidelity* apply to this scenario?

Considerations and discussion:
The emotional responses likely elicited by the event described in this case example must be addressed before moving on to the foundational ethical concerns this encounter presents. Any reader of this case example would no doubt initially focus on the uncivil behaviors exhibited by Juana, the occupational therapist. "Disrespectful and rude" is certainly an accurate characterization of Juana's treatment of her colleagues. Juana's referring to Mr. Garcia as *cholo* (a slang term of disrespect) and the skepticism she voiced about the need for language interpretation were insensitive, bigoted, and clinically inappropriate.

Let's start with by focusing on what's going on with Juana and why. Is this behavior out of character for Juana? Has she ever acted in this way before? Why would she make statements about her ex-husband in the presence of a patient she did not know? Why would Juana refer to Mr. Garcia in a derogatory manner? What might the answers to these questions have to do with Juana's behavior? Anyone who values the ethical principles of fidelity and beneficence would consider Juana's behavior to be absolutely unacceptable.

Some additional background may help shine a light on Juana's behavior:
- Juana has been a clinical specialist in the treatment of head injury for more than a decade. Erin has less than 1 year of experience as a speech-language pathologist. Jim is a contract therapist on a 3-month, contracted assignment, but he has expertise in the treatment of persons with head injuries.
- Juana knows that Carmen transferred to the postconcussion rehabilitation program just before she was to be terminated from her job at another rehabilitation center in the same organization.
- Juana has been assigned as Carmen's mentor since Carmen transferred to this program site more than 2 months ago. Juana has helped the department manager structure a formal learning plan for Carmen. In Juana's assessment, Carmen is seriously lagging in achieving the objectives of her learning plan.
- Although other team members are unaware of it, Juana's very recent divorce left her struggling with her personal finances and the care of her three teenage children. Her ex-husband, who was a

(Continued)

CASE EXAMPLE 8.6. HECTOR: FIDELITY AND EVALUATION *(Cont.)*

college exchange student when they married, recently returned to his home country of Mexico. Juana's ex-husband has not contributed any financial support for their children since his departure. Do any of these intervening circumstances justify Juana's behavior? Likely not.

Let's agree that Juana behaved badly but consider some potentially rational justifications, consistent with the principle of fidelity, that underlie Juana's issues.

- Could Juana be correct that Carmen did not use relevant assessments tools or processes for the occupational therapy evaluation of Mr. Garcia?
  - Juana is a clinical specialist in this area of practice. We can be confident that Juana's clinical judgment regarding appropriate assessments is sound.
- Do we know whether Carmen has demonstrated the clinical competence to evaluate a person in need of postconcussion rehabilitation?
  - Juana is serving in a role that requires her to assess and rate Carmen's clinical performance.
- By what authority did Juana make such bold statements about Carmen's performance?
  - Juana has been assigned as mentor. Juana has a professional duty to critique the assessment tools selected and the documentation Carmen produced.

Juana's primary violations of the ethical principle of fidelity were her disrespectful statements about the patient, her lack of explanation for how Mr. Garcia could have been more appropriately evaluated by an occupational therapist, and her intrusive and disruptive behaviors during an interdisciplinary team meeting. Juana also violated the principle of fidelity by unfairly and publicly questioning the credibility of a colleague, Erin, in this interdisciplinary setting. Juana violated the principle of fidelity by attacking Carmen's performance without discussing the issues with Carmen and also by vociferously denouncing Carmen's work.

A request by Juana to be exempted from care on the basis of a personal bias or personal challenge is one way to honor the principle of fidelity. Because of what appears to be a negative bias, which one can assume was prompted by Juana's spillover feelings about her ex-husband, Juana could have requested to be excused from serving as Carmen's mentor, and she should not have volunteered to participate in this interdisciplinary team meeting. Without question, Juana should not take on the task of reevaluating Mr. Garcia from an occupational therapy perspective. Juana's actions clearly violate any sense of loyalty or freedom from bias, and she should not be allowed to provide evaluation or treatment services to this patient whom she clearly does not respect.

There is more to this scenario that specifically honors the principle of fidelity.

- Carmen, an appropriately credentialed occupational therapist, meets the legal requirements for performing evaluations in an outpatient rehabilitation program. We must assume that Carmen was loyal in fulfilling her assigned job to evaluate Mr. Garcia by selecting and using assessments, and her skills, to do her best.
- Erin, the speech-language pathologist, identified that Mr. Garcia's current comprehension of English could be hampered by the effects of the head injury. Erin acknowledged Mr. Garcia's right to understand the meaningful information being shared by members of the interdisciplinary team.
- Erin also took affirmative action to invite Leona, the physical therapy assistant fluent in Spanish, to act as a interpreter. Erin and Leona honored Mr. Garcia's challenges in comprehending the information so he could adequately participate in formulating his own intervention plan.

(Continued)

CASE EXAMPLE 8.6. HECTOR: FIDELITY AND EVALUATION (*Cont.*)

- Team members attending this meeting could have addressed Juana's behavior when it first occurred early in the meeting. Erin could have ignored or objected to Juana's questioning and certainly could have been insulted. Yet Erin did not appear to take Juana's questioning personally, and she diplomatically and respectfully responded to Juana's objections in a professional manner.
- Jim missed the opportunity to support his colleague, Erin. Jim could have defended Erin's choice or otherwise interrupted and advised Juana to wait to ask her questions until after the meeting. Professional respect and collaboration are expectations consistent with the principle of fidelity.
- We must grant Juana due respect for her role as a clinical specialist. Juana devoted her energy and has made a moral commitment to providing high-quality occupational therapy evaluation and treatment to a vulnerable population. Although it may be difficult to discern, fidelity is likely the core of Juana's concerns.

Additional questions to consider:
- How could Juana have supported her statements (and delivered her opinion of Carmen's work) in ways that better honor the ethical principle of fidelity?
- How could Juana have supported her coworkers and respected the interdisciplinary team process in ways that honor the ethical principle of fidelity?

Ethics and Law

The case studies in this chapter focus on ethical dilemmas and application of ethical principles to dilemmas that an occupational therapy practitioner may encounter while administering assessments and engaging in the totality of the evaluation process. The majority of these case scenarios also referenced a legal standard, cited an applicable law, or described an action that clearly violated an organizational policy or even included fraudulent documentation or billing. It is important to understand that ethics and laws are not the same, yet most laws have, at their core, a value or ethical principle. Laws are enacted for the good of the public and describe what is prohibited and the consequences of violating a specific law (Kornblau, 2019). Unethical behavior may also be illegal. However, strict adherence to laws that are deemed by some to be unjust may in fact be the best and most justifiable path to upholding ethical principles.

Note. A version of this chapter was previously published in *Hinojosa and Kramer's Evaluation and Occupational Therapy: Obtaining and Interpreting Data, 5th Edition,* edited by Paula Kramer and Namrata Grampurohit. Copyright © 2020 by the American Occupational Therapy Association. Reprinted with permission.

REFERENCES

Allen, C. K., Austin, S. L., David, S. K., Earhart, C. A., McCraith, D. B., & Riska-Williams, L. (2007). *Manual for the Allen Cognitive Level Screen–5 (ACLS–5) and Large Allen Cognitive Level Screen–5 (LACLS–5).* ACLS and LACLS Committee.

American Medical Association. (2019). *Current Procedural Terminology: CPT® 2019 professional edition*. Author.

American Psychological Association. (2016). *Ethical principles of psychologists and code of conduct (including 2010 and 2016 amendments)*. https://www.apa.org/ethics/code/

American Speech-Language-Hearing Association. (2020). *National Outcomes Measurement System (NOMS)*. https://www.asha.org/noms/

Ayres, A. J. (1989). *Sensory Integration and Praxis Tests*. Western Psychological Services.

Beauchamp, T. L., & Childress, J. F. (2013). *Principles of biomedical ethics* (7th ed.). Oxford University Press.

Berg, J. W., Appelbaum, P. S., Lidz, C. W., & Parker, L. S. (2001). *Informed consent: Legal theory and clinical practice* (2nd ed.). Oxford University Press.

Bergen, G., Stevens, M. R., & Burns, E. R. (2016). Falls and fall injuries among adults aged ≥65 years—United States, 2014. *Morbidity and Mortality Weekly Report, 65*, 993–998. https://doi.org/10.15585/mmwr.mm6537a2

Bloomer, J. S., & Williams, S. K. (1979). *Bay Area Functional Performance Evaluation* (research ed.). Consulting Psychologists Press.

Braveman, B., & Bass-Haugen, J. D. (2009). Social justice and health disparities: An evolving discourse in occupational therapy research and intervention. *American Journal of Occupational Therapy, 63*, 7–12. https://doi.org/10.5014/ajot.63.1.7

Family Educational Rights and Privacy Act of 1974, Pub. L. 93-380, 20 U.S.C. § 1232g; 34 CFR Part 99.

Fleming, A., & Rucas, K. (2015). Welcoming a paradigm shift in occupational therapy: Symptom validity measures and cognitive assessment. *Applied Neuropsychology: Adult, 22*, 23–31. https://doi.org/10.1080/23279095.2013.822873

Health Insurance Portability and Accountability Act of 1996, Pub. L. 104-191, 42 U.S.C. § 300gg, 29 U.S.C. §§ 1181–1183, and 42 U.S.C. §§ 1320d–1320d9. https://www.govinfo.gov/app/details/PLAW-104publ191

Houston, D., Lang Williams, S., Bloomer, J., & Mann, W. C. (1989). The Bay Area Functional Performance Evaluation: Development and standardization. *American Journal of Occupational Therapy, 43*, 170–183. https://doi.org/10.5014/ajot.43.3.170

Kornblau, B. L. (2019). Understanding the law. In K. Jacobs & G. L. McCormack (Eds.), *The occupational therapy manager* (6th ed., pp. 565–570). AOTA Press.

Law, M. C., & MacDermid, J. (2008). Introduction to evidenced-based practice. In M. C. Law & J. MacDermid (Eds.), *Evidenced-based rehabilitation: A guide to practice* (2nd ed). Slack.

McGourty, L. K. (1978). *Kohlman Evaluation of Living Skills*. Seattle: KELS Research.

Purtilo, R., & Doherty, R. (2011). *Ethical dimensions in the health professions* (5th ed.). Saunders/Elsevier.

Rawls, J. (1971). *A theory of justice*. Belknap Press.

Simon, H. A. (1956). Rational choice and the structure of the environment. *Psychological Review, 63*(2), 129–138. https://doi.org/10.1037/h0042769

Slater, D. Y. (2016). *Reference guide to the Occupational Therapy Code of Ethics*. AOTA Press.

Thomson, L. K., & Robnett, R. (2016). *KELS: Kohlman Evaluation of Living Skills* (4th ed.). AOTA Press.

Veatch, R. M., Haddad, A. M., & English, D. C. (2010). *Case studies in biomedical ethics*. Oxford University Press.

9

Addressing Health Disparities

M. BETH MERRYMAN, PhD, OTR/L, FAOTA

Introduction

Health disparities are "differences in the incidence, prevalence, mortality, and burden of diseases and other adverse health conditions that exist among specific population groups in the United States" (U.S. Department of Health and Human Services [DHHS], National Institutes of Health, National Health, Lung, and Blood Institute, 2017; also see Institute of Medicine, 2002). Broad health-related research has identified the importance of social factors such as *socioeconomic status* (SES; i.e., factors affecting resources to engage and participate in meaningful occupations of daily life; Madsen et al., 2015) and marginalization due to discrimination in measures of health and well-being (American Occupational Therapy Association [AOTA], 2013; Bass-Haugen, 2009).

Occupational therapy practitioners are responsible for upholding the professional AOTA Code of Ethics (the Code). Among the challenges for all health care providers is ensuring access to services. This chapter explores the role of occupational therapy managers to address health care disparity from the perspective of the professional Code. First, the chapter provides foundational information such as terminology and definitions. Then, models that are used to understand health inequality and disparity are presented. Specific ways that health disparity and inequality may be seen in practice are identified, with an emphasis on the role of the manager to establish an environment in which the core values, principles, and standards of conduct of the profession are upheld.

Essential Considerations

HEALTH INITIATIVES

Health inequalities are "avoidable inequalities in health between groups of people within countries and between countries" (World Health Organization [WHO], 2018). *Health disparity* refers to the metric to measure health equity and is a descriptive term for a specific population group difference in access to health care or health status (Gamble & Stone, 2006). An example is a population group that demonstrates reduced health access after controlling for insurance coverage (Braveman, 2014).

A concern that affects health status is the concept of *health literacy,* which refers to a person's "capacity to obtain, communicate, process and understand basic health information and services in order to make appropriate health decisions" (Centers for Disease Control and Prevention [CDC], 2015). This is a concern because health literacy has been demonstrated to influence health outcomes (AOTA, 2017; Schnitzer et al., 2011).

The federal government has established priorities through overarching goals identified in Healthy People 2020, which focuses on improving the health of all groups through elimination of disparities and inequities (DHHS, 2016). This document reflects many of the core values and principles of occupational therapy by emphasizing health status by improving activity participation, emphasizing improved natural and built environments, and promoting participation in everyday activities.

The Agency for Healthcare Research and Quality's *National Healthcare Quality and Disparities Report,* an annual report on quality of health care in the United States, identified improvements in rate of insurance among adults ages 18 to 64 years, specifically among Black and Hispanic adults, and rates of childhood immunization across racial and ethnic groups (DHHS, 2014). However, some areas reflected increased disparity, including hospice care and chronic disease management. Both areas reflect core aspects of occupational therapy practice.

MODELS AND THEORIES TO ADDRESS HEALTH DISPARITY

Several social sciences and occupation-based models inform understanding about the impact of social factors, such as the environment, on client health. In each model described in this section, the role of the environment as part of the relationship between the client and occupational therapy practitioner is emphasized as key to influencing health. Occupational therapy is invested in client health and thus uses models to understand challenges to client behavior change.

Potential occupational therapy interventions include addressing both the person and the environment. For example, an occupational therapy manager committing to an inclusive work environment might research and require staff training on cultural competence and implicit bias, so that staff might more clearly use communication strategies and styles likely to result in client understanding and adoption of important safety considerations (AOTA, 2013). Another example might include institutional efforts to hire occupational therapy practitioners and staff whose sociocultural backgrounds reflect the client population.

Fundamental cause theory

The *fundamental cause theory* was developed by Link and Phelan (1995) to explain why the association between SES and mortality has persisted despite radical changes in diseases, and risk factors are presumed to explain it. The theory posits that those with lower SES continue to have higher rates of cancer and cardiovascular disease because their economic status limits their resources relative to healthy food and reliable transportation. The theory has four aspects:

- Multiple illnesses are potentially affected.
- Multiple risks are present.
- Access and resources can decrease risk and consequence if disease occurs.
- Risk and consequence can be reduced through methods that improve health outcomes.

Stress process model

The *stress process model* (Pearlin, 1989) explores the person–environment interactions relative to individual exposure, response, and recurrence of stress. Pearlin addressed the structural and contextual elements in which behavior occurs and recurs in the form of a habit and the challenges of change. The theory is relevant because it addresses both stressful life events, such as an acute medical crisis, and chronic strain, such as that produced from caregiving over time. The basic premise is that stressors are embedded in the transaction between people and their contexts. This person–environment or ecological model is congruent with the tenets of occupational therapy.

Social–cognitive theory

Social–cognitive theory (Bandura, 2001) posits that learning occurs most effectively through observation of the choices and consequences of others. This theory supports that learning occurs in a social context and that the person and environment influence and are influenced by each other in a bidirectional manner. Personal factors include cognitive, affective, and biological aspects of behavior, whereas environmental influences include social and contextual factors of health.

Transactional perspective

The *transactional perspective* is occupation based and argues that health-promoting theories emphasizing only individual behavior or a systems approach are limiting, because health behavior is more complex (Cutchin & Dickie, 2013; Madsen et al., 2015). This perspective, based on John Dewey's pragmatism and theory of action, argues that the person and context are embedded and of one piece—person, behavior, and occupations cannot be separated from the context in which they will be enacted or performed. The social and cultural aspects of engagement and participation are addressed in this perspective and are crucial in understanding and addressing health behavior and disparity.

Practical Applications in Occupational Therapy

AOTA CODE OF ETHICS, DISPARITY, AND IMPLICATIONS FOR OCCUPATIONAL THERAPY PRACTICE

The Code identifies six principles:

- *beneficence,* or concern for the well-being and safety of clients;
- *nonmaleficence,* or refraining from actions that cause harm;
- *autonomy,* or respect for client self-determination, privacy, confidentiality, and consent;
- *justice,* or the promotion of fairness and objectivity;

- *veracity,* or full, accurate, and nonbiased information; and
- *fidelity,* or to treat with fairness, respect, discretion, and integrity.

The Code also espouses core values, including equality in the treatment of all people free of discrimination and adherence to justice, so that occupational therapy managers establish and work toward a climate where all staff, clients, and family members can effectively function and flourish.

For occupational therapy practitioners and managers, embracing models that reflect the beliefs of occupational therapy—that engagement in occupation promotes and sustains health—is critical. Establishing an environment that is truly inclusive and supports the positive health of all is the objective of occupational therapy managers. Recognizing social and structural barriers to individual engagement and participation and positive health is a critical, ethical role of practitioners and managers.

Occupational justice

Awareness of social inequities led to the term and model of *occupational justice,* which articulates the unique beliefs and contributions of the profession to individual and population health and quality of life (Wilcock & Townsend, 2000). This is done through attention to ways in which occupation is thwarted—by disease, environment, and even society (Townsend & Wilcock, 2004; Wilcock & Townsend, 2000). Among the roots of this contribution were explorations of theories of justice. In turn, this focus on justice led to educating occupational therapy practitioners on ways of righting wrongs, including distributive justice and learning and attending to advocating policies and practices that support engagement and participation in communities of choice—and inclusion—of all members of society. *Distributive justice* generally refers to the just distribution of income, wealth, and opportunities (Sandel, 2009).

Attention to power dynamics and injustice relative to race, gender, and class, such as that espoused by Young (1990) beyond distributive policies, has also been incorporated by occupational scientists. This knowledge has influenced global occupational therapy interest in improving access to resources and necessities of marginalized populations through policy improvements such as better mental health environments (Townsend et al., 2003) and access to HIV care (Braveman & Suarez-Balcazar, 2009). Canadian occupational scientists introduced the notion of *occupational possibilities* (Gerlach, 2015; Rudman, 2012) by applying critical theory and intersectional analysis to understand historical challenges to health and resource access by less powerful, marginalized populations.

Occupational therapy researchers in the areas of public health have used a social justice lens and qualitative research methods to bring to light the lived experiences of marginalized persons with disabilities to influence policy (Magasi & Hammel, 2009). The past decade has seen occupational therapy and science argue not only for justice through individual access to needed therapy but also for global population health in pursuit of occupational justice through attention to occupational possibilities (Rudman & Aldrich, 2017).

Health policy

ACA. In the United States, several health and social policy changes designed specifically to improve access have improved access to occupational therapy services. For example, the enactment of the Patient Protection and Affordable Care Act of 2010 (ACA; P. L. 111-148) enabled access for many people who were shut out of the private health insurance market for structural or social reasons. This included those with preexisting medical conditions and those with complicated and costly conditions who could now access care due to the removal of annual and lifetime caps on essential health benefits. In addition, plans had to accept all applicants without regard to their age, sex, or preexisting medical history. Certain plans needed to meet a minimum threshold and cover essential health care benefits, including mental health and substance abuse treatment and habilitative care.

MHPAEA. The Paul Wellstone and Pete Domenici Mental Health Parity and Addiction Equity Act of 2008 (MHPAEA; P. L. 110-343) was designed to ensure equal coverage and treatment for those seeking mental health and substance use disorder services relative to services for medical conditions (Buchmueller et al., 2007; Centers for Medicare and Medicaid Services, n.d.; Ettner et al., 2016). In addition, some states opted to broaden access to health care for those at income levels traditionally higher than poverty levels through an expansion of Medicaid. Many of these individuals have disabilities and were able to work without fear of losing critical health coverage through Medicaid (Hall et al., 2017).

The ACA also enabled young people with preexisting mental health conditions or substance abuse challenges to receive care until age 26 years on their parents' health policies. Lifetime and annual expense limits were removed, protecting those with devastating conditions that carried exorbitant costs, such as spinal cord injury or complex neonatal intensive care unit conditions, from potential bankruptcy or suffering from lack of needed care. The ACA and MHPAEA were designed to emphasize improved access to needed care. Medicaid waiver programs enable states to increase access and expand care to particular populations, such as children and youth with autism, or adults with serious mental illness (Bilaver & Jordan, 2013).

DISPARITY ISSUES AND THE ETHICAL CONCEPT OF *SOCIAL JUSTICE*

The literature on health disparity focuses on social factors that prevent best practice. The Code requires occupational therapy practitioners to promote fairness in providing services. For the occupational therapy manager, how can fairness be assured in the clinic?

Unconscious bias may lead to subtle differences in health care delivery that can negatively affect client adherence to treatment. Such disparities have been revealed at the system and individual levels (Smedley et al., 2003). An example of an individual-level disparity might be at the practitioner–client level and involve an occupational therapy practitioner's cultural insensitivity to social role or norms that may potentially prevent follow-up, thus limiting the client's access to occupational therapy services. An example of a system-level disparity might be a policy that prevents participation because of religious or ethnic practices, such as a clinic requiring follow-up on Friday afternoons, which prevents some with religious beliefs from either attending or staffing roles.

According to Laveist and Nuru-Jeter (2002), client satisfaction increased among those whose care was race concordant with their provider, implying that attention to sociocultural aspects of care was important to recipients. Client satisfaction may lead to better adherence to treatment, and in this case, a feeling that the provider understands them. Adherence enables the client to receive maximal benefit of therapies, the main objective of a rehabilitation department. Other researchers suggest providing training in cultural competence to improve client perceptions of quality, compliance, and satisfaction (Holden et al., 2014; Saha et al., 1999).

Specific recommendations have been offered relative to system changes, such as allocation of resources to enable training all staff who come in contact with patients and families (Betancourt et al., 2003). The occupational therapy manager, therefore, can address a lack of diverse staff resources by focusing on staff recruitment to ensure that a broad and diverse pool is obtained, and to provide and reinforce ongoing training to assist staff in providing culturally competent care. The manager can also advocate for staff to receive training to identify and address implicit bias that might be reflected in hours of operation, treatment approach, or types of intervention.

In some settings, reimbursement policies may preclude direct service to some populations. Occupational therapy practitioners can work to promote outreach and educational involvement on the part of the rehabilitation staff. Literature shows that some person-level strategies such as education are effective in health promotion. Participation in health fairs, equipment loan programs, and screenings can be a mechanism to provide important health promotion information for those in the community with chronic conditions who would otherwise not have access. Knowledge and awareness of the community influences can guide the health promotion efforts, such as training community leaders and offering outreach at the local community center, school, or church.

Unrealistic productivity demands can sap staff energy to participate in voluntary, off-the-clock, nonrevenue-producing activities. An institutional commitment to the community during work hours demonstrates that fairness regardless of ability to pay is valued. Collaborating with a university occupational therapy program and involving students in both formal fieldwork and outreach can be an effective mechanism to provide important information that would not be available otherwise.

CLIENT DEMOGRAPHICS

Negative health outcomes can result from social factors, such as lower SES; historic marginalization, such as with persons of color; and prejudice against those with illnesses or conditions in which there is a history of stigma, such as HIV/AIDS, serious mental illness, and addictions. There is an increase in people living with complex chronic conditions that likely meet the need for occupational therapy services (Leland et al., 2017). According to the U.S. Census, approximately 56% of the population with health insurance receives it through their employer, with another 19.4% through Medicaid, 17% through Medicare, 16% through individual coverage, and 4.6% through military coverage (Barnett & Berchick, 2017). There is a reported 18.6% increase in Medicaid enrollment during 2013–2015, with

Medicaid and Children's Health Insurance Program now covering 1 in 5 people in the United States (Leonard, 2015). This information reveals that even for those with insurance, 20% meet income and/or disability requirements to receive Medicaid. Despite attempts to improve access to insurance, there is no universal safety net for all citizens, leading to differences in access to occupational therapy services based on health insurance as well as due to lack of insurance.

Occupational therapy practitioners and managers can advocate for occupational therapy's role in the primary care setting, particularly for clients with chronic, complex conditions (AOTA, 2014). Practitioners can assist in supporting clients' self-management through problem-solving aspects of daily life affected by their conditions (Coleman & Newton, 2005). An example of an effective program offered by practitioners in Australia details the relatively minor investment in a 6-week program that yielded improved participation, self-efficacy, and perceived quality of life (O'Toole et al., 2013). A retrospective study conducted in Canada revealed the personal value and cost-savings of home-based versus no care for those with chronic conditions requiring daily management (Health Quality Ontario, 2013). The study also reported fewer emergency room visits and improved ability to perform personal ADLs (e.g., dressing).

PROVIDER DEMOGRAPHICS

A health care workforce that reflects the population served is a desired goal for several reasons. Studies of client satisfaction have indicated higher satisfaction when provider and client are race concordant. Moreover, attention to sociocultural factors can promote adherence to treatment. According to a health care workforce report (Castillo-Page, 2010), between the years 1978 and 2008, 75% of all U.S. medical school graduates practicing medicine were White, 13% were Asian, and 6% were Black/African American. The 2008 data set revealed that, among practicing physicians, 60% were men and 40% were women among the White, Asian, and Hispanic populations, whereas for Black people/African Americans, 45% were men and 55% were women. In the interest of increasing diversity, U.S. medical schools collect applicant and graduate data on an annual basis. Self-reported race and ethnicity may not be linear, because there are opportunities over time for respondents to identify race and ethnicity, and more are identifying as multiracial (Association of American Medical Colleges [AAMC], 2014).

Data for 2015 reveal that the percentage of medical school graduates identifying as Black/African American (6%) and Hispanic/Latino (5%) has remained stable since 2011. Full-time faculty in medical schools has become more diverse in gender, with 39% women, but only 4% of full-time faculty are faculty of color (non-Asian; AAMC, 2016). Data collected between 2005 and 2015 on percentage of medical school graduates planning to work with an underserved population reveal the highest percentage (greater than 50%) reported by Black/African American graduates, and a growth in Hispanic/Latino graduates during this time from 33% to 39% (AAMC, 2016). The data for American Indian/Alaskan Native (37%) and White and Asian (23%) graduates planning to work with underserved populations remained the same during this time period.

TABLE 9.1. Occupational Therapy Provider Demographics

Race/Ethnicity	% U.S. Workforce	% OT Workforce
White	64.4	83.0
Hispanic	16.1	4.0
African American	11.6	4.4
Asian	5.3	6.6

Note. OT = occupational therapy. Data from DHHS Health Resources and Services Administration (2017).

The DHHS Health Resources and Services Administration (2017) revealed that female workers were the majority of 25 of the 30 top U.S. health occupations. All minority groups except Asians were underrepresented in health professions identified as diagnostic and treatment occupations, the category that also includes occupational therapy. Demographics are shown in Table 9.1.

Of the total number of occupational therapy practitioners (*N* = 108,412) in the United States, 90.3% are women, and 9.7% are men. The data indicate that most occupational therapy practitioners are White women. The data also reveal an underrepresentation of occupational therapy practitioners relative to men and persons of color (DHHS Health Resources and Services Administration, 2017). With the knowledge about the impact of social factors on accessing care and following through with treatment recommendations, it is imperative that recruitment and retention strategies emphasize cultural competence. The recommended managerial interventions identified earlier—focused recruitment and mandating ongoing training in cultural competence—can assist departments to meet clinical standards of excellence regardless of staff composition.

Summary

This chapter identified and explored health disparities from the perspective of the code. As the population changes, the workforce must also change to most competently deliver care. The overarching goal of creating an environment that fully supports inclusion is desired. A two-pronged approach includes health care workforce implications relative to recruitment, training, and support and treatment environment implications relative to cultural competence and acknowledgment of the sociocultural aspects of best practice. Case Example 9.1 gives two scenarios to explore how occupational therapy practitioners can address health disparities.

CASE EXAMPLE 9.1. ADDRESSING HEALTH DISPARITIES

Scenario 1
Stating cultural preferences, a male family member of a client with a cognitive impairment admitted to the skilled nursing facility in which you are the manager insists that the client be treated by the only male occupational therapy practitioner on the team. You are concerned because this practitioner is the least experienced with the clinical care needs of this client, and he already has a full caseload.

Questions
1. How might you address the request, using the stress process model in part to guide your reasoning?
2. How could you address the health literacy of the client and family to ensure best practice?
3. Explore your decision regarding how to assign the therapist to this client, applying the Code as your guide.

Scenario 2
A homeless client on the acute rehabilitation unit that you manage must be discharged, and staff is concerned that she has not received full benefit of the rehabilitation treatment for her traumatic brain injury suffered when she fell while intoxicated and was hit by a car. She does not have outpatient coverage, and her life is quite chaotic. Several attempts have been made to have her family attend training sessions to assist her safety and follow-up to prevent readmission, and all have resulted in no-shows. Staff are concerned about safe discharge, but the social worker insists this must occur today.

Questions
1. Consider the case from the perspective of the fundamental cause theory, emphasizing the benefit of ongoing treatment and coordination with the shelter. How would you advocate for additional treatment?
2. Consider the case from the perspective of the stress process model, recognizing that the client may have exhausted family members' support. Explore outreach options based on the Code. How would you advocate for additional time to train shelter staff?
3. As a manager, how could you focus staff recruitment to emphasize interest in social aspects of complex medical conditions?

Note. A version of this chapter was previously published in *The Occupational Therapy Manager, 6th Edition*, edited by Karen Jacobs and Guy L. McCormack. Copyright © 2019 by the American Occupational Therapy Association. Reprinted with permission.

REFERENCES

American Occupational Therapy Association. (2013). AOTA's societal statement on health disparities. *American Journal of Occupational Therapy, 67*, S7–S8. https://doi.org/10.5014/ajot.2013.67S7

American Occupational Therapy Association. (2014). The role of occupational therapy in primary care. *American Journal of Occupational Therapy, 68,* S25–S33. https://doi.org/10.5014/ajot.2014.686S06

American Occupational Therapy Association. (2017). AOTA's societal statement on health literacy. *American Journal of Occupational Therapy, 71*(Suppl. 2), 7112410065. https://doi.org/10.5014/ajot.2017.716S14

Association of American Medical Colleges. (2014). *Diversity in the physician workforce: Facts and figures 2014.* https://www.aamc.org/about-us/mission-areas/health-care/workforce-studies/reports

Association of American Medical Colleges. (2016). *Current trends in medical education.* http://aamc-diversityfactsandfigures2016.org/report-section/section-3/

Bandura, A. (2001). Social–cognitive theory: An agentic perspective. *Annual Review of Psychology, 52,* 1–26. https://doi.org/10.1146/annurev.psych.52.1.1

Barnett, J. C., & Berchick, E. R. (2017). *Health insurance coverage in the United States: 2016.* https://www.census.gov/library/publications/2017/demo/p60-260.html

Bass-Haugen, J. D. (2009). Health disparities: Examination of evidence relevant for occupational therapy. *American Journal of Occupational Therapy, 63,* 24–34. https://doi.org/10.5014/ajot.63.1.24

Betancourt, J. R., Green, A. R., Carrillo, J. E., & Ananeh-Firempong, O. (2003). Defining cultural competence: A practical framework for addressing racial/ethnic disparities in health and health care. *Public Health Reports, 118,* 293–302. https://doi.org/10.1093/phr/118.4.293

Bilaver, L. A., & Jordan, N. (2013). Impact of state mental health parity laws on access to autism services. *Psychiatric Services, 64,* 967–973. https://doi.org/10.1176/appi.ps.201200411

Braveman, P. (2014). What are health disparities and health equity? We need to be clear. *Public Health Reports, 129*(1), 5–8. https://doi.org/10.1177/00333549141291S203

Braveman, B., & Suarez-Balcazar, Y. (2009). Social justice and resource utilization in a community-based organization: A case illustration of the role of the occupational therapist. *American Journal of Occupational Therapy, 63,* 13–23. https://doi.org/10.5014/ajot.63.1.13

Buchmueller, T. C., Cooper, P. F., Jacobson, M., & Zuvekas, S. H. (2007). Parity for whom? Exemptions and the extent of state mental health parity legislation. *Health Affairs, 26,* w483–w487. https://doi.org/10.1377/hlthaff.26.4.w483

Castillo-Page, L. (2010). *Diversity in the physician workforce: Facts and figures 2010.* Association of American Medical Colleges, Diversity Policy and Programs.

Centers for Disease Control and Prevention. (2015). *What is health literacy?* https://www.cdc.gov/healthliteracy/learn/index.html

Centers for Medicare and Medicaid Services. (n.d.). *The Mental Health Parity and Addiction Equity Act (MHPAEA).* https://www.cms.gov/marketplace/private-health-insurance/mental-health-parity-addiction-equity

Coleman, M. T., & Newton, K. S. (2005). Supporting self-management in patients with chronic illness. *American Family Physician, 72,* 1503–1510.

Cutchin, M. P., & Dickie, V. A. (2013). *Transactional perspectives on occupation.* Springer.

Ettner, S. L., Harwood, J. M., Thalmayer, A., Ong, M. K., Xu, H., Bresolin, M. J., . . . Azocar, F. (2016). The Mental Health Parity and Addiction Equity Act evaluation study: Impact on specialty behavioral health utilization and expenditures among "carve-out" enrollees. *Journal of Health Economics, 50,* 131–143. https://doi.org/10.1016/j.jhealeco.2016.09.009

Gamble, V. N., & Stone, D. (2006). U.S. policy on health inequities: The interplay of politics and research. *Journal of Health Politics, Policy and Law, 31,* 93–126. https://doi.org/10.1215/03616878-31-1-93

Gerlach, A. J. (2015). Sharpening our critical edge: Occupational therapy in the context of marginalized populations. *Canadian Journal of Occupational Therapy, 82,* 245–253. https://doi.org/10.1177/0008417415571730

Hall, J. P., Shartzer, A., Kurth, N., & Thomas, K. (2017). Effect of Medicaid expansion on workforce participation for people with disabilities. *American Journal of Public Health, 107,* 262–264. https://doi.org/10.2105/AJPH.2016.303543

Health Quality Ontario. (2013). In-home care for optimizing chronic disease management in the community. *Ontario Health Technology Assessment Series, 13*(5), 1–65.

Holden, K., McGregor, B., Thandi, P., Fresh, E., Sheats, K., Belton, A., . . . Satcher, D. (2014). Toward culturally centered integrative care for addressing mental health disparities among ethnic minorities. *Psychological Services, 11,* 357–368. https://doi.org/10.1037/a0038122

Institute of Medicine. (2002). *Unequal treatment: Confronting racial and ethnic disparities in health care.* National Academies Press.

Laveist, T. A., & Nuru-Jeter, A. (2002). Is doctor–patient race concordance associated with greater satisfaction with care? *Journal of Health and Social Behavior, 43,* 296–306. https://doi.org/10.2307/3090205

Leland, N. E., Fogelberg, D. J., Halle, A. D., & Mroz, T. M. (2017). Occupational therapy and management of multiple chronic conditions in the context of health care reform. *American Journal of Occupational Therapy, 71,* 7101090010. https://doi.org/10.5014/ajot.2017.711001

Leonard, K. (2015). Medicaid enrollment surges across the U.S. *U.S. News and World Report.* https://www.usnews.com/news/articles/2015/02/24/medicaid-enrollment-surges-across-the-us

Link, B. G., & Phelan, J. (1995). Social conditions as fundamental causes of disease. *Journal of Health and Social Behavior, 35,* 80–94. https://doi.org/10.2307/2626958

Madsen, J., Kanstrup, A. M., & Josephsson, S. (2015). The assumed relation between occupation and inequality in health. *Scandinavian Journal of Occupational Therapy, 23,* 1–12. https://doi.org/10.3109/11038128.2015.1075065

Magasi, S., & Hammel, J. (2009). Women with disabilities' experiences in long-term care: A case for social justice. *American Journal of Occupational Therapy, 63,* 35–45. https://doi.org/10.5014/ajot.63.1.35

Mental Health Parity and Addiction Equity Act of 2008, Pub. L. 110–343, 122 Stat. 3765.

O'Toole, L., Connolly, D., & Smith, S. (2013). Impact of an occupation-based self-management programme on chronic disease management. *Australian Occupational Therapy Journal, 60,* 30–38. https://doi.org/10.1111/1440-1630.12008

Patient Protection and Affordable Care Act of 2010, Pub. L. 111–148, § 3502, 124 Stat. 119.

Pearlin, L. I. (1989). The sociological study of stress. *Journal of Health and Social Behavior, 30,* 241–256. https://doi.org/10.2307/2136956

Rudman, D. L. (2012). Governing through occupation: Shaping expectations and possibilities. In G. E. Whiteford & C. Hocking (Eds.), *Occupational science: Society, inclusion, participation* (pp. 100–116). Wiley.

Rudman, D. L., & Aldrich, R. M. (2017). Discerning the social in individual stories of occupation through critical narrative inquiry. *Journal of Occupational Science, 24,* 470–481. https://doi.org/10.1080/14427591.2017.1369144

Saha, S., Komaromy, M., Koepsell, T. D., & Bindman, A. B. (1999). Patient–physician racial concordance and the perceived quality and use of health care. *Archives of Internal Medicine, 159,* 997–1004. https://doi.org/10.1001/archinte.159.9.997

Sandel, M. J. (2009). *Justice: What's the right thing to do?* Farrar, Straus & Giroux.

Schnitzer, A. E., Rosenweig, M., & Harris, B. (2011). Health literacy: A survey of the issues and solutions. *Journal of Consumer Health on the Internet, 15,* 164–179. https://doi.org/10.1080/15398285 .2011.573347

Smedley, B. D., Stith, A. Y., & Nelson, A. R. (Eds.). (2003). *Unequal treatment: Confronting racial and ethnic disparities in health care.* National Academies Press.

Townsend, E., Langille, L., & Ripley, D. (2003). Professional tensions in client-centered practice: Using institutional ethnography to generate understanding and transformation. *American Journal of Occupational Therapy, 57,* 17–28. https://doi.org/10.5014/ajot.57.1.17

Townsend, E., & Wilcock, A. (2004). Occupational justice and client-centered practice: A dialogue in progress. *Canadian Journal of Occupational Therapy, 71,* 75–87. https://doi.org/10.1177/ 000841740407100203

U.S. Department of Health and Human Services, Agency for Healthcare Research and Quality. (2014). *2014 national healthcare quality and disparities report.*

U.S. Department of Health and Human Services, Health Resources and Services Administration. (2017). *Sex, race, and ethnic diversity of U.S. health occupations (2011–2015).*

U.S. Department of Health and Human Services, National Institutes of Health, National Health, Lung, and Blood Institute. (2017). *Health disparities.* https://www.nhlbi.nih.gov/health/educational/ healthdisp/

U.S. Department of Health and Human Services, Office of Disease Prevention and Health Promotion. (2016). *Healthy People 2020.* https://www.cdc.gov/nchs/healthy_people/hp2020.htm

Wilcock, A., & Townsend, E. (2000). Occupational therapy terminology interactive dialogue. *Journal of Occupational Science, 7,* 84–86. https://doi.org/10.1080/14427591.2000.9686470

World Health Organization. (2018). *Social determinants of health: Key concepts.* https://www.who .int/news-room/questions-and-answers/item/social-determinants-of-health-key-concepts

Young, I. M. (1990). *Justice and the politics of difference.* Princeton University Press.

Section 1. Professional Integrity, Responsibility, and Accountability

Ethical Governance

VIRGINIA C. STOFFEL, PhD, OT, FAOTA; PENELOPE MOYERS CLEVELAND, EdD, OT, FAOTA; SHIRLEY WELLS, DrPH, OTR, FAOTA; BRENDA S. HOWARD, DHSc, OTR, FAOTA; and ROGER A. RITVO, PhD

Key Points

- Governance requires leadership. Ethical governance means leading with high standards of ethical conduct when making decisions for an association or organization.
- To enact ethical governance, leaders must know their fiduciary roles and responsibilities.
- A leader must always consider real and apparent conflicts of interest and conflicts of commitment.
- Leaders should seek professional, legal, or other advice when unsure or when sensing that an issue may cause ethical problems.

Introduction

Ethics in governance is about the qualities of leadership and the values expressed by the leaders. Ethics are derived from and based on a particular code of values; in occupational therapy, leaders use the Core Values found in the AOTA Code of Ethics (the Code) to guide their actions. The core values of the American Occupational Therapy Association (AOTA) include altruism, equality, freedom, justice, dignity, truth, and prudence. These core values guide ethical actions in practice as well as in leadership.

Governance encompasses the decisions and advisory processes that leaders use in planning, directing, managing, and evaluating an organization (Governance Today, 2020). Although all members in organizations have a responsibility to lead ethically, this Advisory Opinion focuses more specifically on those who have taken on additional responsibilities in leadership roles, including decision making for the organization. In AOTA, leadership includes the Board of Directors, senior staff, chairs of numerous committees and commissions, and other volunteers who have leadership or decision-making capacity. Additionally, members take part in governance and leadership through elections, responding to surveys regarding the direction of the profession, participating in business meetings and other discussions, and through a myriad of other activities that drive the direction of the organization. Although this Advisory Opinion focuses on leadership within AOTA, these principles may be applied to ethical leadership in any professional association or organization, such as one's state association, regulatory agency, or other professional or community organizations. Throughout this document, the term *organization* is used to refer to any of these groups.

Leaders in volunteer organizations are frequently faced with expectations from members to increase the performance of the organization, but they also must manage limited resources. There are pressures to maintain or expand existing programs, membership benefits, and ideals, but also to lead change and innovation. The result of leadership actions may inadvertently create ethical dilemmas or significant challenges to the profession's values, causing tough choices for volunteers, elected leaders, organizational staff, and/or members. Dilemmas may evolve from conflicts of interest, conflict of commitment (e.g., accepting additional roles that have a negative impact on one's ability to meet current responsibilities), misunderstanding one's fiduciary responsibility, and a variety of other situations that may cause values and ethical principles to come into conflict.

A Framework for Understanding Effective Governance and Leadership

The Association of Governing Boards of Universities and Colleges (AGB; n.d.) presents nine principles within three broad categories for effective governance and leadership. Adapted for AOTA, these principles form a framework guiding ethical governance practices.

CATEGORY 1: UNDERSTAND GOVERNANCE

Each person elected or appointed to a governance role in an organization commits to upholding their *fiduciary responsibilities*: they promise to manage resources in a way that honors the best interests of the organization (Tenenbaum, 2015). Honoring best interests includes being familiar with and upholding the organization's official documents and code of ethics, and carrying out the duties as outlined in their position's description.

Principle 1: Embrace the full scope of your responsibilities
It is critical to immerse oneself in fully understanding the depth and breadth of the leadership position one is assuming as early as possible. The leader must intentionally prepare prior to assuming the role and continue preparing throughout the term of office. The leader should carefully review all materials and engage with others who share governance and management responsibilities. Actively listening, asking critical questions, collaborating in decision making, seeking input from a broad constituency, engaging in ongoing evaluation, and ensuring sustainability are important leadership activities. Principle 1 leadership activities reflect the ethical principles of *beneficence*, a concern for the well-being of others; and *fidelity*, keeping one's commitments to colleagues and others (Beauchamp & Childress, 2019).

Principle 2: Respect the difference between the board's role and the staff's role
An organization's paid staff manage and implement member services in line with the mission and policies. Collaboration between and among organizational leaders, members, and

staff will serve the greatest good and lead to well-informed strategies, communications, and member engagement. Clarifying and respecting boundaries of each may increase satisfaction and reduce any sense of being threatened that can occur. Additionally, organizational leaders must welcome diverse input, promote a culture of respect, and represent the profession to the public. By working collaboratively to impact the profession, volunteers and staff uphold the ethical principle of *fidelity* (Beauchamp & Childress, 2019).

Principle 3: Be an ambassador for the organization and the occupational therapy profession

Advocacy and self-advocacy are considered tools for occupational therapy intervention at the person, community, and population levels. This principle emphasizes the need to communicate clearly to those whom the Association serves; the public; other institutions and professions; and to those engaged in practice, education, research, and policymaking. Clear communication will shed light on occupational therapy's role in improving the accessibility, inclusion, justice, and participation of all persons, communities, and populations in the occupations of everyday life, especially where such occupations hold purpose and meaning leading to health, well-being, and quality of life. In a leadership role, one may serve as an identified spokesperson for the Association and the profession in an identified area of practice important to the health of the community. Qualities of ambassadorship include welcoming those whose perspectives have not been included and overcoming implicit biases that have historically excluded leaders whose diverse life experiences have been less present in the profession's history in the United States. Being an ambassador and advocate for the profession and clients is the role of all Association members, and is consistent with the ethical principles of *beneficence*, caring for the well-being and safety of others; and *autonomy*, respecting a person's right to self-determination, privacy, and consent (Beauchamp & Childress, 2019).

CATEGORY 2: LEAD WITH AUTHENTICITY

It is imperative that every individual who chooses to serve in an organization understands their role in creating a sense of connection to the organization. To provide effective, high-quality services and programs, every leader and member in an organization should ask, "how can we lead with authenticity?"

To lead authentically, leaders have three obligations, individually and collectively (Aulgur et al., 2020), to the organization:

- A *duty of care* requires leaders to use their best judgment to conduct fiscal oversight, manage supervision, assess utilization, and establish reputational goodwill, while maintaining legal standards.
- A *duty of loyalty* compels leaders to place the organization's mission at the forefront of all decision-making activities while avoiding personal gain through a conflict of interest or commitment (whether real or perceived).
- A *duty to abide by laws and a professional code of ethics* charges an organization's leaders with ensuring that the organization complies with governing statutes and is true to and updates its mission, purpose, and internal governing documents.

Authentic leadership is about being oneself and true to one's values and the organization. Authentic leaders take responsibility for their actions and make decisions based on values and principles rather than on short-term success. They use their inner compasses to guide their actions, which enables them to earn the trust of peers and members, creating approachable environments and boosting team performance (Atwijuka & Caldwell, 2017; Lloyd-Walker & Walker, 2011; Raso, 2019).

Principle 4: Lead with integrity

Integrity is the foundation of character and is vital to shaping the capacity to lead. It is about honesty, transparency, and accountability for one's words and actions. It is about the courage to do the right thing, even if it is unpopular or goes against one's political platform. Integrity means being ethical in actions and decisions. Having integrity allows a person to consider all perspectives and relevant information, weigh the potential consequences of actions, and ensure that decisions are consistent with a person's values. Leaders with integrity understand the importance of adhering to a code of ethics and taking responsibility for their actions. Leading with integrity aligns with the core values of *truth*, being faithful to facts and reality; and *justice*, providing objectivity in relationships and fair access to services (AOTA, 2020a); and the ethical principle of *veracity*, being accurate and objective when providing information (Beauchamp & Childress, 2019).

Principle 5: Think independently and act collectively

Authentic leaders must acknowledge they are part of a collective working to address the organization's challenges. They should think for themselves, reach conclusions, and share their perspective diplomatically and productively (Cossin, 2021). Each leader must fully understand what is expected and needed of them and be refocused when they get off track. Leaders must understand how their actions might affect the organization and consider their impact on their decision-making process. Leaders have a responsibility to engage directly with those they seek to serve in ways that ensure that the organization's decisions are made within the context of community assets, needs, preferences, and aspirations (Wallestad, 2021). Individual voice and collective power are essential. They are the mechanism for both earning and maintaining the trust required for the organization's work. This principle of effective governance aligns best with the ethical principle of *fidelity*, in which persons uphold promises and carry out a duty to others (Beauchamp & Childress, 2019).

Principle 6: Champion justice, equity, and inclusion

Authentic and ethical leaders create a sense of belonging or connection to the organization and remove systemic barriers for all members, leaders, and staff. Organizational leaders are accountable for ensuring that the organization creates a welcoming and safe environment where everyone feels respected and valued. Leadership must demonstrate that it cares through appropriate policies and procedures; through visibility, action, and behaviors; and through embracing the strength of diversity and inclusion (Ndalamba et al., 2018).

Ethical leadership is grounded in the principles of trust, equity, and fairness that ultimately promote the common good of the organization. To be fair means offering opportunities without favoritism and condemning improper behavior and manipulation. Organizational leaders must seek input from those with relevant lived experiences and ensure that the information includes the community impacted by the work (Adekanmbi & Ukpere, 2022). An awareness of how systemic inequities have affected society and a willingness to interrogate the organization's role in perpetuating those inequities creates powerful opportunities to deepen the organization's impact, relevance, and advancement of the public good. An equity mindset builds an awareness of systemic inequality and commits the organization to dismantle any barriers that the organization's decisions may have created (Wallestad, 2021).

Leaders who cultivate an inclusive culture ensure that all members of the leadership team are encouraged to bring their perspectives, identity, and life experiences to their volunteerism. They ensure that all leaders share power and responsibility for the organization's work, mission, and purpose. They ensure that every member of the leadership team sees and understands their role in creating an organization's value that strengthens inclusion (Buse et al., 2014). Diversity, equity, inclusion, and belonging are consistent with the ethical principle of *justice*, and the Code, which calls for respect and inclusion of all persons regardless of age, gender identity, sexual orientation, race, religion, origin, socioeconomic status, degree of ability, or any other status or attributes. Leadership is responsible for recruiting, nominating, and appointing new leaders in the organization with the right mix of skills, knowledge, and experiences. Leaders and members actively confront discomfort and perceived obstacles to prioritize diversity, inclusion, and equity.

CATEGORY 3: FACILITATING INNOVATION: THINKING AND ACTING STRATEGICALLY FOR SUSTAINABILITY

Leaders must facilitate innovation at the forefront of their work for the Association and for the profession. The escalating pace of technological advances; the demands on scarce human and financial resources; and entrenched societal problems such as poverty, violence, and disparity have stimulated change in a pervasive way. Occupational therapy addresses the need to provide services to underserved populations, to incorporate new technologies and interventions, and to provide high-quality and low-cost care. Innovation is required to enact these changes. Innovation involves creative and original work to address change where evidence may not be available (Osburg, 2013). The question before leaders is how to design innovative, ethical solutions that are sustainable (Van der Wal & Demircioglu, 2020). Both leaders and followers must engage in behaviors that support, promote, and enable innovative behavior, such as experimentation, risk taking, ingenuity, and creative thinking (Van der Wal & Demircioglu, 2020). Leaders have the power to shape the organizational context and establish a climate for innovation that empowers members, staff, and partners of the organization (Van der Wal & Demircioglu, 2020). Leaders use ethical principles to guide their efforts to lead and participate in transformational change, while monitoring for unintended consequences that over the long term could create ethical dilemmas that future generations may condemn (Groves & LaRocca, 2011).

The expectation of acting ethically while simultaneously engaging in transformative actions may not always align. Risk taking is acceptable when built on a foundation of ethical reasoning so that mistakes can be managed during low-cost pilot testing, and when evaluated progressively for the specific innovation's sustainability (Liedtka & Kaplan, 2019). Leaders and followers are mutually accountable for allowing appropriate and ethical risk taking, where the goal is to change the mindset from struggling with barriers to seizing opportunities with high potential. The intent of innovation is to maximize benefit to the members of the association and to the recipients of services from the profession. The following principles create a culture and climate for ethical innovation and sustainability.

Principle 7: Learn about the mission, constituents, culture, and context

Ethical culture and leadership are the antecedents of innovation (Van der Wal & Demircioglu, 2020). Leaders and followers must work together to engage in the innovation needed for the good of the members, the profession, and the public. Innovation should be central to the mission of the organization, driven by input from its member and organizational partner constituents, and reflective of the organization's culture and context (Blok, 2019). Innovation is an active process in which all members engage and provide feedback needed for maximum sustainability of the organization and the profession. Innovating for the benefit of all members and occupational therapy clients, in alignment with the mission and culture of the organization, is consistent with the ethical principle of *beneficence* (Beauchamp & Childress, 2019).

Principle 8: Ask insightful questions and listen with an open mind

Insightful questions about innovation arise when using the three Ds (Bryden & Gezelius, 2017) of *direction* (type of innovation pursued and its purpose), *distribution* (fair dissemination among members and external constituents), and *diversity* (prioritizing local solutions over standardized, top-down solutions and including client populations in innovation efforts). Leaders should ask questions not only to discern the type of innovation (e.g., process, product), but also to understand the scope of change (e.g., incremental versus disruptive). Leaders also examine sources of innovation for the organization, determining whether these sources should be in-house or external (Osburg, 2013).

Leaders should listen with an open mind and delay criticism that prematurely shuts down the innovation during the early stages of framing problems, generating preliminary ideas, scoping potential solutions, and pilot testing ideas (Liedtka & Kaplan, 2019). Listening with an open mind means welcoming participatory feedback to overcome challenges and being willing to course correct when data indicate the innovation is not working well. Leaders must consistently monitor and adapt the innovation to ensure achieving its full potential (Liedtka & Kaplan, 2019). Making sure the innovation is beneficial and not harmful is consistent with the ethical principles of *beneficence* and *nonmaleficence* (Beauchamp & Childress, 2019).

Principle 9: Focus on what matters most to long-term sustainability

Ethics are an integral part of visioning and strategic thinking. First, visioning starts with organizational values that predetermine the generation of responsible strategies (von

Schomberg, 2013). In occupational therapy, these values include *altruism*, an unselfish concern for the welfare of others, and *justice*, providing services for all. Second, as leaders develop and implement strategies, they must remain focused on keeping processes ethical (Blok, 2019). Leaders must anticipate risks, reflect on desirable outcomes, and engage members and organizational partners (Blok, 2019).

Sustainability of the strategies implemented from visioning involves more than just knowledge. *Sustainability* is defined as "the capacity to endure from an environmental, economic, and social dimension" (Osburg, 2013, p. 18). Sustainability refers to the sustainability of both the organization and the profession, as well as the narrower sustainability related to the specific innovation. Leaders must view innovation as *doing* something new to embrace the complexity of change more fully; this insight about doing fosters innovation ethics, where knowledge and intentions serve as a catalyst for taking responsibility for innovation practices (Blok, 2019). These innovation practices are designed to improve the social desirability, ethical acceptability, and sustainability of innovations. Innovation ethics takes into consideration how problems emerge, thereby influencing how solutions should be developed in an ongoing manner (Blok, 2019). In other words, sustainable innovation for an organization always involves self-criticism, calling all leaders, members, and organizational partners to active involvement in generating responsible action.

Relation to the AOTA Code of Ethics

The nine principles from the AGB (n.d.) reflect the Code, including the core values and ethical principles. Leaders maintain ethical behavior when they act in concert with professional values. See Exhibit 10.1 for ethical standards from the Code related to governance.

Reference to Other AOTA Documents

AOTA's organizational documents contain bylaws, job descriptions for governance officers, and policies and procedures as to how AOTA governance groups act in concert with each other (AOTA, n.d.). Leaders in the Association's governance roles must become familiar with these documents. Occupational therapy practitioners who assume leadership roles in other professional associations and organizations must familiarize themselves with the documents of the organizations in which they lead.

Questions for Reflection

The authors offer the following questions in Table 10.1 for deep reflection on one's own ethical practices for leadership and governance (adapted from AGB, n.d.).

EXHIBIT 10.1.

ETHICAL STANDARDS RELATED TO ETHICAL GOVERNANCE

- Abide by policies, procedures, and protocols when serving or acting on behalf of a professional organization or employer to fully and accurately represent the organization's official and authorized positions.
- Do not engage in conflicts of interest or conflicts of commitment in employment, volunteer roles, or research.
- Do not use one's position (e.g., employee, consultant, volunteer) or knowledge gained from that position in such a manner as to give rise to real or perceived conflict of interest among the person, the employer, other AOTA members, or other organizations.
- Establish a collaborative relationship with recipients of service and relevant stakeholders to promote shared decision making.
- Take steps (e.g., professional development, research, supervision, training) to ensure proficiency, use careful judgment, and weigh potential for harm when generally recognized standards do not exist in emerging technology or areas of practice.
- Treat all stakeholders professionally and equitably through constructive engagement and dialogue that is inclusive, collaborative, and respectful of diversity of thought.
- Demonstrate a level of cultural humility, sensitivity, and agility within professional practice that promotes inclusivity and does not result in harmful actions or inactions with persons, groups, organizations, and populations from diverse backgrounds including age, gender identity, sexual orientation, race, religion, origin, socioeconomic status, degree of ability, or any other status or attributes.

Note. From the Standards of Conduct from the AOTA Code of Ethics.

TABLE 10.1. Questions for Reflection in Governance

Principles	Questions
Principle 1: Embrace the full scope of your responsibilities	• What is your level of engagement during and between meetings? What is the level of engagement of all the members of your team? What do you expect from one another, and how can you promote full and inclusive participation? • How does the work of the team (volunteers and staff) contribute to advancing the mission, vision, and organizational priorities? Are these done in a timely manner?
Principle 2: Respect the difference between the board's role and the staff's role	• What knowledge, skills, or experiences do you have that might be useful to your organization? How might you share those in a way that does not cross the boundaries of the operations of the organization? • When faced with challenging situations, how might collaboration and shared governance approaches be implemented? What responsibilities need to be held separately?

(Continued)

TABLE 10.1. Questions for Reflection in Governance *(Cont.)*

Principles	Questions
Principle 3: Be an ambassador for AOTA and the profession	• How will you serve your Association or organization and the profession as an ambassador, enriching the lives of those whose health, well-being and participation have been unjustly limited? Who are the audiences? Who will you join with or invite to deliver messages of advocacy and self-advocacy? Who else should be at the table? • How might you respond to a constituent who approaches you with a sensitive question? Who might you involve and when might you involve them? What ethical responsibilities might be at play in this situation?
Principle 4: Lead with integrity	• What personal and professional relationships do you have that could interfere with your ability to make decisions in the best interests of the organization? • How do your behaviors, actions, and reputation reflect on the organization in which you serve? • What ethical expectations do you have of your fellow leadership volunteers?
Principle 5: Think independently and act collectively	• How open is the leadership team to dissenting opinions? • What experiences do you bring to your service? What experiences do other volunteers bring? What perspectives are missing? • How do you determine which issues are worth speaking up in favor of or against, regardless of their popularity? When, where, and how will you raise sensitive issues?
Principle 6: Champion justice, equity, and inclusion	• Is the organization's volunteer leadership populated in a way that ensures that power is authorized by and inclusive of the members impacted by the decisions made? • Are leaders doing all they can to listen to what members tell them is most important? • How will the leadership's decision or strategy create more equitable outcomes? Are there ways to avoid systematic inequities?
Principle 7: Learn about the mission, constituents, culture, and context	• What will make the Association and the profession relevant for the next generation? What are the leaders' level of comfort with and capacity for anticipating and bringing about change? What supports are needed to enhance comfort and capacity for change? • How do leaders, members, and organizational partners explore important issues that do not have easy answers? How do the leaders frame questions and work with members and organizational partners to discern answers? How is avoidance of tough issues respectfully addressed so action is facilitated?

(Continued)

TABLE 10.1. Questions for Reflection in Governance *(Cont.)*

Principles	Questions
Principle 8: Ask insightful questions and listen with an open mind	• What questions are appropriate to ask of the leaders, members, and organizational partners? How do leaders address these relevant questions in a respectful and timely way? • How open are the leaders, members, and organizational partners to having ideas and opinions challenged? What assumptions underlie the perspectives of participants in a strategic discussion? Is there civility in discussions that encourages active participation, dissenting views, and listening to all voices?
Principle 9: Focus on what matters most to long-term sustainability	• What decisions are leaders, members, and organizational partners being asked to make regarding change and sustainability? What is the appropriate level of involvement in determining the vision, engaging in strategic planning, and facilitating strategy implementation and evaluation? How does the discovery of risk aversion occur? How are opportunities for appropriate risk taking fully examined? What organizational changes are necessary to support ethical innovation management and risk taking? • How should the strategic priorities for the future be developed? How should leaders, members, and organizational partners be involved in determining strategic priorities? What trends could be the most challenging to the sustainability of the organization? Does the organization have collective experience with such challenges? Who will drive and monitor corresponding innovations to address sustainability?

Next Steps

Decisions made through the governance process are only as good as the ethical actions behind those decisions. Many leadership processes start off with a re-reading of the system's mission and values as a way of reinforcing the reasons for their work and the values that guide these actions. The following points can be helpful to reinforce ethical governance.

BALANCING "BEST INTERESTS"

Leaders in the governance process should always act in the best interests of the organization. However, what may be best for the organization in the shorter term may not be best in the long run. For example, foregoing salary increases for staff may save money in the next 12 to 24 months, but could impact turnover, recruitment, morale, and program effectiveness beyond those dates.

UNDERSTANDING COMPLEXITY

An ever-expanding list of issues and organizational processes fall under the complex governance umbrella. Organizational leaders must provide effective oversight and accountability to those individuals and departments, commissions, task forces, and others to whom it delegates operational responsibility. Understanding the complexity of critical issues in an organization is vital to carrying out one's duties ethically.

Summary

Ethical behavior in governance is based on the same principles as the expected ethical conduct of all members (i.e., the Code). However, volunteer and elected leaders have accepted, by virtue of their position, additional responsibilities. These responsibilities include behaviors that require a higher level of ethical conduct than is expected from members without such responsibilities. Ethical issues are paramount to effective leadership in the profession and are best facilitated when leaders are reflective, authentic, alert, and aware of the multidimensional and complex aspects of what it means to serve as leaders.

Acknowledgment

Kathlyn L. Reed, PhD, OTR, FAOTA, MLIS, authored an earlier version of this Advisory Opinion.

REFERENCES

Adekanmbi, F. P., & Ukpere, W. I. (2022). Perceived workplace fairness, ethical leadership, demographics, and ethical behaviors [Special issue]. *Journal of Governance & Regulation*, *11*(2), 244–256. https://doi.org/10.22495/jgrv11i2siart4

American Occupational Therapy Association. (n.d.). *AOTA organizational documents*. https://www.aota.org/about/leadership-governance/aota-governance-documents

Association of Governing Boards of Universities and Colleges. (n.d.). Principles of trusteeship: Become a highly effective board member. https://agb.org/principles-of-trusteeship/

Atwijuka, S., & Caldwell, C. (2017). Authentic leadership and the ethic of care. *Journal of Management Development*, *36*, 1040–1051. https://doi.org/10.1108/JMD-12-2016-0331

Aulgur, J., Bernstein, R., Aspin, T., & Harrison, Y. (2020). Ethical dilemmas in nonprofit governance: ARNOVA governance section case studies for use in the classroom and practitioner training. *Journal of Nonprofit Education and Leadership*, *10*(3), 304–328. https://doi.org/10.18666/JNEL-2020-V10-I3-10507

Beauchamp, T. L., & Childress, J. F. (2019). *Principles of biomedical ethics* (8th ed.). Oxford University Press.

Blok, V. (2019). Innovation as *ethos*: Moving beyond CSR and practical wisdom in innovation ethics. In C. Neesham & S. Segal (Eds.), *Handbook of philosophy of management* (pp. 1–14). Springer. https://doi.org/10.1007/978-3-319-48352-8_19-1

Bryden, J., & Gezelius, S. S. (2017). Innovation as if people mattered: The ethics of innovation for sustainable development. *Innovation and Development*, *7*, 101–118. https://doi.org/10.1080/2157930X.2017.1281208

Buse, K., Sessler, R., & Bilmoria, D. (2014). The influence of board diversity, board diversity policies and practices, and board inclusion behaviors on nonprofit governance practices. *SIAS Faculty Publications*, *644*. https://digitalcommons.tacoma.uw.edu/ias_pub/644

Cossin, D. (2021). Questions that will help you identify potential conflicts of interest on your board: Part I. *Brain Circuits*. https://www.imd.org/ibyimd/brain-circuits/questions-to-identify-conflict-of-interest-on-your-board/

Governance Today. (2020). *Governance: What is it and why is it important?* https://governancetoday.com/GT/Material/Governance_what_is_it_and_why_is_it_important_.aspx?WebsiteKey=0cf4306a-f91b-45d7-9ced-a97b5d6f6966

Groves, K. S., & LaRocca, M. A. (2011). An empirical study of leader ethical values, transformational and transactional leadership, and follower attitudes toward corporate social responsibility. *Journal of Business Ethics, 103,* 511–528. https://doi.org/10.1007/s10551-011-0877-y

Liedtka, J., & Kaplan, S. (2019). How design thinking opens new frontiers for strategy development. *Strategy & Leadership, 47*(2), 3–10. https://doi.org/10.1108/SL-01-2019-0007

Lloyd-Walker, B. & Walker, D. (2011). Authentic leadership for 21st-century project delivery. *International Journal of Project Management, 29*(4), 383–395. https://doi.org/10.1016/j.ijproman.2011.02.004

Ndalamba, K. K., Caldwell, C., & Anderson, V. (2018). Leadership vision as a moral duty. *Journal of Management Development, 37*(3), 309–319. https://doi.org/10.1108/JMD-08-2017-0262

Osburg, T. (2013). Social innovation to drive corporate sustainability. In T. Osburg & R. Schmidpeter (Eds.), *Social innovation: Solutions for a sustainable future* (pp. 13–22). Springer. https://doi.org/10.1007/978-3-642-36540-9

Raso, R. (2019). Be you! Authentic leadership. *Nursing Management, 50*(5), 18–25. https://doi.org/10.1097/01.numa.0000557619.96942.50

Tenenbaum, J. S. (2015). *Legal duties of association board members.* https://www.asaecenter.org/asae-home/resources/articles/an_plus/2015/december/legal-duties-of-association-board-members

Van der Wal, Z., & Demircioglu, M. A. (2020). More ethical, more innovative? The effects of ethical culture and ethical leadership on realized innovation. *Australian Journal of Public Administration, 79,* 386–404. https://doi.org/10.1111/1467-8500.12423

von Schomberg, R. (2013). A vision of responsible research and innovation. In: R. Owen, J. Bessant, & M. Heintz (Eds.), *Responsible innovation: Managing the responsible emergence of science and innovation in society* (pp. 51–74). Wiley.

Wallestad, A. (2021). The four principles of purpose-driven board leadership. *Stanford Social Innovation Review.* https://doi.org/10.48558/S4ZJ-Q994

Engaging in Business Transactions With Clients

BRENDA S. HOWARD, DHSc, OTR, FAOTA

Key Points

- Selling to or buying from clients may be a conflict of interest.
- Selling products to direct-service recipients requires awareness of and following regulatory and ethical issues regarding business transactions with clients.
- Maintaining the therapeutic relationship and trust is key.

Introduction

Selling equipment and supplies to clients has become a common business activity for many occupational therapy practitioners. However, practitioners must make careful consideration to uphold an objective, professional, and therapeutic relationship with clients who require both goods and services. This relationship may become confusing and unclear when practitioners hold outside interests beyond the therapeutic interaction. Additionally, selling products to recipients of occupational therapy services requires an awareness of the various regulatory and ethical issues that guide how occupational therapy practitioners may engage in this business.

Having a financial interest in a business venture, such as product sales related to occupational therapy intervention, while providing occupational therapy services to the client may be perceived as a conflict of interest. A *conflict of interest* occurs "any time someone in a position of power could be motivated to abuse their position to earn money, make connections, build a reputation, or otherwise promote their personal goals" (Indeed, 2022, p. 1). An ethical conflict of interest occurs when someone's personal motives influence the decisions they make on behalf of a client or the company they work for (Indeed, 2022). *Conflicts of commitment*, or competing obligations, can also occur (Nizet et al., 2021; Scahill et al., 2018). People increasingly handle multiple commitments when on the job. Commitments bind persons to making predetermined decisions based on their relevance to one or more obligations (Nizet et al., 2021). For example, one's business organization and one's client may prompt the practitioner to make a decision that they think will benefit both. Yet having multiple obligations challenges one's ability to make clear decisions and can affect attitudes and actions. Ethical dilemmas can occur when two or more objectives cannot be met at the same time. In some cases, two objectives that start as compatible become incompatible (Nizet et al., 2021). For example, if an occupational therapy practitioner creates a product that they perceive as beneficial to their clients and begins using their position of authority in the therapeutic relationship to encourage clients to purchase the product, they may be guilty of a conflict of commitment (i.e., they have obligations to both the client and the product sales). If their status as a vendor interferes with their judgment as a service provider, they may also be guilty of a conflict of interest. "Compatibility between commitments should not be taken for granted" (Nizet et al., 2021, p. 53).

The ethical issues regarding conflicts of interest when occupational therapy practitioners engage in business transactions with clients may take at least three forms: financial interest, potential harm, and taking advantage of the trust in a therapeutic relationship.

Financial Interest

Occupational therapy practitioners may sell a variety of products, such as adaptive equipment, durable medical equipment, exercise equipment, and educational materials such as books directly to their clients. Less commonly, practitioners may sell alternative medicine items to clients, such as magnets and aromatherapy supplies. Thoughtful reflection on the responses to the following questions can help practitioners determine the appropriateness of selling items to clients. The answers to these questions help clarify whether financial interest in completing this transaction is influencing the therapeutic recommendation.

- What types of products are being sold? Do they have evidence-based benefit for the client?
- If the item is related to a client's therapeutic goals, should the occupational therapy practitioner providing the service be the one to sell the product to the client? Is it sold by others, perhaps at a lower price?
- Does the practitioner hold ownership in the company selling the product? If so, can they provide evidence that the product is the best option, and that it is advantageous for the client to purchase it from them? Does the occupational therapy practitioner provide options for purchasing the product from another company, so that the client has a choice?
- What are the laws in one's location regarding dual relationships and selling items to health care patients and clients?

Occupational therapy practitioners must be versed in the ethics of prudent practice as well as appropriate business laws and behaviors, such as disclosure when dual roles of practitioner and entrepreneur are assumed. For example, objectivity can become clouded if a practitioner prescribes a wheelchair for a client and also sells this equipment to them. Is the practitioner's intention to provide the proper basic wheelchair, or is the practitioner motivated by profit to provide the most expensive wheelchair covered by the client's insurance? Practitioners must not engage in self-dealing, which is when the practitioner makes choices or advises clients based on the practitioner's own direct personal gain rather than on what is best for the client (Indeed, 2022).

Occupational therapy practitioners who regularly sell items to patients and clients need to be aware of the Federal Trade Commission (n.d.) and state consumer protection agency (USA.gov, n.d.) rules and regulations for product safety and liability. In situations in which a practitioner is both a health care service provider and product vendor, clients need to be assured that the practitioner has adhered to these compliance regulations. For example, as a vendor, a practitioner may be required to provide the client with documentation of written warranty information; policies for complaints, questions, returns, and repairs; nondiscrimination policies; a consumer bill of rights; and the Health Insurance Portability and Accountability Act of 1996 (P. L. 104-191) compliance regulations.

Potential Harm

Another area of concern when engaging in business transactions with clients is the potential for harm. What happens if a client is injured from the product an occupational therapy practitioner sold to them? Practitioners could expose themselves to professional liability issues from federal regulatory agencies, such as the Centers for Medicare & Medicaid Services (CMS; 2022). For example, durable medical equipment vendors must meet CMS standards if they want to bill CMS for the equipment (CMS, 2022). Additionally, the product may require specific standards of infection control, such as those regulated by Medicare (CMS, 2018). Practitioners also may be required to meet prevailing industry standards as product vendors, which may require additional state licensure (Howk, 2022). Finally, vendors selling to clients who use Medicare must demonstrate adherence to a variety of rules and regulations, including intake and assessment, educating the client or caregiver in safe care and use of the item, donning or doffing any items that are worn on the body, and follow up (CMS, 2022).

Trust and Taking Advantage of the Therapeutic Relationship

The Standards of Practice for Occupational Therapy support the importance of practicing according to the American Occupational Therapy Association (AOTA), institutional policies, and other relevant documents. When selling products, occupational therapy practitioners may be in a position to use their referral base as a source for potential customers. In such cases, it is critical to use this source objectively, considering the existing trust that clients have in those who provide their therapy. Practitioners have an ethical obligation to inform clients (i.e., disclose) of outside business relationships that may give the appearance of conflict of interest and to assure service recipients that therapeutic decisions are devoid of coercion. Whether financial interest in the business transaction is for direct or indirect monetary gain, practitioners' disclosures must be completely transparent. See Exhibit 11.1 for AOTA Code of Ethics (the Code) standards that apply to conflict of interest.

EXHIBIT 11.1.

ETHICS STANDARDS RELATED TO BUYING AND SELLING GOODS AND SERVICES TO CLIENTS

- Do not exploit any relationship established as an occupational therapy practitioner, educator, or researcher to further one's own physical, emotional, financial, political, or business interests.
- Do not engage in conflicts of interest or conflicts of commitment in employment, volunteer roles, or research.
- Do not use one's position (e.g., employee, consultant, volunteer) or knowledge gained from that position in such a manner as to give rise to real or perceived conflict of interest among the person, the employer, other AOTA members, or other organizations.
- Do not barter for services when there is the potential for exploitation and conflict of interest.
- Do not threaten, manipulate, coerce, or deceive clients to promote compliance with occupational therapy recommendations.
- Do not accept gifts that would unduly influence the therapeutic relationship or have the potential to blur professional boundaries, and adhere to employer policies when offered gifts.
- Do not engage in dual relationships or situations in which an occupational therapy professional or student is unable to maintain clear professional boundaries or objectivity.
- Do not engage in any undue influences that may impair practice or compromise the ability to safely and competently provide occupational therapy services, education, or research.
- Describe the type and duration of occupational therapy services accurately in professional contracts, including the duties and responsibilities of all involved parties.
- Do not use or participate in any form of communication that contains false, fraudulent, deceptive, misleading, or unfair statements or claims.

Source. From the Standards of Conduct from the AOTA Code of Ethics.

Buying Items From Clients

Thus far, this ethics Advisory Opinion has discussed business transactions in which the occupational therapy practitioner is offering goods to the clients. What if the reverse occurs? Clients who attempt to sell goods or services to practitioners or barter for services can inadvertently cause an ethical problem for the practitioner. Although there are no set rules across the United States governing participation in a transaction that a client is offering, the practitioner must be wary of entering into such a relationship, as this constitutes a gray area in the therapeutic relationship. The therapeutic relationship is a one-way relationship, with the client as the beneficiary. The general rule is that if the transaction creates a strain on the therapeutic relationship by crossing professional boundaries and fostering expectations that have no place in the therapeutic relationship, then the transaction ought not occur. The Code offers guidance that practitioners must not exploit the therapeutic relationship in any way, and explicitly states that no bartering for services is ethical in occupational therapy practice.

Relation to the AOTA Code of Ethics

The Code requires that occupational therapy practitioners disclose financial conflicts of interest that may involve clients. Because of the broad spectrum of this topic, several principles from the Code that are applicable to the issue of selling goods and services to clients are listed in Exhibit 11.1.

Tips

- Be aware of legal implications for selling and buying goods and services with clients.
- Understand that buying and selling with clients may rupture the therapeutic relationship.

Next Steps

This Advisory Opinion is not intended to exclude occupational therapy practitioners from entrepreneurial ventures; instead, it is intended to educate them on the numerous issues related to product sales, and the potential ramifications if these ventures are conducted in a manner that is contrary to legal and ethical standards. Practitioners must adhere to current business, professional, and legal standards when conducting business transactions with clients. In the case example, the occupational therapist might have avoided a breach in the therapeutic relationship by disclosing financial interest in the durable medical equipment company and offering a list of other vendors from which the client could make the purchase. Practitioners' behavior is representative of the therapeutic relationships they

CASE EXAMPLE 11.1. FINANCIAL TRANSPARENCY

An **occupational therapy practitioner** who works in a private practice setting is also a partner (part owner) of a durable medical equipment company. The practitioner recommends that a client purchase a certain item to enhance their functional performance in home safety. The occupational therapy practitioner provides the client with the name of their company as a resource for this equipment. They do not tell the client of their financial holdings in this company, nor do they provide a list of other vendors who can supply the same equipment. The client follows the occupational therapy practitioner's instructions and purchases the equipment. The client is dissatisfied because of difficulty using the equipment and a lack of functional improvement. They notice that the occupational therapy practitioner is listed as an owner of the company. The client calls and expresses anger that the occupational therapy practitioner failed to inform them of the practitioner's financial holdings in the company.

Questions
1. What are the ethical issues at stake in this scenario?
2. What further information does the occupational therapy practitioner need to gather?
3. What actions could the occupational therapy practitioner take to salvage the therapeutic relationship, and to avoid this situation in the future?

seek to achieve as well as a demonstration and reflection of the profession of occupational therapy.

Summary

Occupational therapy interventions should be goal directed and focused on the therapeutic relationship, avoiding any perceived or real potential to exploit recipients of service for financial gain. Participating in activities outside of this focus may damage the therapeutic relationship and expose the occupational therapy practitioner to legal liability. Health care providers have an obligation to protect clients from real or perceived abuse, neglect, or exploitation by anyone. Practitioners who operate a private practice and sell therapeutic supplies and equipment to clients must ensure that the items are necessary for the clients' return to function; that the amount charged for products is fair and reasonable according to industry standards and practices; and that disclosures meet all of the legal, federal, and professional requirements.

Acknowledgment

Darryl Auston, MS, OTR/L, authored an earlier version of this Advisory Opinion.

REFERENCES

Centers for Medicare & Medicaid Services. (2018). *Durable medical equipment, prosthetics, orthotics, and supplies (DMEPOS) quality standards.* https://www.cms.gov/Research-Statistics-Data-and-Systems/Monitoring-Programs/Medicare-FFS-Compliance-Programs/Downloads/Final-DMEPOS-Quality-Standards-Eff-01-09-2018.pdf

Centers for Medicare & Medicaid Services. (2022). *Durable medical equipment (DME) center.* https://www.cms.gov/center/provider-type/durable-medical-equipment-dme-center

Federal Trade Commission. (n.d.). *Advice and guidance.* https://www.ftc.gov/

Health Insurance Portability and Accountability Act of 1996, Pub. L. 104-191, 42 U.S.C. § 300gg, 29 U.S.C § 1181–1183, and 42 USC 1320d–1320d9.

Howk, H. (2022). Durable medical equipment licensing requirements. *Wolters Kluwer.* https://www.wolterskluwer.com/en/expert-insights/durable-medical-equipment-licensing-requirements

Indeed. (2022). *What is the definition of conflict of interest?* https://www.indeed.com/hire/c/info/conflict-of-interest?gclid=CjwKCAiAyfybBhBKEiwAgtB7fog1tmam_22XhVy29ybmL2GWZU-vUQoOiD9iQ4k0pxDAwdf5bTRpsCxoCgQMQAvD_BwE&aceid=&gclsrc=aw.ds

Nizet, J., Fatien Diochon, P., & Balachandran Nair, L. (2021). When commitments conflict: Making ethical decisions like a funambulist. *M@n@gement, 24*(1), 44–58. https://doi.org/10.37725/mgmt.v24i1.4497

Scahill, S. L., Tracey, M. S., Sayers, J. G., & Warren, L. (2018). Being healthcare provider and retailer: Perceiving and managing tensions in community pharmacy. *Journal of Pharmacy Practice and Research, 48,* 251–261. https://doi.org/10.1002/jppr.1410

USA.gov. (n.d.). *State consumer protection offices.* https://www.usa.gov/state-consumer

Avoiding Plagiarism in Today's World

BRENDA KORNBLIT KENNELL, MA, OTR/L, FAOTA

Key Points

- Plagiarism can be intentional or unintentional.
- Lack of awareness does not absolve the person from the ethical and legal obligation not to plagiarize.

Introduction

Plagiarism is the "act of using another person's words or ideas without giving credit to that person" (Britannica Dictionary, 2023). Alternative terms include *piracy, theft, stealing, appropriation,* and *thievery.* These words remind us that plagiarism's scope extends beyond the failure to reference a published quote. Plagiarism involves taking someone else's ideas, thoughts, and concepts from any source and making them one's own. This concept encompasses not only material that has been copyrighted and published but also unpublished works, speeches, photographs, drawings, electronic media, presentations or workshops, videotaped or audiotaped materials, and any other information, including social media posts, blogs, and websites.

Intentional and Unintentional Plagiarism

Plagiarism can take several forms. Although it is sometimes a conscious act, *unintentional plagiarism* is the accidental appropriation of the ideas and materials of others because of a lack of understanding of the conventions of citation and documentation. Unintentional confusion of another's ideas with one's own still constitutes plagiarism (Adam et al., 2017; Skandalakis & Mirilas, 2004). Examples of plagiarism are found in Table 12.1.

Relation to the AOTA Code of Ethics

Intentionally claiming the work of others as original violates the ethical principle of veracity, or truthfulness (Beauchamp & Childress, 2019). Even when the action was not intentional, credit for the work or ideas must be accurate. If information is not cited correctly and the reader cannot tell it is outdated or from an unreliable source, an occupational therapy practitioner could provide inappropriate intervention. This incorrect information could affect the well-being of the client and thus violate the ethical principle of beneficence. Exhibit 12.1 contains ethical standards from the AOTA Code of Ethics (the Code) related to plagiarism.

TABLE 12.1. Intentional and Unintentional Plagiarism

Intentional Plagiarism	Unintentional Plagiarism
• Copying entire documents and presenting them as one's own (University of Victoria Libraries, 2013) • Cutting and pasting from the work of others or reproducing sentences verbatim from others, without properly citing the authors • Stringing together the quotes and ideas of others without connecting their work to one's own original work • Actively or intentionally using the words, ideas, or concepts of another without citing the author as the source (Duke University, 2009) • Making only minor changes to the words or phrasing of another's work without properly citing the authors (Washington State University, 2018)	• Misunderstanding paraphrasing, the parameters of common knowledge, or the statute of limitations on the attribution of ideas (University of Victoria Libraries, 2013; Washington State University, 2018) • Having difficulty discerning one's own ideas from the ideas of the many works one has read • Believing that material previously obtained from school, publication, or a presentation is common knowledge or in the public domain and therefore does not require citation

EXHIBIT 12.1.
ETHICAL STANDARDS RELATED TO PLAGIARISM

- Comply with current federal and state laws, state scope of practice guidelines, and AOTA policies and official documents that apply to the profession of occupational therapy.
- Do not engage in illegal actions, whether directly or indirectly harming stakeholders in occupational therapy practice.
- Do not engage in actions that reduce the public's trust in occupational therapy.
- Report potential or known unethical or illegal actions in practice, education, or research to appropriate authorities.
- Record and report in an accurate and timely manner and in accordance with applicable regulations all information related to professional or academic documentation and activities.
- Do not participate in any action resulting in unauthorized access to educational content or exams, screening and assessment tools, websites, and other copyrighted information, including, but not limited to, plagiarism, violation of copyright laws, and illegal sharing of resources in any form.
- Demonstrate responsible conduct, respect, and discretion when engaging in digital media and social networking, including, but not limited to, refraining from posting protected health or other identifying information.
- Do not use or participate in any form of communication that contains false, fraudulent, deceptive, misleading, or unfair statements or claims.

Reference to Other Standards

United States copyright laws require those sharing information to either present only one's own ideas or accurately cite those of others, which makes plagiarism both a legal and an ethical issue (U.S. Copyright Office, n.d.). Copyright laws apply not only to literary works, but to pictorial and graphic works (among others) as well (U.S. Copyright Office, n.d.). Copyright law gives the holder of the copyright the exclusive right to reproduce the work. Under the fair use section of the copyright law, one may reproduce a limited amount of copyrighted material for teaching, scholarship, or research; as long as it is cited, is used for nonprofit educational purposes, and does not affect the value of the work or the ability of the copyright owner to earn income from the work (U.S. Copyright Office, n.d.). Lack of awareness about correct citation of information acquired through electronic media or other sources does not excuse the writer from the obligation to accurately document those sources.

Tips

DIGITAL PLAGIARISM

With the increasing use of electronic media as resources, occupational therapy practitioners, educators, and students face additional challenges in appropriately citing sources when they write a paper, handout, article, or presentation. Increased use of online sources allows individuals to cut and paste content from a variety of websites into a "new" document. This passive or unintentional use of information is called *digital plagiarism* (Copyleaks, 2021; Kauffman & Young, 2015). Artificial intelligence (AI) technology such as ChatGPT can assist people in writing essays and designing handouts or marketing tools. The question arises—Is using AI technology to help with writing a paper or designing a handout plagiarism? It is important to note that AI writing tools can produce awkwardly phrased material that contains factual errors (Quetext.com, 2023). As AI technology becomes more readily available, so does AI detection technology. "While AI content is not usually considered plagiarism in the technical sense of the word, that doesn't mean that using an AI tool guarantees your content to be plagiarism-free even if it passes a plagiarism check. If the content is based on someone else's work, and the tool used paraphrasing to avoid plagiarism detection, it is no different from copy-paste plagiarism" (Quetext.com, 2023, para. 33). Whether or not AI generated material evades detection, claiming AI-generated material as original is unethical.

SOCIAL MEDIA AND PUBLIC DOMAIN

By 2021, 72% of Americans were using social media for social networking, professional networking, media sharing, content production, knowledge and information aggregation, and virtual reality training spaces (AOTA, 2023). People constantly copy, share, and repost messages, photos, quotes, and graphics that they have seen on various sites. They may do this because they thought something was funny or meaningful and they wanted to share it with friends, or they may do it to get attention and "likes" in an effort to increase their own digital media presence. Either way, material may go viral without attributing the originator. This material sharing without attribution may or may not be illegal, but it is still unethical (Think Marketing Magazine, 2021).

Although the internet has certainly simplified the process of research by making information readily available, internet use has resulted in confusion regarding the issues of defining intellectual property and public domain. Public domain is defined as "the state of something that is not owned by a particular person or company and is available for anyone to use" (Merriam-Webster, 2023). Guidelines for what is considered to be in the public domain include works that were created before copyright law was established, those works for which the copyright has expired (usually 75 years), the work of government agencies, and information considered to be general knowledge (Stanford Libraries, 2018).

Most information available to all on the internet is not in the public domain. When in doubt, look for copyright information on the bottom of the web page. Note that electronic information should be assumed to be under copyright unless explicitly stated that it is not. Even work that is free to use generally is copyrighted and needs to be cited. Proper citation is important even when the information is in the public domain, as it establishes the owner and provides a way for others to locate further information on a topic.

PHOTOGRAPHS AND IMAGES

Photographs and images on the internet are assumed to be copyrighted by the creator, the owner, and/or the subject. Occupational therapy practitioners, students, and experienced academicians may inadvertently violate copyright laws by copying an image and using it in a presentation, client education handout, proposal, or other material. It is common belief that material found in search engines, such as Google Images, are in the public domain. In reality, photographs may cost up to a few hundred dollars to use (see Medical Artworks, n.d.). Even those that may be used for free need proper citation. One need only to go to a social media site that houses content images to see examples of occupational therapy evaluation forms, handouts, and intervention plans, many of which have visible copyright stamps. Copyrights must be honored by not using these documents unless permission is obtained from the copyright holder. Doing otherwise is both illegal and unethical.

ACADEMIC RULES AND RESOURCES

All educational institutions have rules against plagiarism reflected in their student guides or handbooks, and many have honor codes as well. Some universities have useful guides for students that help them avoid the pitfalls of plagiarism when preparing papers (e.g., Princeton University, 2023; Purdue University Online Writing Lab, 2022, 2023). The American Psychological Association (APA) also provides helpful plagiarism prevention information (2019). In many universities, plagiarism is grounds for academic suspension or probation and may even lead to expulsion. It is crucial that students learn how to avoid plagiarism when preparing everything from assignments for the classroom to doctoral dissertations to presentations.

CASE EXAMPLE 12.1. REUSING FORMS AND HANDOUTS

Tiffany was recently hired by an outpatient clinic that wants to start a new comprehensive arthritis program. She completed her Level II fieldwork at a hospital where there was a well-developed arthritis program. Tiffany went online to the hospital's website, downloaded their evaluation forms and handouts on joint protection, made a few changes, and reprinted them with the logo of her current employer's clinic. She also wrote a short article for the clinic's webpage about the benefits of an outpatient arthritis program, using data gathered from websites of other successful programs.

Questions
1. Apply an ethical decision-making framework to Tiffany's case. What standards of the Code were potentially violated by Tiffany's actions?
2. If a colleague of Tiffany at her new job found out about her actions, what steps should they take?
3. What are several possible ways that Tiffany could rectify the situation to avoid violating the Code and plagiarism laws?

CASE EXAMPLE 12.2. ACADEMIC COURSE CONTENT

Bob was a newly hired instructor in the occupational therapy assistant program at a local community college. His teaching course load included a class on physical disabilities. Bob prepared his lecture on strokes and included information on neurodevelopmental treatment (NDT) and proprioceptive neuromuscular facilitation that he received while in occupational therapy school and at continuing education courses. To make his PowerPoint more interesting, Bob copied a video from the Neuro-Developmental Treatment Association website. He cited one of his old school textbooks from 20 years ago, but he assumed that the NDT principles were now "general knowledge" and in the public domain in the rehabilitation sciences and that specific citations were not necessary for information from the conferences or websites.

Questions
1. Does Bob need to cite sources when creating his academic PowerPoints for classroom use? Why or why not?
2. Do Bob's actions violate the Code and/or copyright laws? Why or why not?
3. If Bob's supervisor finds out about Bob's actions, what should the supervisor do?

Next Steps

Occupational therapy practitioners and students may take several steps to avoid committing plagiarism. One must always put direct quotes in quotation marks and include the appropriately cited source (Purdue Online Writing Lab, 2022). If authors borrow significant words from the work of another, they must quote those words and give credit to the author who coined them. When paraphrasing statements or borrowing concepts or ideas from another's work, one must include a reference to the source after the adopted information. One should consider introducing the quote or paraphrased language by crediting

CASE EXAMPLE 12.3. UNINTENTIONAL VS. INTENTIONAL PLAGIARISM

Isaac and **Dina** were graduate students working on assignments for one of their occupational therapy courses. Isaac was friends with some students who had graduated 2 years earlier and read their papers to get some ideas. The following week when Isaac wrote his paper, his ideas were strikingly similar to those of the previous students. Dina purchased a paper from a website that said it had received a grade of A, and turned it in as her own work. Both students were surprised when the instructor returned their papers with failing grades and a statement that they must schedule a meeting with the instructor and program director to discuss consequences for their plagiarism.

Questions
1. Did both Isaac and Dina commit plagiarism? Why or why not?
2. What consequences should the students receive for their actions? Should these consequences be the same for both students? Why or why not?

CASE EXAMPLE 12.4. IN-SERVICE PRESENTATION AND PLAGIARISM

Carlotta was required to present an in-service presentation to the therapy staff as part of her Level II fieldwork experience. She gathered information about her topic from web-based sources and copied some slides from one of her classes into her presentation. She omitted some sources from her reference list because she did not know how to format citations for websites, and she assumed that material her professor used in the school was now public domain.

Questions
1. What are some ways in which Carlotta potentially violated copyright laws in this scenario?
2. Did Carlotta violate the Code? Why or why not?
3. What are some steps Carlotta could take to correct this situation?

the author by name in an introductory statement, such as "According to Reilly . . ." (Purdue Online Writing Lab, 2022).

The prevalence of information on the internet, including online journals for disseminating knowledge, has led to new protocols that delineate the proper way to identify online sources of information, including blogs, conference abstracts, and digital books. Those unfamiliar with the standards for citing references should consult such resources as the *Publication Manual of the American Psychological Association* (7th ed.; APA, 2020). Writers should seek out those with more experience in publishing to mentor them in the process of preparing an article or paper correctly.

Additionally, many universities offer web-based resources for preparing citations correctly. Students may be able to use plagiarism prevention tools available from their learning management system to determine whether their papers could be construed as plagiarized. For example, Safe Assign, a plagiarism prevention service available on Blackboard (2023), teaches students proper citation and provides educators with a mechanism for identifying plagiarism.

Summary

Occupational therapy practitioners are expected to demonstrate a high standard of professionalism. This professionalism requires occupational therapists, occupational therapy assistants, and students of occupational therapy at all levels to respect the works of others, as an extension of respect for the author. Practitioners, researchers, educators, and students must be vigilant about avoiding plagiarism. When in doubt, one should cite the source of words, thoughts, and ideas that might have originated from others. Writers must never represent someone else's words, thoughts, or ideas as their own. It is crucial to provide accurate citations and references to all sources, including electronic sources, when preparing in-service or continuing education presentations, facility handouts, or as the author of research or articles, to maintain professional integrity and support appropriate ethical conduct, as delineated in the Code.

Acknowledgments

Brenda Kennell, MA, OTR/L, FAOTA; Brenda Howard, DHSc, OTR, FAOTA; and **Roger Ritvo, PhD, MBA** authored an earlier version of this Advisory Opinion.

REFERENCES

Adam, L., Anderson, V., & Spronken-Smith, R. (2017). "It's not fair": Policy discourses and students' understandings of plagiarism in a New Zealand university. *Higher Education, 74*, 17–32. https://doi.org/10.1007/s10734-016-0025-9

American Occupational Therapy Association. (2023). *AOTA ethics advisory opinion: Ethics and social media.* https://www.aota.org/-/media/corporate/files/secure/practice/ethics/advisory/ethics-and-social-media.pdf

American Psychological Association. (2020). *Publication manual of the American Psychological Association* (7th ed.).

Beauchamp, T. L., & Childress, J. F. (2019). *Principles of biomedical ethics* (8th ed.). Oxford University Press.

Blackboard. (2023). *Blackboard SafeAssign: A plagiarism prevention tool.* https://www.blackboard.com/teaching-learning/learning-management/safe-assign

Britannica Dictionary. (2023). *Public domain.* https://www.britannica.com/dictionary/public-domain

Copyleaks. (2021). *Facts about digital plagiarism.* https://copyleaks.com/blog/facts-about-digital-plagiarism

Duke University, Office of the Dean of Academic Affairs, Trinity College. (2009). *Intentional plagiarism* [Tutorial]. https://plagiarism.duke.edu/intent/

Kauffman, Y., & Young, M. F. (2015). Digital plagiarism: An experimental study of the effect of instructional goals and copy-and-paste affordance. *Computers & Education, 83*, 44–56. https://www.sciencedirect.com/science/article/abs/pii/S0360131514002930?via%3Dihub

Medical Artworks. (n.d.). *Quality medical artwork and 3D animation.* https://www.medicalartworks.com/

Merriam-Webster.com. (2023). *The public domain.* https://www.merriam-webster.com/dictionary/the%20public%20domain

Princeton University. (2023). *Student guide to academic integrity.* https://odoc.princeton.edu/learning-curriculum/academic-integrity#:-:text=academic%20integrity

Purdue University Online Writing Lab. (2022). *Best practices to avoid plagiarism.* https://owl.purdue.edu/owl/avoiding_plagiarism/best_practices.html

Purdue University Online Writing Lab. (2023). *Research and citation resources.* https://owl.purdue.edu/owl/research_and_citation/resources.html

Quetext.c om. (2023). *Is using AI content plagiarism?* https://www.quetext.com/blog/is-using-ai-content-plagiarism

Skandalakis, J. E., & Mirilas, P. (2004). Plagiarism. *Archives of Surgery, 139,* 1022–1024. https://doi.org/10.1001/archsurg.139.9.1022

Stanford Libraries. (2018). *Copyright and fair use: Welcome to the public domain.* https://fairuse.stanford.edu/overview/public-domain/welcome/

Think Marketing Magazine. (2021). *Social media plagiarism: Does it exist? And how to avoid it?* https://thinkmarketingmagazine.com/social-media-plagiarism-does-it-exist-and-how-to-avoid-it/#

University of Victoria Libraries. (2013). *Avoiding plagiarism.* https://www.uvic.ca/library/assets/docs/avoiding-plagiarism-guide.pdf

U.S. Copyright Office. (n.d.). *Copyright law of the United States (Title 17) and related laws contained in Title 17 of the United States code.* https://www.copyright.gov/title17/

Washington State University. (2018). *Plagiarism: What is it?* https://www.wsulibs.wsu.edu/library-instruction/plagiarism/what

Section 2. Therapeutic Relationships

Establishing Professional Boundaries: Where to Draw the Line

LESLIE BENNETT, OTD, OTR/L

Key Points

- Professional boundaries must guide conduct and decision making in all settings, whether paid or volunteer (clinical, educational, and research).
- The primary focus of professional relationships must be on the well-being of the client/student/participant, and professional boundaries must be maintained to achieve that end.
- Occupational therapy practitioners must abide by relevant state, federal, and international laws, as well as state practice acts, organizational policies, and other applicable regulations.

Introduction

The basic tenets of the altruistic occupational therapy profession are helping others and doing no harm. People have the desire to develop relationships for companionship, socialization, and intimacy (Cooper, 2012). However, when one is in a professional rather than a personal relationship, professional *boundaries* must guide conduct and decision making in the clinical or educational setting and in both live and virtual settings. When faced with uncertainty or ethical dilemmas regarding appropriate professional boundaries in the workplace (paid or volunteer positions), practitioners and educators can find guidance in organization policies; state, federal, and international laws; and professional association official documents (e.g., AOTA Code of Ethics [the Code]). Professional association official documents are frequently revised to reflect changes in laws, ethical reasoning, professional practice, shifting organizational priorities, modern developments and technology, and a myriad of other dynamics (Cooper, 2012; National Council of State Boards of Nursing, 2018). See Table 13.1 for definitions of key terms (noted in italics) in relation to professional boundaries.

Professional boundaries set limits and define specific parameters on how occupational therapy practitioners interact with clients, families, students, and other professionals (Collins, 2019). As professionals, practitioners have the responsibility to establish and set clear, appropriate, and professional boundaries. Boundaries establish safe, open, stable,

TABLE 13.1. Key Terms Related to Professional Boundaries

Term	Definition
Boundaries	Physical, psychological, emotional, and/or social limits that provide a framework for healthy and appropriate practitioner–client or practitioner–consumer relationships.
Under-involvement	A situation in which a practitioner neglects the needs of a client, student, or participant by becoming disengaged and inattentive.
Over-involvement	A situation in which a practitioner engages in excessive emotional attachment and blurring of the professional relationship (e.g., sharing personal contact information, flirting, showing favoritism) that results in loss of objectivity and impartiality.
Dual relationships	A situation in which a practitioner is in more than one type of relationship with a client, student or professor, or supervisor or subordinate (e.g., professional role and friend role). Dual relationships can impair the person's ability to remain objective, competent, and effective as a practitioner, educator, student, employer, or employee.
Conflict of interest	A situation in which a person is in a position to derive personal, professional, or financial benefit from actions or decisions made in their official capacity.
Power differential	The inherently greater power and influence that helping professionals have as compared with the people they help, due to the knowledge they possess and the access to services they provide.

and transparent relationships, which will ensure consistent care delivery that builds and maintains trust. Boundaries ensure team coherence and help to establish limits (Collins, 2019; Cooper, 2012).

The continuum of professional behavior related to professional boundaries ranges from under-involved, to helpful, to over-involved (Remshardt, 2012). Staying in the helpful zone involves working with clients and their families or caregivers toward achieving their occupational goals and promoting healthy occupational therapy practitioner and client relationships. The concept of professional boundaries also translates to relationships between faculty educators and students (either in the classroom or on fieldwork), and supervisory relationships between occupational therapy practitioners. A professional may cross a boundary either intentionally or unintentionally, resulting in an unbalanced dynamic that negatively affects the working relationship. Boundary crossing can include developing dual relationships; for example, engaging in romantic relationships with clients, their family members, or students. Boundary crossing may also involve a breach of confidentiality, inappropriate disclosure, inappropriate touch, and/or gift giving, all of which all lead to an imbalance of power. The existence of power differentials can impair judgment and impact trust and the sense of safety between the occupational therapy practitioner and their various stakeholders (e.g., clients, colleagues, students, subordinates).

Under-involvement occurs when a practitioner neglects the needs of the client by be-coming disengaged. Perhaps the practitioner seems bored, is not attentive to client input or response, or ignores protocols and safety measures. Practitioners need to be continually alert and focused on their work to deliver the quality care that clients and their families or caregivers deserve. In academia, faculty could be perceived as being inattentive to student issues and concerns related to their studies or fieldwork. Conducting oneself in this man-ner could place a client in an unsafe situation.

Over-involvement occurs when a practitioner demonstrates behavior that exceeds the generally accepted boundaries of the practitioner–client relationship. Over-involvement may include engaging in personal conversations or requesting personal advice from a cli-ent or family member or caretaker. For faculty members, over-involvement may include participating with students in social activities not related to curricular, professional, or university events. When practitioners' or educators' actions do not follow the usual or cus-tomary standards of professional conduct, they could potentially be in violation of organi-zational policies; the Code; or local, state, federal, or international laws (National Council of State Boards of Nursing, 2018).

Occupational therapy practitioners need to be alert to circumstances in which they find themselves in different roles with the same person (e.g., friend and client, lover and family member of a client). In academia, educators must avoid engaging in relationships with stu-dents that could lead to conflicts of interest and impact professional judgment and objectiv-ity. When two roles coincide, there is potential for conflicting allegiances and a loss of the practitioner's or educator's ability to maintain the best interests of their client or student.

Occupational therapy practitioners often share intimate moments with their clients and can develop close personal relationships with them without realizing it. The primary focus of occupational therapy practice must be on the well-being of the client, student, other subordinate, or colleague at all times; and occupational therapy practitioners must maintain professional boundaries to achieve that end. When practitioners or educators are faced with ethical dilemmas and cannot find solutions in their state practice acts, or-ganizational policy manuals, or association documents, they may need to seek additional resources from supervisors and ethics committees to find support. Additional resources are provided below to help guide practitioners as they negotiate questions regarding pro-fessional boundaries.

Relation to the AOTA Code of Ethics

Exhibit 13.1 contains ethical standards from the Code related to professional boundaries.

Reference to Other Standards

It is important that occupational therapy practitioners refer not only to professional codes of conduct but also to their state practice acts, organizational policies, and local laws and

EXHIBIT 13.1.

ETHICAL STANDARDS RELATED TO PROFESSIONAL BOUNDARIES

- Do not exploit any relationship established as an occupational therapy practitioner, educator, or researcher to further one's own physical, emotional, financial, political, or business interests.
- Do not engage in conflicts of interest or conflicts of commitment in employment, volunteer roles, or research.
- Do not use one's position (e.g., employee, consultant, volunteer) or knowledge gained from that position in such a manner as to give rise to real or perceived conflict of interest among the person, the employer, other AOTA members, or other organizations.
- Do not engage in sexual activity with a recipient of service, including the client's family or significant other, while a professional relationship exists.
- Do not accept gifts that would unduly influence the therapeutic relationship or have the potential to blur professional boundaries, and adhere to employer policies when offered gifts.
- Do not engage in dual relationships or situations in which an occupational therapy professional or student is unable to maintain clear professional boundaries or objectivity.

Source. From the Standards of Conduct from the AOTA Code of Ethics.

guidelines to help negotiate questions related to professional boundaries. When in doubt, one should ask before the boundary lines are blurred.

Tips

- Communication
  - Be assertive.
  - Be open and up-front about boundaries.
  - Ask yourself:
    - What are the client's needs?
    - What is my role, and am I within my role in taking this action?
    - What impact will my actions have on other members of the staff? Clients? Family? Students?
    - What are my overt or covert motivations?
    - Which rules or policies are relevant to this decision?
- Self-awareness
  - Be aware of what your needs and issues are (examine your own patterns of behavior).
  - Ensure that your emotional needs are being met outside of work.
  - Monitor your own behaviors and feelings (Cooper, 2012).

CASE EXAMPLE 13.1. SUPERVISOR AND STUDENT RELATIONSHIPS

Camryn is a Level II occupational therapy fieldwork student from New York City who is assigned to a remote hospital in North Dakota. Camryn's fieldwork supervisor, Sam, is a recent graduate who also came from a big city to this small town. Sam senses Camryn's loneliness, and they become friends, enjoying beers after a long day and working out at the gym together. Sam's intentions are good—they are trying to make a difficult situation better for their student. However, the development of a friend relationship between a supervisor and someone they are supervising and evaluating places them in an awkward situation.

Questions

1. What are the ethical issues at stake in this scenario?
2. Who are the stakeholders who may be harmed in this scenario?
3. What should Sam do to avoid a conflict of interest?
4. What should Camryn do to advocate for themself?

CASE EXAMPLE 13.2. DATING AND ROMANTIC RELATIONSHIPS

Taylor is a 35-year-old occupational therapist who works with adults in an outpatient setting. One of their clients is Aron, a 37 year old who was injured in a skydiving accident that resulted in C6 incomplete quadriplegia.

Taylor has been working with Aron for 1 month, and Aron has achieved dressing and bathing independence as well as the ability to use the commode with minimal assistance. As Aron's self-esteem has improved, they have begun to flirt with Taylor and eventually ask them out on a date. Taylor is unsure about what they should do, because they don't want to hurt Aron's feelings and senses that they see them as a "safe" first date to try out their new body image.

Questions

1. What are the ethical issues at stake in this scenario?
2. What further information does Taylor need to gather?
3. What are the power dynamics in this situation, and how do they play into crossing ethical boundary lines?
4. How can Taylor avoid unethical practice in this case?

Summary

Occupational therapy practitioners and educators must understand the importance of maintaining professional boundaries and conducting themselves so they stay in the helpful zone. Whether one is working with clients, colleagues, or subordinates; engaging in research; or teaching as a faculty member in academia, one must adhere to professional boundaries to maintain ethical practice. It is essential that practitioners abide by relevant state, federal, and international laws, as well as state practice acts, organizational policies, and other applicable regulations. The Code, as well as other professional documents, can provide guidance in the face of ethical dilemmas related to delineating acceptable professional boundaries.

Acknowledgments

Ann Moodey Ashe, MHS, OTR/L, and **Loretta Jean Foster, MS, COTA/L,** authored an earlier version of this Advisory Opinion.

REFERENCES

Collins, J. (2019). *Knowing your ethical boundaries.* https://www.drjimcollins.com/knowing-your-ethical-boundaries/

Cooper, F. (2012). *Professional boundaries in social work and social care: A practical guide to understanding, maintaining and managing your professional boundaries.* Jessica Kingsley Publishers.

National Council of State Boards of Nursing. (2018). *A nurse's guide to professional boundaries.* http://ncsbn.org/public-files/ProfessionalBoundaries_Complete.pdf

Remshardt, M. A. (2012). On the horizon: Do you know your professional boundaries? *Nursing Made Incredibly Easy, 10*(1), 5–6. https://journals.lww.com/nursingmadeincrediblyeasy/_layouts/15/oaks.journals/downloadpdf.aspx?an=00152258-201201000-00003

Culturally Responsive Care

BRENDA KORNBLIT KENNELL, MA, OTR/L, FAOTA; CRISTINA REYES SMITH,
OTD, OTR/L, FAOTA; WAYNE L. WINISTORFER, MPA, OTR, FAOTA;
RENA B. PUROHIT, JD, OTR/L; and SHANESE L. HIGGINS, DHSc, OTR/L, BCMH

Key Points

- Culturally responsive care is key to effective therapeutic interactions and outcomes.
- Ethical considerations dictate that cultural responsiveness be considered in recruitment, preparation, and management of the occupational therapy workforce.
- Cultural competence is a career-long journey, requiring continuous improvement and accountability.
- Efforts to improve cultural competence require individual and organizational engagement.
- Occupational therapy practitioners must enter into the therapeutic relationship with an awareness of their own culture and cultural biases, knowledge about other cultures, and skills in cross-cultural communication and intervention (Wells et al., 2016).

Definitions

- *Culturally responsive care* refers to intentional and consistent attention to respecting and understanding a patient's experiences, values, beliefs and preferences. Culturally responsive care improves the quality of care (San Diego Foundation, 2023).
- *Cultural competency* is "a developmental process in which one achieves increasing levels of awareness, knowledge, and skills along a continuum, improving one's capacity to work and communicate effectively in cross-cultural situations" (U.S. Department of Health and Human Services [DHHS], n.d., para. 4).
- *Cultural humility* is "a reflective process of understanding one's biases and privileges, managing power imbalances, and maintaining a stance that is open to others in relation to aspects of their cultural identity that are most important to them" (DHHS, n.d., para. 5).
- *Cultural negotiation* is determination of a mutually acceptable way to address the client's cultural needs and the health care environment and processes (Wisconsin Technical College, n.d.). For example, before an outpatient clinic discharges a client for missed or late appointments, they should investigate whether a client's culture views being on

time as a relative concept. Cultural needs should be accommodated when feasible and if they do not adversely affect the treatment plan (Wisconsin Technical College, n.d.).

Introduction

Cultural competence is widely viewed as a foundational pillar for reducing disparities through culturally sensitive and unbiased quality care. When patients are valued for all aspects of their identity, background, and experiences, they feel safe, understood, and, most importantly, valued. As the U.S. population becomes increasingly more diverse, occupational therapy practitioners and students should be proactive in providing culturally responsive care by educating themselves regarding the cultural differences they will encounter and how best to respond to the cultural needs of colleagues and clients alike. Table 14.1 depicts the results of the 2020 U.S. census, indicating a wide diversity and a slight decrease in the White, non-Hispanic population since 2010 (Jones et al., 2021).

Ward and Batalova (2023) report that since 2021, there have been approximately 45.3 million immigrants in the United States, comprising 13.6% of the U.S. population; and 22% of the U.S. population reported speaking a language other than English at home. This means that

> health care providers must be aware of pertinent cultural factors that affect health-care provision and decision making . . . Because the patient population has changed to reflect a more integrated world, understanding some of the customs, preferences, and communication styles of others helps in providing safer, more personalized interactions and will improve satisfaction levels for everyone involved. (Cherry & Stuart, 2011, p. 1)

Occupational therapy practice holds therapeutic use of self as one of the cornerstones of the profession. This cornerstone provides a fundamental foundation for practitioners from which to view their clients and their occupations and facilitate the occupational therapy

TABLE 14.1. U.S. Census Bureau 2020 Demographic Makeup of the Population

Demographic	Percentage of Population
White, non-Hispanic	57.8
Hispanic or LatinX	18.7
Black, non-Hispanic	12.1
American Indian and Alaskan Native	1.1
Asian	6.0
Native Hawaiian or Other Pacific Islander	0.2
Some other race	15.1
Multiracial	10.2

Sources. Jensen et al. (2021); Jones et al. (2021).

process. The effective development and management of a therapeutic transactional relationship requires recognizing and honoring the client's *context*. The *Occupational Therapy Practice Framework: Domain and Process* defines *context* as the environmental and personal factors that are specific to each client (e.g., persons, group, population) that influence engagement and participation. *Personal factors are* the unique features of a person that make up the particular background of the person's life and living. Personal factors include customs, beliefs, activity patterns, behavioral standards, and expectations accepted by the society or cultural group of which a person is a member. The occupational therapy practitioner provides services incorporating professional reasoning, empathy, and a client-centered, collaborative approach. Attention to the client's personal factors is a key component to effective therapeutic use of self and culturally responsive care.

Unconscious bias includes subtle, involuntary assumptions or judgments that are based on people's prior experiences and culture. This can include *affinity bias* when people have an unconscious preference for others similar to themselves (Avarna Group, n.d.). *Implicit bias,* which is based on how one views and categorizes specific groups of people, can affect the relationships between the practitioner and the client and caregivers. Bias can create barriers to treatment, including overlooking necessary interventions or not providing appropriate recommendations or referrals based on presumed noncompliance (American Occupational Therapy Association [AOTA], 2021). Unconscious and implicit bias can lead to *microaggressions*—conscious or unconscious behaviors or words that "unintentionally disempower someone based on a marginalized identity (real or perceived)" (Avarna Group, n.d.). Although these behaviors may seem small and subtle, the recipient of the actions or words can be deeply affected, especially when microaggressions are chronic or ongoing (Avarna Group, n.d.). Microaggressions can impact occupational performance. For example, if a practitioner assumes a client won't understand or comply with a home program because of perceived lack of intellect based on the client's race or socioeconomic status, that practitioner is committing a microaggression (AOTA, 2021).

Providing culturally responsive care is not just avoiding bias. It also means respecting and including clients' cultural beliefs and practices. This may involve what is used or not used in treatment interventions, such as types of food, toys, or clothing. Practitioners may need to learn how to don a sari or use chopsticks in order to help their clients with ADLs. Clients may reject certain foods based on cultural beliefs about the properties of food, such as not eating cold foods in the postpartum period. The timing of treatment may be affected by religious observances or cultural patterns (e.g., the preference to bathe first thing in the morning or the custom of praying at certain times of day). Respecting religious strictures such as not touching an adult of the opposite gender except one's spouse, or using the right hand for eating and the left hand for personal hygiene, can be challenging when a practitioner views the situation through the lens of, "why is that client's spouse dressing or feeding them?" Culturally responsive care includes considering who is involved in planning, decision making, and client or caregiver education. Occupational therapy practitioners can show caregivers how to help a family member be more independent, but in some cultures, it is considered to be the responsibility of family members to care for others with disabilities.

Culture is not limited to race, religion, and ethnic origin. Cultural groups can be related to gender identity, marital status, English competency, ability status, literacy levels, or socioeconomic status. A pediatric practice with signs and handouts that use language about mothers and fathers is not inclusive for single parents or same-gender or non-binary parents. Printed or verbal instructions that use professional jargon or colloquial terminology may be unclear to clients and caregivers who are non-native English speakers, or to people from different parts of the United States.

Relation to the AOTA Code of Ethics

The ethical principle of *beneficence* guides occupational therapy practitioners to demonstrate a concern for the well-being and safety of persons. Culturally responsive care includes respecting and honoring the preferences and wishes of the clients and providing evaluation and intervention that is specific to the needs of the service recipient. Honoring preferences may present ethical concerns when the service recipient's needs, wishes, beliefs, or values differ from those of the occupational therapy practitioner. Ethically, practitioners should collaborate with clients and other relevant persons when planning intervention and making decisions. In some cultures, relevant persons may include extended family members, chosen family, cultural elders or leaders, or religious practitioners. The occupational therapy practitioner may be faced with a situation where other people are encouraging a client to refuse services or to incorporate their own cultural practices into the intervention, which reflects the ethical principle of *autonomy*. To make informed, autonomous decisions about an intervention, a client or caregiver must understand the risks and benefits involved in following or declining recommendations. A client cannot make an informed decision if there are communication barriers such as limited English proficiency, deficits in literacy or health literacy, hearing impairment, or aphasia; therefore, the occupational therapy practitioner must address these barriers. Likewise, if a client cannot use the resources or participate in interventions due to issues regarding funding, scheduling, mobility, accessibility, or transportation, the occupational therapy practitioner should address these barriers as well. A practitioner also impedes the client's ability to provide informed consent if they do not communicate effectively due to their own values or bias, or if they are committing microaggressions. If for any reason an occupational therapy practitioner feels unable to accommodate the cultural differences and needs of a client, the practitioner should follow the policies of their employer in making other arrangements for the client to be served or should refer the client to another practice.

Ethical dilemmas can be further complicated by the unequal distribution of power in the relationship between the client and practitioner. "The power differential is the inherently greater power and influence that helping professionals have as compared to the people they help" (Barstow, 2015, para. 1). It is important to understand the potential impacts of the power differential, as clients and families faced with medical decisions can be over- or under-influenced by the health care system and providers (Barstow, 2015). See Exhibit 14.1 for ethical standards from the AOTA Code of Ethics (the Code) related to culturally responsive care.

EXHIBIT 14.1.
ETHICAL STANDARDS RELATED TO CULTURALLY RESPONSIVE CARE

- Respect and honor the expressed wishes of the recipients of service.
- Establish a collaborative relationship with recipients of service and relevant stakeholders to promote shared decision making.
- Adhere to organizational policies when requesting an exemption from service to an individual or group because of self-identified conflict with personal, cultural, or religious values.
- Provide appropriate evaluation and a plan of intervention for recipients of occupational therapy services specific to their needs.
- Respect the client's right to refuse occupational therapy services temporarily or permanently, even when that refusal has the potential to result in poor outcomes.
- Refer to other providers when indicated by the needs of the client.
- Provide information and resources to address barriers to access for persons in need of occupational therapy services.
- Facilitate comprehension and address barriers to communication (e.g., aphasia; differences in language, literacy, health literacy, or culture) with the recipient of service, student, or research participant.
- Do not engage in communication that is discriminatory, derogatory, biased, intimidating, insensitive, or disrespectful or that unduly discourages others from participating in professional dialogue.
- Treat all stakeholders professionally and equitably through constructive engagement and dialogue that is inclusive, collaborative, and respectful of diversity of thought.
- Demonstrate a level of cultural humility, sensitivity, and agility within professional practice that promotes inclusivity and does not result in harmful actions or inactions with persons, groups, organizations, and populations from diverse backgrounds, including age, gender identity, sexual orientation, race, religion, origin, socioeconomic status, degree of ability, or any other status or attributes.

Note. From the Standards of Conduct from the AOTA Code of Ethics.

Reference to Other AOTA Documents

AOTA's Diversity, Equity, and Inclusion Toolkit (n.d.) includes many resources such as PDF documents, word banks and glossaries, articles, recordings, evaluation and assessment resources, and links to external resources. Some of the resources include:

- Occupational Therapy's Commitment to Diversity, Equity, and Inclusion (AOTA official document)
- Links to implicit association self-tests in health professions education
- Links to unconscious bias training
- Disability inclusion toolkit

Other AOTA official documents can help practitioners understand the role of context, including culture; the standards for quality occupational therapy practice; and the effects of illiteracy and health disparities on health care services. These include:

- *Occupational Therapy Practice Framework: Domain and Process*
- Standards of Practice for Occupational Therapy
- AOTA's Societal Statement on Health Disparities
- AOTA's Societal Statement on Health Literacy

Reference to Other Standards

DHHS publishes national standards on culturally and linguistically appropriate services (CLAS) to enable health care practitioners and organizations to "provide effective, equitable, understandable and respectful quality care and services that are responsive to diverse cultural health beliefs and practices, preferred languages, health literacy, and other communication needs" (DHHS, n.d., para. 1). CLAS should be employed by all members of an organization (regardless of size) at every point of contact. CLAS helps meet the six aims for improving health care quality: the delivery of care that is (1) safe, (2) effective, (3) patient-centered, (4) timely, (5) efficient, and (6) equitable. Providing CLAS means practicing cultural competency and cultural humility (DHHS, n.d.).

Tips

To provide culturally responsive care, follow these tips:

- Practitioners should complete cultural awareness and cultural humility training, and include self-reflection to identify implicit or unconscious bias. Ancillary and support staff and occupational therapy fieldwork students should participate in this training as well.
- When mistakes or microaggressions occur, practitioners should acknowledge them and make plans for self-improvement.
- Printed material should reflect clear language that is accessible from a health literacy perspective, gender-neutral, and free from jargon. Practitioners should use graphics that are representative of diverse patient populations.
- Practitioners should respect culture-specific attitudes and incorporate them into the occupational therapy intervention plan and decision-making processes.
- Practitioners should provide interpreter services if the client and caregivers do not speak or read English.
- Clients' preferred healing practices and practitioners must be respected.

CASE EXAMPLE 14.1. CULTURAL HUMILITY IN PEDIATRIC SERVICES

Susan is a busy occupational therapy practitioner working in pediatric home care. She is having a difficult time determining the ethical course of action while working with a family. The following factors caused conflicts for Susan:

- The family is difficult to schedule because Susan's availability does not line up with their cultural and religious needs, and Susan admits that this starts the relationship off poorly, with both parties feeling like the other is inflexible.
- There are many issues surrounding what is permitted within the home, including types of food and toys. Multiple times Susan brings equipment in only to learn it is not allowed, which requires her to re-plan on the spot.
- Susan feels as though the parents want to do everything for their child, and her attempts to foster the child's independence are met with resistance.
- Susan recognizes that she is having difficulty connecting with the parents, but she has been trained to work with people from various cultures and prides herself on being compassionate and treating everyone equally.

Susan feels that it might be best if another practitioner from the same culture works with this family. Unfortunately, there is a shortage of occupational therapy staff and there will likely be a delay in finding a new practitioner.

Questions
1. What power dynamics might exist within this relationship between the practitioner and family?
2. Which standards from the Code are relevant to this scenario?
3. What would it look like if Susan practiced cultural humility in this situation? And how does this differ from cultural competence?
4. What course of action do you recommend for Susan?

Next Steps

- Commit to taking courses related to culturally responsive care and cultural humility in practice; for example, take a course on language access.
- Create or advocate for training activities for cultural responsiveness within the workplace.
- Survey the community and workplace or organization in which you practice, and identify opportunities to support clients and address any health care initiatives that address identified gaps in service.
- Regularly (e.g., quarterly) review scholarly resources that highlight current trends in practice through a culturally responsive practice lens; for example, look up current trends in practice and cultural considerations for community-based behavioral health with children and adolescents.
- Actively acknowledge systemic issues affecting underrepresented groups and populations, and be aware of how these affect both practitioners and clients.

CASE EXAMPLE 14.2. CULTURALLY RESPONSIVE THERAPEUTIC USE OF SELF

Sasha is a relatively new occupational therapy practitioner, having graduated just about a year ago. Sasha is working in a community that has many people considered to be of a historically marginalized background. Although Sasha is not from this specific area, or the state, they identify as belonging to this historically marginalized group, Sasha is providing direct intervention on a secured acute care behavioral health unit. This is their second encounter with **Kendra**. Sasha notices that Kendra seems slightly frustrated during the session and is not fully engaging in the activity. Sasha does not understand why, as the choice of activity is based on their understanding and personal experience of the culture and what are considered meaningful tasks and roles within the marginalized group. This information is based on evidence-based research and current best practice trends learned while in school, which was not that long ago. Following the treatment session, Sasha meets with the case manager, who informs them that Kendra requested to be dismissed from occupational therapy because she didn't feel the intervention was relevant to her and wasn't helping her achieve goals for discharge.

Questions
1. What is the difference between ethnocentrism and cultural humility?
2. How can occupational therapy practitioners move from cultural awareness to cultural humility?
3. What did Sasha need to do differently to employ best evidence-based practice and culturally responsive and humble care with Kendra?
4. What is the next step of the occupational therapy process for Sasha and Kendra?

CASE EXAMPLE 14.3. RESPECTING CULTURAL TRADITIONS IN HEALTH CARE

When the regular home health occupational therapist is out sick, **Terry** comes to treat **Mr. Guillermo,** a 68-year-old Salvadoran man who recently had shoulder surgery. When Terry arrives at the home, Mr. Guillermo is short of breath and dizzy. Without any introduction, Terry checks Mr. Guillermo's vital signs and reviews his medication list. Terry brusquely addresses the client, pronouncing his name as "gill-rah-mo." "Your blood pressure is over 200! How long have you been feeling like this?" he demands. Mr. Guillermo hesitates and then invites Terry to sit down at the table with him. Terry continues to pepper him with questions: "Have you been taking your blood pressure medication? Are you following your diet restrictions?" Mr. Guillermo finally replies, "I take the medication sometimes when I don't feel too good. The doctor told me to eat less fried foods and salt, but the *yerbero* [herbalist] wants me to eat more avocado and garlic, so I made fresh guacamole and tortilla chips. That drink is lemon tea, which he recommended to help cool my blood pressure." Terry decides not to do any exercises for Mr. Guillermo's shoulder, but instead focuses on client education and review of the home program. Mr. Guillermo admits he has not been doing his home exercises every day, because his *sobandero* [healer] comes to his house 3 times a week. Terry emphasizes the importance of following the physician's orders; taking medication as prescribed; following dietary restrictions on fried foods, fat, and sugar; and limiting sugary drinks. Mr. Guillermo says he will, and Terry leaves the home.

At the end of the day Terry returns to the Home Health Agency office and says, "Please don't send me back to see Mr. Guillermo. He is uncooperative and lazy, and he is a heart attack waiting

(Continued)

CASE EXAMPLE 14.3. RESPECTING CULTURAL TRADITIONS IN HEALTH CARE *(Cont.)*

to happen. Instead of following the recommendations of his doctor and OT, he's listening to some Mexican quack." The director replies, "Don't worry, Terry. Mr. Guillermo has asked that you not be sent to his house again. He said he won't work with you because you were rude and dismissive, and disrespectful of his culture. We would also like you to sign up for the next training on diversity, equity, and inclusion [DEI] and culturally responsive care and review our policies on cultural humility."

Questions
1. In what ways did Terry disrespect Mr. Guillermo and his culture?
2. What standards from the Code did Terry violate?
3. What could Terry do to learn more about Latino cultures in general, and Mr. Guillermo's cultural priorities specifically?
4. How can an occupational therapy practitioner work collaboratively with a *yerbero* (herbalist), *sobandero* (similar to a massage therapist), and other healers?

Summary

Providing culturally responsive care begins with learning about clients' cultures and demonstrating respect for their beliefs and practices. Culturally responsive care includes promoting health literacy, addressing social determinants of health, developing awareness of potential provider implicit or unconscious bias, and ameliorating potential systemic and other barriers to care. These barriers to care can include decreased access to care; poor quality of care; and client satisfaction due to client factors, such as preferred language, geographic location, gender and gender identity, sexual orientation, religious beliefs, values, and so forth.

Training in cultural humility and self-reflection to identify unconscious bias can reduce the potential for actions or words that offend, exclude, or disempower clients, caregivers, or colleagues. Acknowledging bias or microaggression can help occupational therapy practitioners and clients repair and improve the therapeutic relationship, and lead to improved outcomes. Respecting the autonomy of the client and their family or caregivers facilitates a cohesive team to address the client's needs.

REFERENCES

American Occupational Therapy Association. (n.d.). *Diversity, equity, and inclusion resource library*. https://www.aota.org/practice/practice-essentials/dei/diversity-equity--inclusion-toolkit-resource-library

American Occupational Therapy Association. (2021). *AOTA's guide to addressing the impact of racial discrimination, stigma, and implicit bias on provision of services*. https://www.aota.org/-/media/corporate/files/practice/dei/addressing-guide-racial-discrimination.pdf

Avarna Group. (n.d.). *Diversity, equity, & inclusion (DEI) vocab*. https://theavarnagroup.com/

Barstow, C. (2015). *The power differential and why it matters so much in therapy*. https://www.goodtherapy.org/blog/power-differential-why-it-matters-so-much-in-therapy-1009154

Cherry, C., & Stuart, J. (2011). *Pocket guide to culturally sensitive health care.* F. A. Davis.

Jensen, E., Jones, N., Rabe, M., Pratt, B., Medina, L., Orozco, K., & Spell, L. (2021, August 12). *The chance that two people chosen at random are of different race or ethnicity groups has increased since 2010.* U. S. Census Bureau. https://www.census.gov/library/stories/2021/08/2020-united-states-population-more-racially-ethnically-diverse-than-2010.html

Jones, N., Marks, R., Ramirez, R., & Ríos-Vargas, M. (2021). *2020 census illuminates racial and ethnic composition of the country.* U.S. Census Bureau. https://www.census.gov/library/stories/2021/08/improved-race-ethnicity-measures-reveal-united-states-population-much-more-multiracial.html

San Diego Foundation. (2023). *What is culturally responsive care?* https://www.sdfoundation.org/news-events/sdf-news/what-is-culturally-responsive-care/#:~:text=Culturally%20responsive%20care%20is%20defined,how%20this%20shapes%20their%20experiences.%E2%80%9D

U.S. Department of Health and Human Services. (n.d.). *National culturally and linguistically appropriate services standards.* https://thinkculturalhealth.hhs.gov/clas/standards

Ward, N., & Batalova, J. (2023). *Frequently requested statistics on immigrants and immigration in the United States.* Migration Policy Institute. https://www.migrationpolicy.org/article/frequently-requested-statistics-immigrants-and-immigration-united-states

Wells, S. A., Black, R. M., & Gupta, J. (2016). Model for cultural effectiveness. In S. A. Wells, R. M. Black, & J. Gupta (Eds.), *Culture and occupation: Effectiveness for occupational therapy practice, education, and research* (3rd ed., pp. 65–79). AOTA Press.

Wisconsin Technical College. (n.d.). *Nursing fundamentals: Culturally responsive care* [Chapter 3.8]. https://wtcs.pressbooks.pub/nursingfundamentals/chapter/3-8-culturally-responsive-care/

Social Justice, Occupational Justice, and Ethical Practice

BRENDA S. HOWARD, DHSc, OTR, FAOTA

Key Points

- Social justice is concerned with the equitable distribution of resources and opportunities. Occupational justice is concerned with the right for all persons to engage in occupations needed to survive, find meaning, and connect with their communities. Both types of justice relate to social inclusion.
- Social justice and occupational justice are fundamentally human rights issues.
- Social justice acknowledges that inequities are caused by societies, and societies can choose to amend their actions to correct injustices.
- Occupational justice addresses the right for all persons to participate in occupations to promote health and well-being.
- Occupational therapy practitioners can work toward social justice by taking an attitude as a learner, creating collaborative partnerships, and learning to advocate for change.

Introduction

Justice has been a core value of the American Occupational Therapy Association (AOTA) for decades (AOTA, 1993). *Social justice* is defined as "ethical distribution and sharing of resources, rights, and responsibilities between people recognizing their equal worth" (Wilcock & Townsend, 2014, p. 542). Social justice includes the concepts of equity of opportunity and reduction of inequalities. It focuses on social relationships (Wilcock & Townsend, 2014). Social justice acknowledges two things: that inequities exist because they are created by societies, and that societies could change these inequities if they chose to do so (Hocking, 2017). Social justice approaches to righting inequities include (1) procedural justice—providing for rights during the process of resolution of differences; (2) distributive justice—giving equal rights and responsibilities for goods, services, and privileges; and (3) restorative justice—rehabilitating perpetrators of injustice and providing restitution to survivors (Townsend & Whiteford, 2005). Social justice, specifically distributive justice, in the health care system "refers to providing equal health care services for all individuals, regardless of their personal characteristics"

(Habibzadeh et al., 2021, p. 2). The concept of social justice is intertwined with human rights, including the right to the occupations of work, education, leisure, and cultural life (Chichaya et al., 2020; Hocking, 2017). Social justice focuses on equity; it is thought of as occurring on a societal level (Hammell, 2017). Equity creates conditions by which all persons have opportunities to have their needs met (Hammell, 2017).

Similar to social justice, *occupational justice* focuses on equity and fairness, but is more specific to occupational engagement, enablement, and empowerment (Wilcock & Townsend, 2014). The World Federation of Occupational Therapists (WFOT; 2019) defines occupational justice as "The right for all people to engage in occupations they need to survive, define as meaningful, and that contribute positively to their own well-being and the well-being of their communities" (p. 1). Occupational justice includes addressing the many reasons people may be prohibited from some occupations, including socioeconomic status; culture and class; and personal characteristics such as age, gender, race and ethnicity, disability status, and others (Wilcock & Townsend, 2014). Although occupational justice is sometimes thought of as occurring on the individual level (Hammell, 2017; Wilcock & Townsend, 2014), social determinants of health, health disparities, and societal structures that exclude some people from participation play an important role in a person's access to occupation (Braveman & Bass-Haugen, 2009; Crawford & Turpin, 2018; Hocking, 2017; Milliken et al., 2018).

There are causal and correlational relationships between poverty and health and their social determinants. Chronic health conditions, illiteracy, health illiteracy, unemployment, underemployment, food and nutrition scarcity, limited transportation, and lack of social and community supports are just some of the personal, contextual, and social differences that people experience (Synovec & Aceituno, 2020). Occupational therapy practitioners have a role in addressing these social determinants of health with clients. The Participatory Occupational Justice Framework (POJF), introduced by Townsend & Whiteford (2005), focuses on both person-level and systems-enabling approaches to providing access to occupation. The POJF discusses six nonlinear processes by which occupational justice occurs: (1) analyze and coordinate resources; (2) negotiate a justice framework; (3) analyze occupational injustices; (4) negotiate program designs, outcomes, and evaluations; (5) evaluate client-specific strengths, resources, and challenges; (6) and plan, implement, and evaluate client-specific services (Townsend & Whiteford, 2005). Social inclusion is the intended outcome of the POJF process (Whiteford et al., 2018). Townsend & Whiteford (2005) purport that occupational justice "expresses ethical, moral, and civic concerns that participation in daily life should contribute to rather than undermine health, empowerment, and quality of life" (p. 116). Social justice and occupational justice are two sides of the same coin, addressing both the social and occupational needs of humans (Wilcock & Townsend, 2014).

Injustice Issues

Occupational therapy practitioners encounter many injustices, from the personal level to the systems level, on a daily basis. On the personal level, autonomy and safety are sometimes at odds, and one of the reasons can be disparities. The client may not have the financial means, insurance backing, or support systems to be safe at home following a major health event. How might an occupational therapy practitioner respect the client's autonomy when home is not a "safe" option? This predicament is a question that ethicists and the health care team often debate (Milliken et al., 2018). At the heart of this discussion is the concept of "dignity of risk"—does the team afford the client the dignity of assuming the risk of an unsafe situation, if it gives them the autonomy they desire? Even just one team meeting discussing these issues can bring into focus the injustices of an entire health care system and expose larger societal problems (Milliken et al., 2018). Also at the individual level, a paternalistic approach of "doing to" a client rather than affording the client the dignity of choice violates the occupational rights of clients. For example, clients with dementia have been placed in front of televisions, with no choice in which program they watched, instead of being offered activities. Morgan-Brown et al. (2019) found that an institutional attitude that did not allow for occupational participation and choice violated "the needs and the human rights of residents with dementia, as full citizens, to engage in everyday occupations and social networks" (p. 405).

At the organizational or population level, occupational injustice occurs when some populations are restricted from experiencing occupations at liberty, "deliberately or through taken-for-granted social exclusion from participation, at any point across the lifespan, in the occupations typical of their community" (Nilsson & Townsend, 2010, p. 65). These restrictions may occur as a result of discrimination due to critical differences, including race (Rivas-Quarneti et al., 2018) and disability (Chichaya et al., 2020). For example, an inaccessible school playground demonstrates the assumption that children with mobility or sensory issues will not want to use it; or worse, these children haven't even been considered. Another injustice issue at the organizational level is fair allocation of resources and processes. With limited resources, practitioners must consider factors such as cost, resource utilization, and client adherence to intervention protocols and the proper use of assistive technology by the end user (Grajo & Boisselle, 2018; Packham & VanderKaay, 2018).

The occupational therapy practitioner must consider that ways of understanding issues of injustice extend beyond a Western worldview (Butler, 2022; Chattopadhyay et al., 2017; daSilva & Oliver, 2022) or the views of the dominant culture (Beagan et al., 2022). These differences in ways of understanding and thinking must be considered not only in regard to the therapeutic relationship, but also in regard to the health care team. Current client-centered practice models implicitly assume that team members hold "dominant group" views (Beagan et al., 2022). Team leaders and health care professionals should consider how to facilitate equitable distribution of professional power to colleagues who experience social differences related to being members of marginalized groups (e.g., people who experience social realities of racism, ableism, heterosexism, religious differences; Beagan et al., 2022).

Bringing About Social and Occupational Justice

Occupational therapy practitioners can be swept along by unjust forces, reacting to moral distress, and experiencing burnout (Durocher et al., 2016; Penny et al., 2014), or they can choose to be prepared and proactive, and to act with an advocacy mindset on both personal and systemic levels (Cassady et al., 2014; Frank & Muriithi, 2015; Naidoo & Van Wyk, 2023; Yao et al., 2020). The key to addressing issues of injustice lies in enabling fair and equitable access to opportunities and resources, including occupational therapy services, so that people can engage in occupations that are necessary, desired, and meaningful (daSilva & Oliver, 2022; Hemphill, 2015). Practitioners can take meaningful action by promoting community health, providing prevention and chronic disease management education, focusing on reducing health risk behaviors, and advocating for clients in all settings (Cassady et al., 2014; Naidoo & Van Wyk, 2023). Practitioners have an ethical obligation to address disparities when encountered in practice at the individual level, as well as looking at the contexts in which disparities occur and the social causes of inequities at the population level (Grajo & Boiselle, 2018; Synovec & Aceituno, 2020; Townsend & Whiteford, 2005). Advocating for social justice at the population level may require practitioners to become involved in policy formation and change (Chichaya et al., 2020; Yao et al., 2020). Policy change may involve equipping and educating people in local communities to advocate for themselves (Cassady et al., 2014; Frank & Muriithi, 2015). The ultimate goal in this process is occupational participation and social inclusion (Hocking, 2017; Hammell, 2022).

The process for being prepared for advocacy must begin with entry-level occupational therapy education. Social justice is a professional value that should be included in professional socialization for the health professions (Habibzadeh et al., 2021). Professional education should include opportunities for students to create programs that promote social justice in community settings with academic assignments, service learning, and/or fieldwork experiences (Naidoo & Van Wyk, 2023). VanSchalkwyk et al. (2019) recommend using a *transformative learning* pedagogical approach. This approach advocates for "the process of using a prior interpretation to construe a new or revised interpretation of the meaning of one's experience in order to guide future action" (VanSchalkwyk et al., 2019, p. 548). In other words, transformative learning enables learners to transform fixed assumptions into inclusive, open, reflective, and changeable perspectives. If educators want students to become practitioners who enact change, they must teach students about the process of how transformation happens, not just what they should think (VanSchalkwyk, et al., 2019).

Relation to the AOTA Code of Ethics

The core value of *justice* specifically addresses the concepts of social justice and occupational injustice. *Social justice* includes the concept of addressing unjust inequities that limit opportunities for participation in society. *Occupational justice* means full inclusion in everyday meaningful occupations for persons, groups, or populations. Exhibit 15.1 contains the standards related to social justice in the AOTA Code of Ethics (the Code).

EXHIBIT 15.1.
ETHICAL STANDARDS RELATED TO SOCIAL JUSTICE

- Inform employers, employees, colleagues, students, and researchers of applicable policies, laws, and official documents.
- Provide information and resources to address barriers to access for persons in need of occupational therapy services.
- Report systems and policies that are discriminatory or unfairly limit or prevent access to occupational therapy.
- Treat all stakeholders professionally and equitably through constructive engagement and dialogue that is inclusive, collaborative, and respectful of diversity of thought.
- Demonstrate a level of cultural humility, sensitivity, and agility within professional practice that promotes inclusivity and does not result in harmful actions or inactions with persons, groups, organizations, and populations from diverse backgrounds including age, gender identity, sexual orientation, race, religion, origin, socioeconomic status, degree of ability, or any other status or attributes.

Note. From the Standards of Conduct from the AOTA Code of Ethics.

Reference to Other AOTA Documents

AOTA has a number of official documents addressing issues of social and occupational justice to support occupational therapy practitioners when addressing injustices. Some examples include societal statements on community violence, health disparities, and disaster response; and professional policies on affirming gender diversity and identity, affirming sexual orientation, and sustainability and climate change (AOTA, n.d.-a). The AOTA website also contains many practice resources giving guidance for working with persons and populations experiencing disparities (AOTA, n.d.-c). One example of these resources is the Diversity, Equity, and Inclusion (DEI) Learning Modules that include a DEI resource library, word bank, and toolkit with substantial resources including case studies and theoretical frameworks (AOTA, n.d.-b). *Occupational Therapy's Commitment to Diversity, Equity, and Inclusion* discusses the relationship of these topics to the profession (AOTA, 2020). Lastly, the *Occupational Therapy Practice Framework: Domain and Process* discusses the role of occupational therapy practitioners related to this area of practice, including therapeutic use of self (i.e., empathy, cultural humility), occupational justice, and advocacy.

Reference to Other Standards

WFOT (2019) has published a statement on human rights. This statement supports occupational therapy practitioners in advocating for occupational justice by stating, "Occupational therapists are obligated to enact our client-centered aspiration by collaborating with those experiencing abuses and with diverse partners to eradicate abuses that undermine occupational justice" (p. 1). WFOT has also provided a toolkit with resources for advocating for occupational justice for persons, organizations, and populations (WFOT, 2020). Additionally, the World Health Organization (2023) offers a comprehensive toolkit on social determinants of health, health practice, and health equity.

Tips

- Occupational therapy practitioners and students should equip themselves for acting on behalf of persons, groups, and populations experiencing social and occupational injustice.
- Occupational therapy practitioners should work to equip persons, groups, and populations with the skills to advocate for themselves.
- Occupational therapy educators should develop curricula that equip entry-level practitioners to become advocates and change agents.
- Occupational therapy practitioners can advocate for social and occupational justice at the person level by ensuring equitable distribution of resources, including occupational therapy services.
- Occupational therapy practitioners can advocate for social and occupational justice at the community and population levels through addressing contexts and becoming involved in policy formation and change.

CASE EXAMPLE 15.1. SERVICES FOR PEOPLE WITH LIMITED RESOURCES

Jackie was a 39-year-old woman who sustained a right cerebral vascular accident (CVA) because of a previously undiagnosed pancreatic growth that caused severe hypertension. Prior to the CVA, she had been employed in sales at a large home repair store chain. She was single and lived alone and was thus responsible for all home management tasks. Jackie received comprehensive inpatient rehabilitation, including occupational, physical, and speech therapy, and she was referred for further outpatient services after her discharge from the hospital. Jackie received services for approximately 1 month, at which time her employer notified her by mail that they were terminating her employment and canceling her health care insurance. Although she had applied for disability insurance and Medicaid, Jackie had not yet been approved. Jackie did not have the financial resources to self-pay for her therapies, so she discharged herself from outpatient physical therapy, occupational therapy, and speech therapy.

Questions
1. What are the ethical principles and standards in question in this scenario?
2. Apply an ethical problem-solving framework to this case.
3. What steps should the occupational therapy practitioner take to address Jackie's needs?
4. Choose one possible solution to this ethical problem. What would be the possible outcomes? What issues would remain outstanding?

CASE EXAMPLE 15.2. CENTER FOR UNSTABLY HOUSED PEOPLE

An entry-level occupational therapy **doctoral student** was completing a capstone in a center for unstably housed persons to create and teach a life skills group. The student was leading an education session about the importance of showering and doing laundry and noticed people glancing at each other and glancing down with knowing smiles. The student asked what the participants were thinking, and they responded that the student was naive; showers at the shelter were often cold; showers could only be used at certain times of day; safety in the showers and in the laundry room was an issue, with theft and assaults common; and there was inconsistent access to soap, shampoo, and laundry detergent. Following the group session, the student discussed the issues with the program director at the center. The director stated that they relied on two semi-annual toiletry donation drives to obtain supplies, and that supplies often ran low before the next donations were due.

Questions

1. What are the occupational justice and social justice issues in this scenario?
2. What are some possible solutions to sustainably source the supplies needed?
3. How would these solutions reflect ethical practice and the principles of occupational and social justice?

CASE EXAMPLE 15.3. FACILITY POLICIES VS. SOCIAL JUSTICE

An outpatient rehabilitation clinic has a policy of "three strikes and you're out"—clients are terminated from therapy services if they miss three appointments. An **occupational therapy assistant** notices that clients from underserved populations often have unstable transportation, and therefore frequently miss appointments or arrive late to appointments. The occupational therapy assistant also notes that the clinic has a policy of providing access to services for all and brings up the conflict with the supervisor who states, "if clients miss frequently, we have to discharge them to make way for clients who are going to show up. Besides, it's our paying clients who keep the lights on."

Questions

1. What ethical principles and standards from the Code are at stake in this scenario?
2. Apply an ethical decision-making framework. What options does the occupational therapy practitioner have?
3. Which of these options would bring about the greatest result for social and occupational justice for clients?

Next Steps

Occupational therapy practitioners should adopt an attitude as learners and demonstrate cultural humility (Murray-Garcia & Tervalon, 2014) when advocating for and engaging with others. Persons, communities, organizations, and populations may hold beliefs and values of health and wellness that differ from those of the occupational therapy practitioner.

The work of advocacy for social and occupational justice requires critical thinking and reflection to consider one's personal values compared to and in contrast with the needs of those for whom one is advocating. Thinking of oneself as a learner rather than an expert will enable solidarity, humility, and culturally relevant advocacy (Cassady et al., 2014).

Summary

As a core value in occupational therapy practice, justice informs ethical practice on a daily basis. When an occupational therapy practitioner sees that a person, group, or population is being treated inequitably and advocates for needed resources and occupational engagement, that practitioner has held to the values of the profession. It is through these micro and macro acts of boldness, creativity, and empathy that occupational therapy will continue to transform into a more equitable, inclusive, and accessible profession to meet the diverse needs of our society.

Acknowledgment

Ann Moodey Ashe, MHS, OTR/L, authored an earlier version of this Advisory Opinion.

REFERENCES

American Occupational Therapy Association. (n.d.-a). *AOTA official documents.* https://www.aota.org/practice/practice-essentials/aota-official-documents

American Occupational Therapy Association. (n.d.-b). *Diversity, equity, and inclusion in OT.* https://www.aota.org/practice/practice-essentials/dei

American Occupational Therapy Association. (n.d.-c). *Practice: Trusted resources to elevate your practice.* https://www.aota.org/practice

American Occupational Therapy Association. (1993). Core values and attitudes of occupational therapy practice. *American Journal of Occupational Therapy, 47,* 1085–1086. https://doi.org/10.5014/ajot.47.12.1085

American Occupational Therapy Association. (2020). Occupational therapy's commitment to diversity, equity, and inclusion. *American Journal of Occupational Therapy, 74*(Suppl. 3), 7413410030. https://doi.org/10.5014/ajot.2020.74s3002

Beagan, B. L., Sibbald, K. R., Pride, T. M., & Bizzeth, S. R. (2022). Client-centered practice when professional and social power are uncoupled: The experiences of therapists from marginalized groups. *Open Journal of Occupational Therapy, 10*(4), 1–14. https://doi.org/10.15453/2168-6408.1955

Braveman, B., & Bass-Haugen, J. (2009). From the desks of the guest editors—Social justice and health disparities: An evolving discourse in occupational therapy research and intervention. *American Journal of Occupational Therapy, 63,* 7–12. https://doi.org/10.5014/ajot.63.1.7

Butler, M. (2022). A partnership of principles: Ethical reasoning as a foundation for occupational therapy practice. *New Zealand Journal of Occupational Therapy, 69*(1), 3–9. https://search.informit.org/doi/abs/10.3316/informit.432484228310398

Cassady, C., Meru, R., Chan, N. M. C., Engelhardt, J., Fraser, M., & Nixon, S. (2014). Physiotherapy beyond our borders: Investigating ideal competencies for Canadian physiotherapists working in resource-poor countries. *Physiotherapy Canada, 66*(1), 15–23. https://doi.org/10.3138/ptc.2012-54

Chattopadhyay, S., Myers, C., Moxham, T., & DeVries, R. (2017). A question of social justice: How policies of profit negate engagement of developing world bioethicists and undermine global bioethics. *American Journal of Bioethics, 17*(10), 3–14. https://doi.org/10.1080/15265161.2017.1365185

Chichaya, T. F., Joubert, R. W. E., & McColl, M. A. (2020). Voices on disability issues in Namibia: Evidence for entrenching occupational justice in disability policy formulation. *Scandinavian Journal of Occupational Therapy, 27*(1), 14–27. https://doi.org/10.1080/11038128.2018.1496273

Crawford, E., & Turpin, M. J. (2018). Intentional strengths interviewing in occupational justice research. *Scandinavian Journal of Occupational Therapy, 25*(1), 52–60. https://doi.org/10.1080/1103 8128.2017.1322635

daSilva, A. C. C., & Oliver, F. C. (2022). Social participation as a possible way forward for social and occupational justice. *Cadernos Brasileiros de Terapia Ocupacional, 30*(Special Ed.), e3081. https://doi.org/10.1590/2526-8910.ctoAO233130812

Durocher, E., Kinsella, E. A., McCorquodale, L., & Phelan, S. (2016). Ethical tensions related to systemic constraints: Occupational alienation in occupational therapy practice. *OTJR: Occupation, Participation and Health, 36*(4), 216–226. https://doi.org/10.1177/1539449216665117

Frank, G., & Muriithi, B. A. K. (2015). Theorising social transformation in occupational science: The American civil rights movement and South African struggle against apartheid as "occupational reconstructions." *South African Journal of Occupational Therapy, 45*(1), 11–20.

Grajo, L. C., & Boisselle, A. K. (2018). Infusing an occupational justice perspective to technology use in occupational therapy practice. *Open Journal of Occupational Therapy, 6*(3), 1–3. https://doi.org/10.15453/2168-6408.1543

Habibzadeh, H., Jasemi, M., & Hosseinzadegan, F. (2021). Social justice in health system: A neglected component of academic nursing education: A qualitative study. *BMC Nursing, 20*(16), 1–9. https://doi.org/10.1186/s12912-021-00534-1

Hammell, K. R. W. (2017). Critical reflections on occupational justice: Toward a rights-based approach to occupational opportunities. *Canadian Journal of Occupational Therapy, 84*, 47–57. https://doi.org/10.1177/0008417416654501

Hammell, K. W. (2022). Securing occupational rights by addressing capabilities: A professional obligation. *Scandinavian Journal of Occupational Therapy, 29*(1), 1–12. https://doi.org/10.1080/11038 128.2021.1895308

Hemphill, B. (2015). Social justice as a moral imperative. *Open Journal of Occupational Therapy, 3*(2), Article 9. https://doi.org/10.15453/2168-6408.1150

Hocking, C. (2017). Occupational justice as social justice: The moral claim for inclusion. *Journal of Occupational Science, 24*(1), 29–42. https://doi.org/10.1080/14427591.2017.1294016

Milliken, A., Jurchak, M., & Sadovnikoff, N. (2018). When societal structural issues become patient problems: The role of clinical ethics consultation. *The Hastings Center Report, 48*(5), 7–9. https://doi.org/10.1002/hast.894

Morgan-Brown, M., Brangan, J., McMahon, R., & Murphy, B. (2019). Engagement and social interaction in dementia care settings. A call for occupational and social justice. *Health and Social Care in the Community, 27*, 400–408. https://doi.org/10.1111/hsc.12658

Murray-García, J., & Tervalon, M. (2014). The concept of cultural humility. *Health Affairs (Project Hope), 33*, 1303. https://doi.org/10.1377/hlthaff.2014.0564

Naidoo, D., & Van Wyk, J. M. (2023, April 13). Competencies required to deliver a primary healthcare approach in the occupational therapy: A South African perspective. *Occupational Therapy International*, Article 4965740. https://doi.org/10.1155/2023/4965740

Nilsson, I., & Townsend, E. (2010). Occupational justice—Bridging theory and practice. *Scandinavian Journal of Occupational Therapy, 17*(1), 64–70. https://doi.org/10.3109/11038120903287182

Packham, T., & VanderKaay, S. (2018). Ethics and evidence in occupational therapy. *Occupational Therapy Now, 21*(2), 11–12.

Penny, N. H., Ewing, T. L., Hamid, R. C., Shutt, K. A., & Walter, A. S. (2014). An investigation of moral distress experienced by occupational therapists. *Occupational Therapy in Health Care, 28*, 382–393. https://doi.org/10.3109/07380577.2014.933380

Rivas-Quarneti, N., Movilla-Fernández, M., & Magalhães, L. (2018). Immigrant women's occupational struggles during the socioeconomic crisis in Spain: Broadening occupational justice conceptualization. *Journal of Occupational Science, 25*(1), 6–18. https://doi.org/10.1080/14427591.2017.1366355

Synovec, C., & Aceituno, L. (2020). Social justice considerations for occupational therapy: The role of addressing social determinants of health in unstably housed populations. *Work, 65*, 235–246. https://doi.org/10.3233/WOR-203074

Townsend, E., & Whiteford, G. (2005). A participatory occupational justice framework: Population-based processes of practice. In F. Kronenberg, S. S. Algado, & N. Pollard (Eds.), *Occupational therapy without borders: Learning from the spirit of survivors* (1st ed., pp. 110–126). Elsevier Limited.

VanSchalkwyk, S., Hafler, J., Brewer, T., Maley, M., Margolis, C., McNamee, L., . . . Davies, D. (2019). Transformative learning as pedagogy for the health professions: A scoping review. *Medical Education, 53*, 547–558. https://doi.org/10.1111/medu.13804

Whiteford, G., Jones, K., Rahal, C., & Suleman, A. (2018). The participatory occupational justice framework as a tool for change: Three contrasting case narratives. *Journal of Occupational Science, 25*, 497–508. https://doi.org/10.1080/14427591.2018.1504607

Wilcock, A. A., & Townsend, E. (2014). Occupational justice. In B. A. Boyt Schell, G. Gillen, & M. Scaffa (Eds.), *Willard & Spackman's occupational therapy* (12th ed., pp. 541–552). Wolters Kluwer/Lippincott Williams & Wilkins.

World Federation of Occupational Therapists. (2019). *Position statement: Occupational therapy and human rights* (Rev.). https://www.wfot.org/resources/occupational-therapy-and-human-rights

World Federation of Occupational Therapists. (2020). *Advocacy toolkit.* https://wfot.org/resources/advocacy-toolkit

World Health Organization. (2023). *Social determinants of health.* https://www.who.int/health-topics/social-determinants-of-health#tab=tab_1

Yao, D. P. G., Inoue, K., Sy, M. P., Bontje, P., Suyama, N., Yatsu, C., . . . Ito, Y. (2020). Experience of Filipinos with spinal cord injury in the use of assistive technology: An occupational justice perspective. *Occupational Therapy International, 6696296.* https://doi.org/10.1155/2020/6696296

Balancing Client Rights and Practitioner Values

ASHLEY WAGNER, OTD, OTR∕L

Key Points

- Occupational therapy practitioners are never obligated to put themselves in danger.
- Moral objection to another individual's identity or occupational roles, rituals, or routines is not an ethical reason to terminate the therapeutic relationship or abandon professional civility.
- Ethical occupational therapy practitioners engage in self-reflection and address any personal values that may limit their ability to fulfill professional responsibilities prior to and during ethical dilemmas.

Introduction

Occupational therapy practitioners come to the profession with a variety of backgrounds, experiences, and beliefs. However, regardless of personal values, every practitioner is expected to uphold and prioritize the profession's unifying core values of altruism, equality, freedom, justice, dignity, truth, and prudence. These core values are meant to guide every professional interaction and ethical decision of the practitioner. Yet situations may arise where a practitioner finds themselves questioning whether respecting a client's right to client-centered, collaborative care, or honoring similar rights of students and colleagues, may put the practitioner in conflict with their own personal values. In such scenarios, the practitioner may even worry about exposing themselves to physically unsafe situations or moral injury. Moral injury occurs in the clinical, administrative, or academic realm when an occupational therapy practitioner finds they have either performed or witnessed actions that drastically violate their deeply held, personal beliefs (Griffin et al., 2019). Moral injury may result in symptoms similar to those of depression or post traumatic stress (Griffin et al., 2019). Therefore, situations where practitioners are at risk of moral injury cannot be disregarded as harmless or trivialized.

Occupational therapy practitioners are never ethically obligated to put themselves in physical danger to deliver client care or fulfill professional responsibilities. If an occupational therapy practitioner finds themselves in a situation where they may experience physical harm, they may immediately remove themself from the situation. Once in a place of safety, the practitioner should attempt to collaborate as appropriate with the client or other individual to mitigate future danger. If collaboration does not yield a reasonable resolution, it can be ethical for the practitioner to pursue termination of the relationship following the guidelines of their organization.

Recognizing the impact of implicit racial, gender, and other biases on health care decisions and how practitioners interpret health care situations, the ethical occupational therapy practitioner must engage in reflective practices both before and during times of imminent threat. This reflection can ensure that the practitioner is not misinterpreting the context and over-representing the potential threat of an environment during their analysis of safety (Marcelin et al., 2019; Ricks et al., 2021). These reflections should include identifying and acknowledging implicit biases and practicing the skills needed for cultural humility, especially during times of stress or conflict (Marcelin et al., 2019; Ricks et al., 2021). Reflection of potential bias could include discussions with an objective mentor, reviewing organizational and professional standards, and training on cultural humility or inclusion (Wade, 2015).

Occupational therapy practitioners should be cautioned that the much more common but benign discomfort that often accompanies ethical uncertainty or dilemmas is not equivalent to the potentially significant impact of moral injury, which places the practitioner at high risk for no longer being able to participate in their profession due to disruptive symptoms of depression or anxiety and burnout (Durocher & Kinsella, 2021; Tigard, 2019). Therefore an ethical practitioner will engage in earnest, intensive self-reflection and tolerate the unpleasant but temporary discomfort of moral distress in order to avoid the long-term mental health harm associated with moral injury (Wade, 2015).

Moral objection to another individual's identity or occupational roles, rituals, or routines is not an ethical reason to terminate the therapeutic relationship or abandon professional civility. Even in those rare situations when an occupational therapy practitioner has proactively reflected, mitigated their limitations, and still finds themselves in a situation where they are at risk of moral injury and need to step away from a situation, the practitioner is bound to the code of ethics and the ethical standards of the profession as they navigate that transition. The practitioner must take all reasonable steps to mitigate the harm to the clients, students, or colleagues involved while removing themself from the situation; or, if they determine such personal limitations will be ongoing, removing themselves from their professional position. This process of stepping away from professional relationships or from professional positions must be completed in a collaborative manner with clients, following organizational guidelines for such a transition; and with diligence to prioritize the well-being of the client or other involved individuals, as well as the team effectiveness.

Relation to the AOTA Code of Ethics

See Exhibit 16.1 for ethical standards from the AOTA Code of Ethics (the Code) related to client rights versus practitioner values.

EXHIBIT 16.1.

ETHICAL STANDARDS RELATED TO BALANCING CLIENT RIGHTS WITH PRACTITIONER VALUES

- Respect and honor the expressed wishes of recipients of service.
- Do not inflict harm or injury to recipients of occupational therapy services, students, research participants, or employees.
- Do not abandon the service recipient, and attempt to facilitate appropriate transitions when unable to provide services for any reason.
- Adhere to organizational policies when requesting an exemption from service to an individual or group because of self-identified conflict with personal, cultural, or religious values.
- Recognize and take appropriate action to remedy occupational therapy personnel's personal problems and limitations that might cause harm to recipients of service.
- Do not engage in actions or inactions that jeopardize the safety or well-being of others or team effectiveness.
- Demonstrate a level of cultural humility, sensitivity, and agility within professional practice that promotes inclusivity and does not result in harmful actions or inactions with persons, groups, organizations, and populations from diverse backgrounds including age, gender identity, sexual orientation, race, religion, origin, socioeconomic status, degree of ability, or any other status or attributes.

Note. From the Standards of Conduct from the AOTA Code of Ethics.

Tips

- Proactive self-reflection to identify and address biases or accommodate beliefs will help prevent many ethical dilemmas where a practitioner must balance the rights of others against their own personal values.
- Following organizational guidelines and taking all reasonable steps to avoid harm to others or perceived client abandonment will aid the practitioner when it is necessary to step away from a situation to prevent physical danger or true moral injury to themselves.

Summary

Occupational therapy practitioners are never ethically obligated to put themselves in danger of physical or moral injury. However, moral objection to another individual's identity or occupational role, rituals, or routines is not an ethically justifiable reason to terminate a therapeutic relationship or to act with incivility. All practitioners are required to practice proactive self-reflection to identify when their personal values may conflict with their ability to uphold the core values of the occupational therapy profession and, once those limitations are recognized, to address those limitations in a way that prioritizes client, student, or colleague well-being without putting those individuals at risk of harm or abandonment.

CASE EXAMPLE 16.1. CONFLICT OF VALUES AND UNSAFE ENVIRONMENT

Keisha, an occupational therapist working in home care, meets her new patient **Rafaella,** who recently had a hip replacement as a result of long-standing rheumatoid arthritis. Rafaella is currently estranged from her husband, who has been abusive in the past. On the second visit, Keisha notices a large bruise on Rafaella's neck, which Rafaella has attempted to cover up with a scarf. Keisha inquires as to how Rafaella got bruised, and Rafaella responds that she fell out of bed, but she seems withdrawn and does not make eye contact while speaking. Keisha is concerned about the situation and suspects abuse.

As Keisha continues to treat Rafaella, they establish a therapeutic relationship, and Rafaella discloses that her husband continues to stop by when he is intoxicated and can become physically abusive. Keisha encourages Rafaella to file a police report and get a restraining order. Rafaella adamantly refuses this advice, stating that she still loves her husband and would not want to get him into trouble. Keisha questions her ability to continue treating Rafaella because she does not feel that she can support Rafaella's choice to remain in an abusive relationship.

One day, while Keisha is treating Rafaella, Rafaella's estranged husband arrives with alcohol on his breath, is verbally abusive, and staggers around the house. Keisha notices a gun in his waistband. The husband confronts Keisha and orders her to leave, yelling that he will shoot if she returns. Keisha feels that she cannot continue to treat Rafaella in her home because she fears for her own safety. Keisha also fears for Rafaella, but she feels she has done all she can to encourage Rafaella to seek assistance from the police.

Questions

1. How might Keisha balance Rafaella's right to autonomy and client-centered, collaborative care against Keisha's personal values regarding relational health and safety for her client?
2. What aspects of this case should Keisha document in her initial assessment?
3. Is Keisha ethically obligated as an occupational therapy practitioner to stay in the home with Rafaella in this scenario?
4. Is Keisha ethically obligated to continue working with Rafaella in her home once the situation described in the scenario is resolved?

CASE EXAMPLE 16.2. TRIGGERING SYMBOL

An **occupational therapy assistant** arrives in a hospital room and finds that the patient has a swastika tattooed on their forehead. The occupational therapy assistant is Jewish, a descendent of Holocaust survivors, and has extremely negative associations with this symbol. The occupational therapy assistant immediately leaves the room and finds their supervisor to talk about their concerns. The supervisor is sympathetic but states that the occupational therapy assistant cannot refuse to treat the patient.

Questions

1. Does the occupational therapy assistant have an ethical obligation to treat the patient? Why or why not?
2. Is it ethical for the supervisor to require the occupational therapy assistant to treat this patient? Why or why not?

Acknowledgments

Lea Cheyney Brandt, OTD, OTR/L, and **Donna F. Homenko, PhD, RDH,** authored an earlier version of this Advisory Opinion.

REFERENCES

Durocher, E., & Kinsella, E. A. (2021). Ethical tensions in occupational therapy practice: Conflicts and competing allegiances. *Canadian Journal of Occupational Therapy*, *88*, 244–253. https://doi .org/10.1177/00084174211021707

Griffin, B. J., Purcell, N., Burkman, K., Litz, B. T., Bryan, C. J., Schmitz, M., . . . Maguen, S. (2019). Moral injury: An integrative review. *Journal of Traumatic Stress*, *32*, 350–362. https://doi.org/10.1002/ jts.22362

Marcelin, J. R., Siraj, D. S., Victor, R., Kotadia, S., & Maldonado, Y. A. (2019). The impact of unconscious bias in healthcare: How to recognize and mitigate it. *Journal of Infectious Diseases*, *220*(Suppl. 2), S62–S73. https://doi.org/10.1093/infdis/jiz214

Ricks, T. N., Abbyad, C., & Polinard, E. (2021). Undoing racism and mitigating bias among healthcare professionals: Lessons learned during a systematic review. *Journal of Racial and Ethnic Health Disparities*, *9*, 1990–2000. https://doi.org/10.1007/s40615-021-01137-x

Tigard, D. W. (2019). The positive value of moral distress. *Bioethics*, *33*, 601–608. https://doi .org/10.1111/bioe.12564

Wade, M. E. (2015). Handling conflicts of personal values. *Ethics Inquiries*. https://www.coun-seling.org/docs/default-source/ethics/ethics-columns/ethics_april_2015_personal-values .pdf?sfvrsn=1e24522c_4

Section 3. Documentation, Reimbursement, and Financial Matters

Ethical Considerations for Productivity, Billing, and Reimbursement

LESLIE BENNETT, OTD, OTR/L

Key Points

- Productivity standards and reimbursement requirements are a source of tension in occupational therapy practice.
- When occupational therapy practitioners face discrepancies and potential ethical or legal violations, they have an ethical responsibility to act.

Introduction

Productivity is the measurement standard by which most occupational therapy practitioners account for their time, and it reflects workload expectations of the practice environment. Contemporary occupational therapy practice requires practitioners to focus on objective, quantifiable, functional outcomes and to generate "units of service" for reimbursement purposes. It is a delicate balance between focusing on the quality of care provided to clients and maintaining productivity rates (Cote et al., 2022).

Workload expectations and productivity measurement are legitimate management tools used to ensure appropriate staffing resources for service delivery, and to maximize reimbursement to achieve economic sustainability. Service delivery models, productivity standards, and the practices and methods used to report reimbursement services must be reasonable and adhere to prevailing ethical and legal standards. In October 2019, the Patient-Driven Payment Model was introduced into the health care system (Centers for Medicare & Medicaid Services [CMS], 2023b). Under this model, the patient's medical diagnosis is tied to the amount and type of services they will most likely need. Although this model focuses on decreasing the emphasis on productivity, its unintended impact is that billable units of therapy services no longer drive reimbursement. Therefore, institutions and facilities have looked for ways to offset this changing system. One way they have done so is to decrease the number of therapy practitioners they employ (CMS, 2023b).

In today's environment, health and human services are influenced by complex business models. Labor accounts for a significant percentage of health care costs, so efforts to rein in escalating expenses have emphasized productivity management as an essential tool to positively affect net revenue. However, increasing costs, coupled with diminishing reimbursement and emphasis on efficiency, produce a dynamic challenge for occupational therapy practitioners (Cote et al., 2022). In particular, practitioners are challenged to maintain higher caseloads to offset decreased per-client reimbursement, yet manage direct and indirect (e.g., documentation) client-related care in less time than previously available, while still meeting quality standards for appropriate clinical services. These challenges are not unique to occupational therapy practice and have been reported by other therapy service providers (American Occupational Therapy Association [AOTA] et al., 2014).

As a result, AOTA, in collaboration with the American Speech-Language-Hearing Association (ASHA) and the American Physical Therapy Association (APTA), developed a *Consensus Statement on Clinical Judgment in Health Care Settings* (AOTA et al., 2014). The Consensus Statement reinforces the importance of ethical practice, understanding and complying with Medicare and other payer system guidelines, and the need for independent clinical judgment when determining appropriate client care. Resources are also included to guide practitioners in taking action if a problem arises.

Occupational therapy practitioners have a legal and ethical obligation to conform to the productivity standards set by their organization, yet they also have a professional duty to critically examine whether those expectations are congruent with ethical guidelines, legal standards, and requirements of the payer. If the organizational expectations conflict with ethical and legal guidance, administrative directives should not take priority over the practitioner's clinical judgment and the best interests of the client. However, efforts to comply with such directives can result in moral distress or ethical dilemmas for occupational therapy practitioners (Bennett et al., 2019; Cote et al., 2022; Smith-Gabai et al., 2018). Ethical reasoning knowledge and skills can assist practitioners in their professional responsibility to identify, analyze, and take action to resolve ethical dilemmas in these situations.

THE ISSUES

Some of the most frequent questions that occupational therapy practitioners have posed to AOTA focus on the challenges and dilemmas they have encountered in striving to meet employers' expectations while practicing efficiently, legally, and ethically. Occupational therapy practitioners work in environments in which productivity expectations and business practices often drive service delivery models and daily schedules. Further, current reimbursement models emphasize practitioner productivity along with measurable performance outcomes (Gergen Barnett, 2017). Administrative policies, practice standards, available labor resources, environmental conditions, technology systems, payment sources, and the fluid, real-time decision making for daily scheduling all influence how caseloads are managed and prioritized.

Bushby et al. (2015) published a systematic review of literature related to sources of ethical tension in occupational therapy practice. Their findings reinforced that resource and system issues, including conflicting values, discharge planning, decision making, and goal setting have been among the most frequent sources of ethical tension in practice. Emphasizing productivity and measuring performance without considering the demand on providers has led to burnout and moral distress (Bennett et al., 2019; Cote et al., 2022; Furniss, 2019).

Ethical challenges related to productivity, billing, and reimbursement may include, but are not limited to:

- being directed to charge for services not provided
- treating clients in groups when reimbursement guidelines do not allow such configurations
- using students or other service extenders to provide "billable" service when not permissible within the applicable regulations
- being directed to rate clients' functional performance as more impaired than is supported by objective data
- providing services that are not medically necessary (overtreatment)
- coercing participation in services despite the client's objections
- being required to meet productivity standards that are not realistically achievable in the typical workday
- feeling forced to comply with employer directives in order to "keep the job" rather than "do the right thing" (i.e., being asked to document off clock)
- deciding whether to report a coworker, manager, or organization when violations are suspected or verified.

PROFESSIONAL RESPONSIBILITY

Despite the significant challenges of reimbursement policies, there is no justification for engaging in illegal or unethical behavior while providing, reporting, or billing for occupational therapy services, even if one's intentions are good. Occupational therapy practitioners cannot ignore their ethical and professional duty to be informed about billing requirements, nor can they rely solely on others, such as supervisors or administrators, to ensure compliance. Individual practitioners who do not comply with regulatory requirements for reimbursement may face legal jeopardy and are at risk of losing their license. Other potential negative consequences for practitioners that may result from unethical practice include criminal charges, professional disciplinary action, and scandal or blemish on their professional reputation.

Although many health care organizations, such as hospitals, rehabilitation centers, long-term-care facilities, and home health agencies have compliance programs and dedicated professionals to keep up to date with federal, state, and other requirements, practitioners must verify the source and accuracy of payer processes and administrative directives that affect their practice and payment for services. Certainly, the best, first step is to work internally within the formal structure of the organization. If that is not effective, reporting should be considered. *Compliance Reporting*, developed by AOTA, ASHA, APTA, and the National Association for the Support of Long-Term Care (n.d.), outlines considerations and steps to take in reporting fraud, abuse, and other non-compliance incidents.

Adverse actions for offending practitioners can include exclusion from participation in federal, state, or private programs that provide reimbursement for services. Consequences may also include termination of employment and loss of right to work if a practitioner's state license is suspended or revoked. In severe cases, fines are levied, and incarceration can result (U.S. Department of Health & Human Services, Office of Inspector General, n.d.). In addition, organizations governing occupational therapy practice share information about adverse final actions, so disciplinary action could also be taken by the National Board for Certification in Occupational Therapy® or by the AOTA Ethics Commission if the practitioner is within the jurisdiction of these professional organizations.

Reporting fraudulent or unethical activity requires moral courage and may result in negative professional repercussions or jeopardize one's professional employment, even when reporting is the right course of action (Markkula Center for Applied Ethics, 2015). In an untenable environment, an occupational therapy practitioner may decide to leave their job, particularly if violations are frequent, violations are not addressed or are not resolved, or the practitioner's ethical obligations are constantly challenged. The possible negative consequences for the individual who makes these difficult personal decisions cannot be discounted (Smith-Gabai et al., 2018).

When retaliation is a credible threat, practitioners should investigate whistle-blower protections and mechanisms to report anonymously before taking action. Many organizations have whistle-blower protection programs, as well as policies and procedures to guide employees when they believe they have observed financial improprieties, ethical violations, or other illegal activity. Whistle blowing takes moral courage, as the person who seeks to report harmful or illegal actions of their organization may themselves suffer retaliation, marginalization, or even termination from employment while trying to do the right thing (Markkula Center for Applied Ethics, 2015), but the long-term yield of doing the right thing should provide enduring relief. In situations in which whistle blowing results in a finding of fraud, the whistleblower may reap a financial reward for assisting in identifying the dishonest conduct (CMS, 2021).

At the federal level, the Civil Actions for False Claims Act (2015) provides the opportunity to redress adverse employment consequences and offers a potential, substantial monetary reward if the proper legal procedures related to whistle blowing are followed. This law allows a private person to sue a person or company who is knowingly submitting false bills to the federal government. The act also protects qui tam plaintiffs (i.e., whistleblowers) who are "demoted, suspended, threatened, harassed, or in any other manner discriminated against in the terms and conditions of employment" for actions done in furtherance of filing a claim under the Act. This provision allows reinstatement; double back pay; interest on back pay; and special damages, such as reimbursement for litigation costs and reasonable attorneys' fees.

Despite a whistleblower's good intentions, the risks associated with reporting must not be minimized. The whistleblower must understand the differentiation between legal and illegal practices and gather substantial information and evidence before filing a complaint. Nonetheless, although doing nothing may be an option, occupational therapy practitioners must consider the potential damage to their self-esteem and personal integrity, as well as the moral distress that may result from not taking action and remaining in an adverse and unethical work environment.

Relation to the AOTA Code of Ethics

The AOTA Code of Ethics (the Code) directly addresses ethical issues related to productivity, billing, and reimbursement. It is the obligation of every occupational therapy practitioner to follow these ethical standards. Exhibit 17.1 contains standards from the Code related to productivity, billing, and reimbursement.

EXHIBIT 17.1.

ETHICAL STANDARDS RELATED TO PRODUCTIVITY, BILLING, AND REIMBURSEMENT

- Comply with current federal and state laws, state scope of practice guidelines, and AOTA policies and official documents that apply to the profession of occupational therapy.
- Abide by policies, procedures, and protocols when serving or acting on behalf of a professional organization or employer to fully and accurately represent the organization's official and authorized positions.
- Do not engage in actions that reduce the public's trust in occupational therapy.
- Report potential or known unethical or illegal actions in practice, education, or research to the appropriate authorities.
- Bill and collect fees justly and legally in a manner that is fair, reasonable, and commensurate with services delivered.
- Ensure that documentation for reimbursement purposes is done in accordance with applicable laws, guidelines, and regulations.
- Do not follow arbitrary directives that compromise the rights or well being of others, including unrealistic productivity expectations, fabrication, falsification, plagiarism of documentation, or inaccurate coding.

Note. From the Standards of Conduct from the AOTA Code of Ethics.

Resources for Ethical Productivity, Billing, and Reimbursement Practices

There are many printed and video resources available regarding productivity, billing, and reimbursement. Some examples include:

- *AOTA Practice Essentials*: Provides tools and educational materials regarding billing, productivity, and reimbursement. https://www.aota.org/practice/practice-essentials
- *U.S. Department of Health and Human Services, Office of Inspector General*:
  800-447-8477, TTY: 800-377-4950
  https://oig.hhs.gov/fraud/report-fraud/

- *Safe Hotline—Ethics Reporting Service*: Anonymous and confidential service to report potential fraud, ethics violations, and other concerns. https://tinyurl.com/3j6pvj93
- *Office of the Inspector General*: 2008 Advisory Opinion related to "prompt pay" discounts https://tinyurl.com/52t22kd6
- *Centers for Medicare and Medicaid Services*:
  800-633-4227, TTY: 877-486-2048
  Medicare Beneficiary Contact Center, PO Box 39, Lawrence, KS 66044
- *Individual insurance carriers, other third-party payers, or health plan sponsors*
  Note. Most entities have reimbursement policies and procedures that outline coding methodology, industry-standard reimbursement logic, and regulatory requirements. Inquire directly to the specific company when reimbursement information or clarification is required. Most policies and procedures can be found on the payer's website.
- *State agencies regulating the insurance industry*:
  Office of the Insurance Commissioner (Commissioner of Insurance) or (state) Department of Insurance
  https://content.naic.org/state-insurance-departments
- *State, district, or territorial authority responsible for regulating the occupational therapy profession*: State Licensure Laws & Regulation: https://www.aota.org/career/state-licensure
- OT Practice *magazine, October 2018*: "An OT/OTA Team's Experience Reporting Illegal Skilled Nursing Facility Billing: Relying on Core Values, AOTA, and the OIG to Persevere" https://www.aota.org/Publications-News/otp/Archive/2018/illegal-billing.aspx

---

CASE EXAMPLE 17.1. BILLING GROUP TREATMENT AT THE HIGHER INDIVIDUAL RATE

Blake and **Parker** were occupational therapy practitioners at an outpatient pediatric clinic that used *Current Procedural Terminology (CPT®)* codes (CMS, 2023a), most of which are based on 15-minute increments of direct, 1-to-1 service. Blake learned that Parker routinely treated up to 5 children at a time during a single 1-hour session, and billed and documented for 4 *CPT* codes per child. This practice meant that Parker billed up to 20 units (5 children × 4 *CPT* codes) which is up to 5 hours of direct 1-to-1 time during a 1-hour treatment time.

Parker justified this practice by stating that they were not reporting their treatment time as "group" treatment but were grouping children appropriately by common treatment needs or goals and that the children were working on individual activities. Parker indicated that the children were lined up on therapy balls or seated at a kidney-shaped table while working on exercises or on their handwriting program or fine motor skills. Parker divided their time among the children to ensure that all of them were working on their activities. Blake felt that this was not accurate billing and did not reflect what services were provided. Blake believed it was not legal or ethical to bill for 5 hours of treatment during 1 actual hour, and that simultaneous treatment required billing as a group.

(Continued)

CASE EXAMPLE 17.1. BILLING GROUP TREATMENT AT THE HIGHER INDIVIDUAL RATE *(Cont.)*

Blake thought that Parker's practice may have been an intentional act of deceit for the purpose of receiving greater reimbursement for the clinic and winning a bonus for having the best productivity but had some doubts and did not want to judge a colleague without knowing all the facts. Blake wondered how best to address this issue with Parker.

Questions

1. What is the proper procedure for billing services done simultaneously?
2. What standards from the Code did Parker violate?
3. What is Blake's best course of action without knowing whether the clinic supports Parker's billing practices?

CASE EXAMPLE 17.2. UNREALISTIC PRODUCTIVITY EXPECTATIONS

Jing began working in a skilled nursing facility (SNF) after working in an acute care hospital for 6 years. Jing made the switch in order to spend more time with the residents being served, instead of doing evaluations on patients who left the next day. Expected productivity for the occupational therapy staff in the hospital was 50%, as patients were often unavailable due to pain, other therapies, physicians being in the room, or tests being conducted. Jing was surprised to learn that the expected productivity in the SNF was 90% for occupational therapists and 95% for occupational therapy assistants. As an occupational therapy assistant, this meant Jing had to bill for 7.6 hours or at least 31 units (using *CPT* codes) in an 8-hour day to achieve productivity. To come close to this level, Jing started to do all documentation after clocking out at the end of the day. Jing also skipped lunch or breaks several times a week and limited water intake to avoid having to use the restroom, in order to achieve productivity. After 2 months, Jing complained to the Rehab Manager about the unrealistic productivity. The Rehab Manager replied, "If you don't like it, you can leave. I can get another occupational therapy assistant here tomorrow who will do the job." At the state occupational therapy association's conference later that month, Jing met several occupational therapy practitioners who had previously worked for the same SNF company. They told Jing that there had been several complaints about the productivity standard over the last 3 years and that the complaining staff were all terminated. The previous Rehab Manager had left the company after being told to "get the staff to bill however necessary to achieve productivity standards." After talking to friends and family, Jing decided to resign from the SNF and seek employment elsewhere.

Questions

1. What standards were violated by the SNF company and the Rehab Manager?
2. What avenues of recourse are available to Jing?
3. What would you do if you were asked to maintain an unrealistic productivity standard?

Summary

Productivity demands and reimbursement issues can be sources of tension in the workplace. The realities and challenges of the current clinical service delivery environment do not supersede occupational therapy practitioners' ethical and legal obligations to be knowledgeable about and compliant with applicable standards and regulations. Occupational therapy practitioners have responsibilities as employees in an organization to meet reasonable productivity requirements and bill for services accurately and appropriately. In addition, practitioners have an overarching ethical duty to advocate for safe, effective, appropriate services for clients.

Discordance between productivity demands and reimbursement issues is an ongoing challenge and may lead to unresolved conflict or provoke ethical angst. Some difficult decisions may be required. When discrepancies and potential violations are identified, occupational therapy practitioners have an ethical responsibility to consider taking action. Ignoring violations is not an appropriate ethical response. Silence is implicit consent, and inaction allows harm to continue.

Using ethical reasoning and accessing the available resources from AOTA and elsewhere to resolve conflicts can help practitioners meet this professional obligation.

Acknowledgments

Deborah Y. Slater, MS, OT/L, FAOTA; Wayne L. Winistorfer, MPA, OTR; and **Linda S. Scheirton, RDH, PhD,** authored earlier versions of this Advisory Opinion.

REFERENCES

American Occupational Therapy Association, American Physical Therapy Association, American Speech-Language-Hearing Association, & National Association for the Support of Long Term Care. (n.d.). *Compliance reporting.* https://www.asha.org/siteassets/uploadedfiles/compliance-reporting.pdf

American Occupational Therapy Association, American Physical Therapy Association, & American Speech-Language-Hearing Association. (2014). *Consensus statement on clinical judgment in health care settings.* https://www.aota.org/-/media/corporate/files/practice/ethics/apta-aota-asha-consensus-statement.pdf

Bennet, L. E., Jewell, V. D., Scheirton, L., McCarthy, M., & Muir, B. C. (2019). Productivity standards and the impact on quality of care: A national survey of inpatient rehabilitation professionals. *Open Journal of Occupational Therapy, 7*(4), 1–11. https://doi.org/10.15453/2168-6408.1598

Bushby, K., Chan, J., Druif, S., Ho, K., & Kinsella, E. A. (2015). Ethical tensions in occupational therapy practice: A scoping review. *British Journal of Occupational Therapy, 78,* 212–221. https://doi.org/10.1177/0308022614564770

Centers for Medicare and Medicaid Services. (2021). *Medicare fraud and abuse: Prevent, detect, report.* https://www.cms.gov/Outreach-and-Education/Medicare-Learning-Network-MLN/MLNProducts/Downloads/Fraud-Abuse-MLN4649244.pdf

Centers for Medicare and Medicaid Services. (2023a). *List of CPT/HCPCS codes.* https://www.cms.gov/medicare/regulations-guidance/physician-self-referral/list-cpt/hcpcs-codes

Centers for Medicare and Medicaid Services. (2023b). *Patient driven payment model.* https://www.cms.gov/medicare/payment/prospective-payment-systems/skilled-nursing-facility-snf/patient-driven-model

Civil Actions for False Claims Act, 31 U.S. Code § 3730 (2015). https://www.law.cornell.edu/uscode/text/31/3730

Cote, A., Duffy, J., Watson, J. L., & Smith, R. A. (2022). The relationship between OT practitioner productivity requirements and quality care measures in nursing homes. *American Journal of Occupational Therapy, 76*(Suppl. 1), 7610510160. https://doi.org/10.5014/ajot.2022.76S1-PO160

Furniss, J. (2019). Federal health care programs and outcomes. In K. Jacobs & G. McCormack (Eds.), *The occupational therapy manager* (6th ed., pp. 277–284). AOTA Press.

Gergen Barnett, K. A. (2017). In pursuit of the fourth aim in health care: The joy of practice. *Medical Clinics of North America, 101*(5). https://doi.org/10.1016/j.mcna.2017.04.014

Markkula Center for Applied Ethics. (2015). *Whistle blowing in the public sector.* https://www.scu.edu/government-ethics/resources/what-is-government-ethics/whistle-blowing-in-the-public-sector/

Smith-Gabai, H., Kuzminski, S., & Eldridge, E. (2018). Surveying moral distress among skilled nursing facility practitioners. *OT Practice, 23*(18), 24–25.

U.S. Department of Health & Human Services, Office of Inspector General. (n.d.). *Fraud and abuse laws.* https://oig.hhs.gov/compliance/physician-education/fraud-abuse-laws/

Organizational Ethics

DEBORAH YARETT SLATER, OT, MSOT, FAOTA, and
BRENDA S. HOWARD, DHSc, OTR, FAOTA

Key Points

- Essential characteristics of organizational ethics include balancing regulatory and financial pressures with a focus on the client–practitioner relationship.
- Sources of ethical tension in organizations include challenges to professional codes of ethics, and conflicting values and allegiances.
- Despite power differentials and interprofessional team differences, the organization should not jeopardize the trust that is essential to the client–practitioner relationship.

Introduction

Occupational therapy practitioners face a variety of ethical challenges in the increasingly complex workplace. These challenges may be specific to the organization or system but may also include inequities in society. Organizational trends include a business orientation with a regulatory and reimbursement focus; inadequate staff to provide safe, appropriate, effective services; questionable resource allocation; and the need to address cultural diversity and social drivers of health as they impact client outcomes (Durocher & Kinsella, 2021; Lahey et al., 2020; McArdle et al., 2023; McDuffie et al., 2023; Tammany et al., 2019). Although practitioners work in many different types of organizations, this Advisory Opinion focuses primarily on health care organizations such as hospitals, outpatient clinics, skilled nursing facilities, and home health agencies.

Interest in organizational ethics related to the health care environment began in the 1990s in the United States but gained strength in 1992 when the Joint Commission for Accreditation of Healthcare Organizations added an organizational ethics requirement to its standards (Borges Paraizo & Bégin, 2020). Hospitals were mandated to adopt a code of conduct to address hospital admissions, advertising, client billing, and relations with staff and other health care practitioners, including educational institutions (Borges Paraizo & Bégin, 2020).

Although traditional ethics focuses on individuals, *organizational ethics* typically focuses on group behavior of people in the organization (e.g., clinicians and nonclinical workers, clients, administrators, institutions) and diverse interests that may conflict (Phelan, 2020). "The interplay among hierarchy, management and policy in current health care systems suggests that an organizational ethics lens is indispensable for appraising ethical problems" (Phelan, 2020, p. 183). Organizational ethics programs can identify conflicts between the organization's values and its decisions. They can do so in a transparent and fair manner to reach consensus on challenging decisions such as those related to resource scarcity and allocation, as well as balancing client needs with other institutional issues (Lahey et al., 2021). These programs can also provide support to leaders within the system as they make these decisions and policies.

Ethics at the Organizational Level

Ethics in organizations are often complicated by business pressures. In a study of ethical problems faced by practitioners during their first 5 years of practice, investigators identified issues, including productivity, billing, compromised care as a result of cost containment or socioeconomic status, and moral distress in therapeutic relationships (Howard et al., 2022). Ethical tensions have often resulted from pressures to do more with less. Organizations have been expected to improve quality and expand access while reducing costs (Balak et al., 2019). However, these pressures do not excuse organizations from their primary purpose of caring for people. When an occupational therapy practitioner works for an organization, they cannot hide behind the policies or administration of the institution; one's professional code and values must continue to guide practice.

Ethics for the Occupational Therapy Practitioner Within an Organization

For occupational therapy practitioners, multiple and sometimes conflicting allegiances to clients, colleagues, team members, and employers, as well as systemic barriers to care, can result in ethical tensions that are challenging to resolve (Durocher & Kinsella, 2021). The practitioner may be in the challenging position of balancing respect for client rights with supporting their organization's policies and procedures and financial viability. Practitioners are not immune to market-based pressures in health care. Most clinicians are familiar with the pressure to do more with less, whether manifested in lack of human or financial resources or in increased productivity standards (Balak et al., 2019). Constraints on time and money will continue to exist; therefore, practitioners must understand how to handle these problems ethically while addressing the needs of the clients and the communities they serve (Durocher & Kinsella, 2021). Practitioners may work in an organization, but they also belong to a profession with core values based on the concepts of altruism, equality, freedom, justice, dignity, truth, and prudence.

Occupational therapy practitioners, like most health care practitioners, may experience ethical tensions related to client autonomy, global inequities, and multiple but conflicting allegiances. Ethical conflicts could include client autonomy vs. safety concerns, client vs.

practitioner values, intercollegial differences, practitioner values vs. employer directives, and regulatory mandates (Durocher & Kinsella, 2021). The organization in which a practitioner works often acts as a domain that influences their behavior. As an employee, the practitioner subsumes a level of accountability to that organization's culture, standards, and financial viability. Although the focus of accountability is often limited to the dynamic of the practitioner–client relationship, service delivery is influenced by relationships external to this dyad. The practitioner may be placed in situations in which it is difficult to protect and maintain the client–practitioner relationship. In some circumstances, practitioners are pressured to provide services that conflict with their personal or professional code of ethics to support decisions made by individual physicians, other team members, or within the organization (Durocher & Kinsella, 2021).

The conflict that arises from the occupational therapy practitioner's conflicting allegiances often leads to lack of trust between clients and practitioners. Due to the nature of the power differential between practitioner and client, trust is a necessary component of the therapeutic relationship (Goold, 2001). In the client–practitioner relationship, the practitioner has more power, and how one uses that power can quickly enhance or degrade the trust of a client who is vulnerable. Practitioners have an ethical duty to advocate for the client's needs and well-being, fulfilling the ethical principle of *beneficence*, and to protect them from harm, fulfilling the principle of nonmaleficence (Beauchamp & Childress, 2019). This duty also reinforces the ethical concept of client–practitioner collaboration and shared decision making (Phelan, 2020).

Systemic and Global Issues

Larger systemic or global issues can include limited or unequal access to occupational therapy services for individuals and groups due to their sociopolitical or socioeconomic status. Difficulty in accessing related financial and/or social services may also affect appropriate and necessary health care intervention. Occupational therapy practitioners often feel a duty to address the inequities generated by global issues as well as those due to failures of the health systems where they work, sometimes going beyond their usual roles. Within the organization, practitioners may magnify issues in clinical reports to maximize funding, advocate for clients beyond their role expectations by contacting other professionals to assist with access to financial and social services, provide free advice when a client cannot access care, and appeal to higher-level administrators who are in decision-making roles. These strategies may decrease the practitioner's feeling of being powerless. Conflicting values among one's personal and professional life, as well as differences in values from other team members, can be additional sources of ethical angst (McArdle et al., 2023). The goal of organizations to meet individual as well as comprehensive societal needs may, at times, seem to conflict with the practitioner's responsibility to the client. When this conflict occurs, the practitioner is often presented with a dilemma regarding whether to support the organization's goals or the client's rights. A practitioner encounters an ethical dilemma when a morally correct course of action requires them to support both the organization and the client, but they cannot do both because the supporting actions are mutually exclusive (Doherty & Purtilo, 2016).

Managing Organizational Ethics and Moral Distress

Ethical tensions contribute to moral distress and ethical dilemmas, and they have significant personal, professional, and practice implications (Durocher & Kinsella, 2021). Closer alignment between institutional values and organizational decisions (e.g., through integrating organizational ethics programs into leadership decision-making processes) can decrease moral distress and increase staff and client satisfaction (Lahey et al., 2020). Depending on the institution, organizational ethics programs can develop out of existing clinical ethics programs; with ethics consultants or the ethics committee integrated with senior leadership to offer expertise on an as-needed or standing basis (Lahey et al., 2021). An organizational ethics program can bridge the gap between leadership and frontline staff by making the decision-making process explicit and promoting shared understanding (Lahey et al., 2020). In addition, clinical ethicists can bring to light flawed structures and processes within the organization and ensure that all relevant perspectives are heard.

Resource allocation and scarcity can also contribute to moral distress experienced by leaders and managers. Moral distress occurs when there are no constructive solutions or support in a morally challenging situation. Therefore, it is important for the organization to address moral distress by supporting staff at multiple levels (Hertelendy et al., 2022). "Tensions can be especially intense for clinical leaders who are responsible for both patients and staff" (Hertelendy et al., 2022, p. 392). The most effective approach is transparency and alignment of personal, professional, and organizational values, as well as honest communication (Hertelendy et al., 2022). Addressing the impact of stressful events on staff should include opportunities to debrief and express their feelings. It is important for employees to see these situations as organizational or workplace concerns rather than as personal failures (Hertelendy et al., 2022). Additional strategies can include employing shared decision making, creating interdisciplinary ethics teams, providing psychological support, and reinforcing moral leadership, with a goal of creating an ethical organizational culture. A preventive approach to looking at precursors to moral distress rather than consequences is most likely to be effective (Hertelendy et al., 2022). However, research shows that focusing on changing the organizational culture through a team-based approach to communication, debriefing, and ethics discussions reinforces that moral distress is an organizational concern rather than an individual's isolated burden (Hertelendy et al., 2022).

An ethical work climate where organization, leadership, and individual values are aligned can be key in creating a morally resilient workplace and supporting job satisfaction (Hertelendy et al., 2022). A strong indicator of the need to change an organization's culture is a disconnect between the mission and values of its culture and the daily decisions and behaviors of its staff (Nelson et al., 2020). This gap affects staff morale, quality of care provided, and the organization's reputation in the community; it also supports the need for change (Nelson et al., 2020). Characteristics of an organizational ethics culture in need of improvement include minimal or absent leadership support for ethical behavior, little supervisory reinforcement of ethical conduct, and limited staff commitment to support colleagues who behave ethically (Nelson et al., 2020).

Occupational therapy managers can be effective role models, setting policies and procedures that reflect professional standards within their departments and facilitating ongoing ethical learning with diverse resources (Slater, 2019). Because quality is the common denominator between practitioners and the organization (Nelson et al., 2020), and is an emerging focus of the payment system (Centers for Medicare & Medicaid Services, n.d.), occupational therapy practitioners have an opportunity to promote their value in meeting those benchmarks. Practitioners who are frustrated with unrealistic productivity standards or other potentially unethical directives, can have a conversation with supervisors or higher-level leaders that focuses on recognizing the value of quality—not just to the client, but also to the practitioner and organization. Data routinely collected in occupational therapy evaluations and subsequent interventions can measure client improvement in key quality and safety areas such as falls prevention, functional cognition, and discharge to the community. These areas must be tracked and submitted by the organization as quality benchmarks that determine reimbursement (Nelson et al., 2020). Practitioners can provide objective data, such as daily time studies, to address the negative impact of unrealistic productivity requirements on the ability and quality of client interventions to reach these mandated targets, while supporting the value of their practice within the organization. However, a practitioner facing an ethically challenging work environment may eventually have to make hard decisions about whether to stay, to actively seek change, or to leave. Personal and other considerations may influence this decision. If the practitioner can gain support from colleagues and approach leadership with objective strategies and rationale to change the root causes of ethical distress, the outcome may benefit all parties concerned (Durocher & Kinsella, 2021).

Relation to the AOTA Code of Ethics

Ethical principles related to organizational ethics include *beneficence, autonomy*, and *nonmaleficence*. See Exhibit 18.1 for applicable standards from the AOTA Code of Ethics.

Reference to Other AOTA Documents

An occupational therapy practitioner is obligated to follow the American Occupational Therapy Association's (AOTA's) Standards of Practice for Occupational Therapy, including those established for professional responsibilities, service delivery, and throughout the occupational therapy process. Likewise, AOTA's Standards for Continuing Competence outline obligations of the practitioner to stay up to date on knowledge, professional reasoning, interpersonal skills, performance skills, and ethical practice.

EXHIBIT 18.1.
ETHICAL STANDARDS RELATED TO ORGANIZATIONS

- Abide by policies, procedures, and protocols when serving or acting on behalf of a professional organization or employer to fully and accurately represent the organization's official and authorized positions.
- Inform employers, employees, colleagues, students and researchers of applicable policies, laws, and official documents.
- Respect the practices, competencies, roles, and responsibilities of one's own and other professions to promote a collaborative environment reflective of interprofessional teams.
- Respect and honor the expressed wishes of recipients of service.
- Establish a collaborative relationship with recipients of service and relevant stakeholders to promote shared decision making.
- Proactively address workplace conflict that affects or can potentially affect professional relationships and the provision of services.
- Ensure that documentation for reimbursement purposes is done in accordance with applicable laws, guidelines, and regulations.
- Do not follow arbitrary directives that compromise the rights or well-being of others, including unrealistic productivity expectations, fabrication, falsification, plagiarism of documentation, or inaccurate coding.
- Respect the client's right to refuse occupational therapy services temporarily or permanently, even when that refusal has potential to result in poor outcomes.
- Report systems and policies that are discriminatory or unfairly limit or prevent access to occupational therapy.

Note. From the Standards of Conduct from the AOTA Code of Ethics.

Reference to Other Standards

Employees should refer to their organization's policies and procedures, and to their licensing board regarding any regulations pertaining to organizational ethics. Employees should also be aware of requirements of payers, certification agencies, and accrediting bodies as appropriate for their setting.

Tips

- Reflect on and uphold personal and professional values.
- Consider whether personal and professional values agree with each other or are in conflict, and determine which values will take precedence.
- Be confident in occupational therapy's contributions to and role in the organization.
- Work collaboratively with colleagues and support each other to address and resolve ethical issues interrelated with larger social issues.

- Advocate strongly for policy changes by documenting risk to clients under current policies.
- Facilitate transparent and open conversations with clients and colleagues that acknowledge systemic barriers.

CASE EXAMPLE 18.1. ORGANIZATIONAL LOYALTY VS. CLIENT AUTONOMY

An **occupational therapist** has received a referral to see a client on the cardiac floor of a community hospital. When the therapist enters the room to complete the evaluation, the client refuses occupational therapy services. The therapist continues to attempt to see the client over the course of the next week. On all occasions, the client refuses to participate in occupational therapy. During each visit the therapist explains to the client and their family the importance of occupational therapy services, why the physician has referred the client for treatment, and the risks of minimal activity after cardiac surgery. In addition, the therapist speaks with nursing staff to determine whether the client has been seen by a psychiatrist to rule out depression or any other emotional state that may be affecting their participation. The nurse refers the therapist to a report compiled by the psychiatrist, which indicates that the client is slightly depressed but has full decision-making capacity and is therefore able to make decisions related to their health care. The therapist decides to call the physician to report that they will be discharging the client from services because of the client's informed refusal of treatment. During this discussion, the physician states that the client will need to continue treatment and the therapist should "not allow the client to refuse services," and then abruptly hangs up the phone. When the therapist arrives to work the next day, there is another written physician referral on the scheduling desk for the client that states, "Evaluate and treat for occupational therapy services; do not allow the client to refuse." The referral is accompanied by a note from the Rehabilitation Director, stating that the therapist must see this patient today.

Questions
1. What ethical issues are in conflict for this occupational therapist?
2. What may be some of the organizational consequences for failing to follow this physician's order? Conversely, what are some of the ethical consequences for following the order?
3. Apply an ethical decision-making framework to this scenario. What options does the occupational therapist have?
4. Choose an option and reflect on the potential outcome. What positive and negative outcomes might occur as a result of the selected option?

Summary

Occupational therapy practitioners have an ethical responsibility to maintain the integrity of the client–practitioner relationship in the face of organizational pressures. Whether they maintain this relationship by respecting clients' autonomy or advocating for their rights and needs regarding care, practitioners must be aware of their responsibilities to the well-being of the client. In addition, the practitioner has a responsibility to advocate for and support an ethical environment within the organization, to the extent they can do so, thus minimizing or even avoiding conflicts between professional codes of ethics and the workplace, while benefiting positive client outcomes.

Acknowledgment

Lea Cheyney Brandt, OTD, MA, OTR/L, wrote an earlier edition of this Advisory Opinion.

REFERENCES

Balak, N., Broekman, M. L. D., & Mathiesen, T. (2019). Ethics in contemporary health care management and medical education. *Journal of Evaluation in Clinical Practice, 26*, 699–706. https://doi.org/10.1111/jep.13352

Beauchamp, T. L., & Childress, J. F. (2019). *Principles of biomedical ethics* (8th ed.). Oxford University Press.

Borges Paraizo, C., & Bégin, L. (2020). Organizational ethics in health settings. *Revista Ciência & Saúde Coletiva Jour, 25*(1), 251–259. https://doi.org/10.1590/1413-81232020251.28342019

Centers for Medicare & Medicaid Services. (n.d.). *Quality payment program overview.* https://qpp.cms.gov/about/qpp-overview

Doherty, R. F., & Purtilo, R. B. (2016). *Ethical dimensions in the health professions* (6th ed.). Elsevier/Saunders.

Durocher, E., & Kinsella, E. A. (2021). Ethical tensions in occupational therapy practice: Conflicts and competing allegiances. *Canadian Journal of Occupational Therapy, 88*, 244–253. https://doi.org/10.1177/00084174211021707

Goold, S. (2001). Trust and the ethics of health care institutions. *Hastings Center Report, 31*(6), 26–33. https://doi.org/10.2307/3527779

Hertelendy, A., Gutberg, J., Mitchell, C., Gustavsson, M., Rapp, D., Mayo, M., & vonSchreeb, J. (2022). Mitigating moral distress in leaders of healthcare organizations: A scoping review. *Journal of Healthcare Management, 67*, 380–402. https://doi.org/10.1097/jhm-d-21-00263

Howard, B., Govern, M., Haney, M., Ottinger, H., Earls, A., Retter, A., & Rippe, T. (2022). Encounters with ethical problems during the first 5 years of practice in OT. *American Journal of Occupational Therapy, 76*(Suppl. 1), 7610510158. https://doi.org/10.5014/ajot.2022.76S1-PO158

Lahey, T., DeRenzo, E., Crites, J., Fanning, J., Huberman, B. J., & Slosar, J. P. (2020). Building an organizational ethics program on a clinical ethics foundation. *Journal of Clinical Ethics, 31*, 259–267. https://doi.org/10.1086/JCE2020313259

Lahey, T., Reeves, S., Desjardins, I., & Nelson, W. (2021). Organizational ethics support for health care leaders during the COVID-19 pandemic and beyond. *Journal of Hospital Ethics, 7*(2), 58–64. https://myhcds.dartmouth.edu/s/1353/images/gid8/editor_documents/events/virtual_events/2021/lahey_et_al_oe_and_covid.pdf

McArdle, H., Barlott, T., McBryde, C., Shevellar, L., & Branjerdporn, N. (2023). Navigating ethical tensions when working to address social inequities. *American Journal of Occupational Therapy, 77*, 7701205160. https://doi.org/10.5014/ajot.2023.050071

McDuffie, K., Patneaude, A., Bell, S., Adiele, A., Makhija, N., Wilfond, B., & Opel, D. (2022). Addressing racism in the healthcare encounter: The role of clinical ethics consultants. *Bioethics, 36*(3), 313–317. https://doi.org/10.1111/bioe.13008

Nelson, W. A., Taylor, E., & Walsh, T. (2020). Building an ethical organizational culture. *The Health Care Manager, 39*(4), 168–174.

Phelan, P. S. (2020). From the editor: Organizational ethics for U.S. health care today. *AMA Journal of Ethics, 22*(3), E183–E186. https://doi.org/10.1001/amajethics.2020.183

Slater, D. Y. (2019). Organizational ethics. In K. Jacobs & G. L. McCormack (Eds.), *The occupational therapy manager* (6th ed., pp. 539–545). AOTA Press.

Tammany, J. E., O'Connell, J. K., Allen, B., & Brismée, J.-M. (2019). Are productivity goals in rehabilitation practice associated with unethical behaviors? *Archives of Rehabilitation Research and Clinical Translation, 1*(1–2), 100002, 1–9. https://doi.org/10.1016/j.arrct.2019.100002

Section 4. Service Delivery

Ethical Considerations for Emerging Technology-Based Interventions

ASEEL DALTON, PhD, LLM, RPh, and BARBARA ELLEMAN, OTD, MHS, OTR/L

Key Points

- Emerging technologies provide new opportunities for client-centered interventions but come with the risks associated with lack of evidence, the need for competence, the potential for added expense, and possible threats to privacy.
- Educational and training opportunities for emerging technology-based interventions ensure the sustainability of an ethical client-centered practice.
- When considering emerging technology interventions, the occupational therapy practitioner should weigh possible outcomes against cost and available evidence.

Introduction

The development of emerging technology-based interventions has caused occupational therapy practitioners to adapt and accommodate the use of these new interventions. Such intervention techniques have warranted serious consideration of the potential for ethical concerns. Health technology can include medical devices, adaptive equipment, assessments, and other services (Masselink, 2018). Technology utilized by occupational therapy practitioners varies widely and can include simple, low-tech measures such as an adaptive tool for handwriting or dressing, or more complex, high-tech options such as biometric access to open a door, virtual environments to practice new skills, or exoskeletons and artificial intelligence (AI) to assist with participation in daily tasks (Liu, 2018; O'Brien & Conners, 2022). Despite the variation in complexity, practitioners often incorporate technology interventions as a means to improve a client's participation in meaningful, goal-oriented occupations (Crabtree & Katz, 2017).

In her 2012 Presidential Address at the American Occupational Therapy Association's (AOTA's) Annual Conference & Expo, then-President Florence Clark shared, "The information revolution is changing the world" (p. 646), and occupational therapy must adjust, not only to survive and thrive but also to evolve practice (Clark, 2012). The rapid emergence of new technologies brings both challenges and opportunities. Occupational therapy practitioners must adjust and evolve quickly to address the impact of emerging technologies on practice (Hills et al., 2016; Liu, 2018). The challenge to remain knowledgeable and proficient amid the ever-evolving technology landscape is accompanied by the opportunity to create new roles and advocate for innovative solutions that address client needs and improve occupational performance (Liu, 2018). However, the decisions that involve selecting the most appropriate, safe, and effective technology interventions should be made with consideration of the best available research evidence, judicious clinical reasoning, sound judgment, clinician experience, and in collaboration with the client to address individual goals.

Occupational therapy practitioners have long embraced the concept of *evidence-based practice*. Practitioners should incorporate clinical expertise combined with the best available research evidence to inform intervention decisions in collaboration with the client. Careful consideration should also be given to the ethical impact of clinical decisions. Professional codes of ethics may be used to assist practitioners in making ethical decisions about less traditional aspects of clinical practice such as new or emerging technology-based interventions. When considering emerging technology, practitioners must consider not only what is medically justified, but also what contributes to "inclusion, participation, safety, and well-being for all recipients in various stages of life, health, and illness" (AOTA, 2021b, p. 1). The unique perspective of the occupational therapy profession must be considered as part of the discussion when developing health policies that govern the use of, and equitable access to, health technologies to meet the population and individual needs (Braveman, 2015; Stover, 2016; World Health Organization [WHO], 2022).

Emerging Technology-Based Interventions

Technology is an integral part of everyday occupations and therefore inherent to the practice of occupational therapy (Smith, 2017). Technology interventions are defined in the *Occupational Therapy Practice Framework: Domain and Process*, align with the Occupational Therapy Scope of Practice, and are identified in the AOTA Code of Ethics (the Code). The integration of technology interventions has enabled the inclusion and participation of clients while maintaining and improving their independence and well-being (Marston et al., 2015; WHO, 2022). The type of technology interventions available to clients varies widely and may include assistive devices utilized to improve participation in daily tasks, such as one-handed can openers or magnetic zippers; environmental or assistive technologies to support access such as smart home devices, electric wheelchairs, or exoskeletons; therapeutic tools or devices to support skill acquisition and practice, such as virtual reality games, robotics, or training gloves; or technologies to support success in occupational performance, such mindfulness applications of artificial intelligence (Smith, 2017). Constant change and frequent updates are inherent to the use of technology-based tools. Some of the more rapidly emerging technology interventions involve AI, automation technology, virtual reality, 3D printing, and robotics. As these and other developing technologies become more advanced and intertwined, thoughtful consideration must be given to the ethical challenges that accompany each.

ARTIFICIAL INTELLIGENCE

Artificial intelligence (AI) is one area of technology experiencing constant change and rapid growth. AI involves a computer program's ability to perform reasoning, learning, sensory interaction, and adaptation tasks that are most frequently attributed to human intelligence (Rigby, 2019). AI advancements in the areas of machine learning, natural language processing, and robotics have exploded and present unlimited potential for use in health-related fields such as occupational therapy (Rigby, 2019). Artificial intelligence can already be found embedded in technologies and computer applications to support client engagement and compliance, and to create plans of care and individualized interventions (Davenport & Kalakota, 2019). As the use of AI continues to advance and the applications within occupational therapy continue to emerge, consideration should be given to transparency, autonomy, and collaboration related to how health care decisions are made; accountability for recommendations and ongoing use; risk versus benefit for clients and practitioner; and client education and training.

SMART HOME TECHNOLOGIES AND AUTOMATION

Smart home technologies allow the automation of processes and tasks such as management of lighting, groceries, or appliances (to name a few) connected in a way that can increase independence. In addition to ease, these technologies offer options for older adults and individuals living with disabilities to live independently or with remote support (Liu, 2018; Sime et al., 2021). This independence, however, may involve remote monitoring by caregivers or storage of personal information such as medical or financial information, which could impact privacy (Sime et al., 2021). In line with the use of smart home technologies is automation of everyday tasks, such as driving. Automated and semi-automated cars offer potential for independence and freedom for individuals who are unable to operate a standard vehicle. As technology in this area advances, consideration will need to be given to educating and training both the client and the occupational therapy practitioner, the safety of the client and others, and accountability for outcomes.

VIRTUAL REALITY

Virtual reality provides a simulated environment where individuals use specialized equipment to interact with 3D images in a "realistic" manner. Virtual reality offers the opportunity to increase client engagement, follow through, and acquisition of new skills. Virtual reality is widely used in occupational therapy; however, the opportunities for new developments and sophistication exist as virtual reality becomes immersed with other new technologies (Liu, 2018). Privacy, weighing the risks and benefits to clients, the cost, ongoing training and equipment, and judicious evaluation of client acceptance and adoption are important considerations.

3D PRINTING

3D printing allows occupational therapy practitioners and family members to create customized health supplies, supports, and aids that are cost-effective (Liu, 2018). Many of these health care items are now commercially available, or designs can easily be located in 3D printing repositories for free or for a nominal fee. When considering specialized supports, positioning aids, or mobility devices, judicious consideration should be given to the training and competence of the individual making the clinical decisions and creating the device; safety and risk versus benefit to the client; education to the client; and ongoing monitoring, maintenance, and replacement of the device.

ROBOTICS

Robotic technologies aid in completing complex movements or tasks with the assistance of, or independently for clients. Robotics have been recommended for use in rehabilitation through robotic gloves or exoskeletons or supports to provide assisted movement (Kim et al., 2017; Liu, 2018). Robotic interventions are often paired with other technologies such as virtual reality or AI. The nature of the robotic devices and level of technology involved often come with a high price tag. Practitioners should consider the effectiveness of robotic devices, their own knowledge and competence, the cost of and access to the device, including repair and maintenance, and the client's knowledge when making clinical decisions.

Considerations for Emerging Technology

Despite the potential benefits of technology, barriers to adoption can preclude its consistent use. Both clients and occupational therapy practitioners vary in their level of comfort and familiarity with technology-based interventions (Smith, 2017). Even familiar users often report a lack of knowledge and training as major barriers to continued use, whereas non-users report barriers related to the expense of the products or technology (Hwang et al., 2022). The potential benefits to clients must be carefully weighed against the lack of research. Educational and extensive training opportunities are required to promote the use of technology-based interventions by occupational therapy practitioners, while highlighting their usefulness to achieve client-centered, customized approaches.

Emerging technology-based interventions offer the potential to improve care quality and cost savings across health and social care (Maguire et al., 2018). However, considerations related to equitable access to the use of technology is warranted. Given the scarcity of conclusive evidence to validate the effectiveness and safety of some emerging technologies, occupational therapy practitioners must evaluate new technologies and address the challenges related to their use while also considering ethical standards as part of developing a client-centered treatment plan.

Relation to the AOTA Code of Ethics

The Code requires that personnel adhere to standards of conduct. The Preamble to the Code specifically refers to "emerging technologies that can present potential ethical concerns in practice, research, education, and policy." Reference to applicable standards of conduct can assist practitioners in evaluating and making decisions about whether to incorporate emerging technologies into their practice. Exhibit 19.1 contains ethical standards from the Code related to emerging technology-based interventions.

In order to ensure the sustainability of an ethical client-centered practice, occupational therapy practitioners need to carefully examine their own motivations, driving forces, and rationale (e.g., financial gain and innovative interventions versus client benefit) if they choose to use emerging technology-based interventions that seem to have little evidence for treatment efficacy.

EXHIBIT 19.1.

ETHICAL STANDARDS RELATED TO EMERGING TECHNOLOGY-BASED INTERVENTIONS

- Comply with current federal and state laws, state scope of practice guidelines, and AOTA policies and official documents that apply to the profession of occupational therapy.
- Respect and honor the expressed wishes of recipients of service.
- Establish a collaborative relationship with recipients of service and relevant stakeholders to promote shared decision making.
- Do not engage in actions or inactions that jeopardize the safety or well-being of others or team effectiveness.
- Provide appropriate evaluation and a plan of intervention for recipients of occupational therapy services specific to their needs.
- Use, to the extent possible, evaluation, planning, intervention techniques, assessments, and therapeutic equipment that are evidence based, current, and within the recognized scope of occupational therapy practice.
- Fully disclose the benefits, risks, and potential outcomes of any intervention; the occupational therapy personnel who will be providing the intervention; and any reasonable alternatives to the proposed intervention.
- Provide occupational therapy services, including education and training, that are within each practitioner's level of competence and scope of practice.
- Provide information and resources to address barriers to access for persons in need of occupational therapy services.
- Take steps (e.g., professional development, research, supervision, training) to ensure proficiency, use careful judgment, and weigh potential for harm when generally recognized standards do not exist in emerging technology or areas of practice.
- Engage in collaborative actions and communication as a member of interprofessional teams to facilitate quality care and safety for clients.

Note. From the Standards of Conduct from the AOTA Code of Ethics.

Occupational therapy practitioners have an ethical obligation to be fully transparent in disclosing their ability to provide certain interventions and to avoid practice in areas of limited competence (i.e., professional limitations). They also have an ethical obligation to ensure that equipment is safe and effective for use with clients. Practitioners must not inflict or cause harm to a client by using an intervention that does not have a reasonable expectation of benefit or that they are not competent to administer. In addition, practitioners must consider that, by virtue of their trust in the therapeutic relationship, consumers may be biased to accept recommendations about innovative technology to address their condition. Therefore, practitioners must think carefully when introducing new technologies in order to weigh the potential for harm versus the benefit to the client. Relevant ethical questions include the following:

- Does the client (and/or caregiver) fully understand the risks and benefits, effectiveness, and safety factors associated with a new, nontraditional intervention when evidence is not available or is limited? Some risks may be unknown.
- Has existing, relevant research been shared with the client (and/or caregiver) regarding the proposed utilization of an emerging technology-based treatment?
- What considerations should direct the ethical decision-making process when evidence is limited, or the research does not demonstrate effectiveness?

Ethical reasoning and transparency can assist in communication and autonomous decision making with the client when there is minimal or no evidence for a treatment. Occupational therapy practitioners have an ethical obligation to provide interventions that they can reasonably expect to benefit clients; improve their quality of life; and have a safe, effective outcome. Practitioners should take action to prevent any foreseeable harm that could be caused by using an intervention for which safety or the potential for harm has not been determined. Moreover, any potential undue influence that pertains to financial incentives associated with providing these new technology-based interventions must be avoided.

Clients have the right to privacy and the right to make their own decisions on the basis of individual values, interests, and preferences, even if these decisions are not in alignment with occupational therapy practitioner recommendations. It is important to distinguish between the concepts of *informed consent* and *consent to treat*. Informed consent is a client's right to full disclosure of what is to be expected in terms of objectives or goals, plan of care, and the known or unknown risks or benefits associated with therapy services in order to make decisions on the basis of that information. Consent to treat refers to a client's autonomous decision to receive services by volitionally engaging in treatment. It is a professional and ethical mandate to obtain consent to treat from a client before initiating the evaluation and any subsequent services. Because technology-based interventions may be at an experimental stage, clients may not want to try them. Conversely, a client may want to try an intervention that the practitioner is not yet convinced is safe or appropriate. Emerging technology-based interventions should be monitored until best practice, evidence-based, valid, and reliable outcome measures demonstrate definitive positive or negative results.

Ethical decision making related to emerging technology warrants consideration of transparency and vulnerability. To ensure transparency, occupational therapy practitioners should provide full disclosure of the risks and benefits of emerging technology-based interventions, including lack of research, if applicable; or the rationale for why they are proposing to use a particular device or modality.

The concept of *vulnerability* applies to clients with disabilities or their caregivers. Vulnerability involves issues of trust and the therapeutic relationship between practitioner and client. Clients in need of and receiving services are at a very vulnerable point in their lives and must trust in the honesty of a practitioner–client relationship to protect their well-being. Parents or other family members of individuals with a disability may be vulnerable because they are willing to seek and try any available intervention that they believe may help their loved one improve occupational performance skills. In some circumstances, all customary therapeutic options have been exhausted, and when a new technology intervention becomes available, even if it is untried, family members may be in danger of being exploited as they seek positive outcomes. Consequently, they may find themselves susceptible to costly interventions or technology equipment as they seek to leave no stone unturned to benefit their loved one, regardless of financial stress.

Reference to Other AOTA Documents

AOTA's Occupational Therapy Scope of Practice official document is an excellent resource guide for reference when an emerging or nontraditional intervention is introduced to clinical practice. This document can provide practice domain guidance. However, AOTA official documents do not replace the legal language in state practice acts.

Reference to Other Standards

- Official documents do not replace the legal language in state practice acts.
- Occupational therapy practitioners have a professional and ethical obligation to be familiar with and comply with state licensure laws (or applicable state regulations) that govern appropriate practice conducted by a practitioner. Licensure laws legally define the profession's scope of practice or domain, and each state has jurisdiction, authority, and power to enforce the legally defined scope of occupational therapy practice in that state. However, language in state practice acts tends to be quite general, so practitioners may need to seek interpretation from the licensure board to assist in decisions about whether particular emerging technology interventions are within their scope of practice. The links to each state regulatory board are available through the Licensure section of AOTA's website (AOTA, 2023).
- The National Board for Certification in Occupational Therapy (NBCOT®) provides practice standards and a code of conduct to which all certified occupational therapy practitioners must adhere (NBCOT, 2023).

CASE EXAMPLE 19.1. PARENT OF PEDIATRIC CLIENT AND 3D PRINTING

An **occupational therapist** who works with pediatric clients is approached by the parent of a client who has a diagnosis of cerebral palsy. The parent shares a video of a child with a similar diagnosis using a 3D printed mobility aid for assisted upper-extremity movement and tells the therapist they plan to print the device and would like the therapist to train the child in use of the mobility aid.

Questions
1. What are the ethical issues at stake in this scenario?
2. What additional information does the occupational therapy practitioner need to gather?
3. What actions could the practitioner take?

CASE EXAMPLE 19.2. PRODUCT PROMOTION

An **occupational therapy practitioner** in practice is approached by a product developer of a robotic glove to promote its use with clients who are in rehabilitation following a stroke. The developer offers to supply the practice with robotic gloves at no cost, providing the practitioners use the gloves with every patient recovering from stroke as a standard intervention.

Questions
1. What are the ethical issues at stake in this scenario?
2. What additional information does the occupational therapy practitioner need to gather?
3. What actions could the practitioner take?

Next Steps

Ensuring competence is a professional responsibility, as is familiarity with applicable current research, to provide state-of-the-art intervention to the extent possible. However, if no evidence exists in the literature, additional professional resources should be sought and used (e.g., ethical reasoning, critical thinking skills, professional resources). Professionals can maintain current competency through additional specialty training; certification, if available; or continuing education to deliver services competently and adequately. However, in some cases, emerging technology-based interventions have not demonstrated sufficient or conclusive evidence of effectiveness, and organized training may not be available. What should the decision-making process be when training is limited or altogether absent? The following questions may facilitate the ethical and scope-of-practice reasoning process when limited evidence and guidelines are available for emerging technology interventions:

• Was this body of knowledge contained in the practitioner's core occupational therapy educational curriculum?

- Does the practitioner have adequate education and competence to provide this intervention on the basis of past education or current related continuing education?
- Has the practitioner sought professional feedback from other practitioners who may have used new and non traditional interventions, and if so, what has their experience and feedback been as reported from patients who opted to use new technology-based interventions?

Summary

New and emerging technologies or interventions can have positive applications for occupational therapy clients but can also pose ethical challenges to occupational therapy practitioners seeking to integrate them into their practice. Practitioners must understand the level of education and training required to use these technologies and interventions competently from a legal and ethical perspective. Practitioners have an ethical obligation and professional responsibility to seek evidence and research related to the latest technologies in clinical practice, and to remain up to date in terms of their continued education and/or training in order to help them make appropriate clinical decisions in collaboration with clients.

The rapid onset of new technology offers new and promising ways for occupational therapy clients to participate in everyday occupations. While occupational therapy practitioners have an obligation to promote benefit for the good of their clients by encouraging and promoting the therapeutic use of technology in their practice, they must do so with judicious clinical reasoning and sound judgment after carefully considering the available evidence and in alignment with client goals.

Acknowledgment

Paige M. Johns, OTD, OTR/L, authored an earlier version of this Advisory Opinion.

REFERENCES

American Occupational Therapy Association. (2023). *Licensure.* https://www.aota.org/career/state-licensure

Braveman, B. (2015). Population health and occupational therapy. *American Journal of Occupational Therapy, 70,* 700109001. https://doi.org/10.5014/ajot.2016.701002

Clark, F. (2012). Beyond high definition: Attitude and evidence bringing OT in HD-3D. *American Journal of Occupational Therapy, 66,* 644–651. https://doi.org/10.5014/ajot.2012.666002

Crabtree, J. L., & Katz, L. W. (2017). Emerging areas of practice. In K. Jacobs & N. MacRae (Eds.), *Occupational therapy essentials for clinical competence* (3rd ed., pp. 715–731). Slack.

Davenport, T., & Kalakota, R. (2019). The potential for artificial intelligence in healthcare. *Future Healthcare Journal, 6*(2), 94–98. https://doi.org/10.7861/futurehosp.6-2-94

Hills, C., Ryan, S., Smith, D. R., Warren-Forward, H., Levett-Jones, T., & Lapkin, S. (2016). Occupational therapy students' technological skills: Are 'generation Y' ready for 21st century practice? *Australian Occupational Therapy Journal, 63*, 391–398. https://doi.org/10.1111/1440-1630.12308

Hwang, N. K., Shim, S. H., & Cheon, H. W. (2022). Use of information and communication technology by South Korean occupational therapists working in hospitals: A cross-sectional study. *International Journal of Environmental Research and Public Health, 19*, 6022. https://doi.org/10.3390/ijerph19106022

Kim, G., Lim, S., Kim, H., Lee, B., Seo, S., Cho, K., & Lee, W. (2017). Is robot-assisted therapy effective in upper extremity recovery in early stage stroke? A systematic literature review. *Journal of Physical Therapy Science, 29*, 1108–1112. http://doi.org/10.1589/jpts.29.1108

Liu, L. (2018). Occupational therapy in the fourth industrial revolution. *Canadian Journal of Occupational Therapy, 85*, 272–283. https://doi.org/10.1177/0008417418815179

Maguire, D., Evans, H., Honeyman, M., & Omojomolo, D. (2018, June). *Digital change in health and social care*. The King's Fund. https://www.kingsfund.org.uk/sites/default/files/2018-06/Digital_change_health_care_Kings_Fund_June_2018.pdf

Marston, H. R., Woodbury, A., Gschwind, Y. J., Kroll, M., Fink, D., Eichberg, S., . . . Delbaere, K. (2015). The design of a purpose-built exergame for fall prediction and prevention for older people. *European Review of Aging and Physical Activity, 12*, 13. https://doi.org/10.1186/s11556-015-0157-4

Masselink, C. E. (2018). Considering technology in the occupational therapy practice framework. *Open Journal of Occupational Therapy, 6*(3). https://doi.org/10.15453/2168-6408.1497

National Board for Certification in Occupational Therapy. (2023). *Professional conduct*. https://www.nbcot.org/professional-conduct

O'Brien, J., & Conners, B. (2022). *Introduction to occupational therapy* (6th ed.). Elsevier.

Rigby, M. J. (2019). Ethical dimensions of using artificial intelligence in healthcare. *American Medical Association Journal of Ethics, 21*(2), 121–124. https://doi.org/10.1001/amajethics.2019.121

Sime, M. M., Bissoli, A. L., Lavino-Júnior, D., & Bastos-Filho, T. F. (2021). Usability, occupational performance and satisfaction evaluation of a smart environment controlled by infrared oculography by people with severe motor disabilities. *PLoS ONE, 16*(8), e0256062. https://doi.org/10.1371/journal.pone.0256062

Smith, R. O. (2017). Technology and occupation: Past, present, and the next 100 years of theory and practice. *American Journal of Occupational Therapy, 71*, 7106150010. https://doi.org/10.5014/ajot.2017.716003

Stover, A. D. (2016). Client-centered advocacy: Every occupational therapy practitioner's responsibility to understand medical necessity. *American Journal of Occupational Therapy, 70*, 7005090010. https://doi.org/10.5014/ajot.2016.705003

World Health Organization. (2022). *Global report on assistive technology: Summary*. https://www.who.int/publications/i/item/9789240049178

Ethical Considerations in Telehealth

ASEEL DALTON, PhD, LLM, RPh, and MARITA HENSLEY, COTA/L

Key Points

- Telehealth improves access and delivery of health care services, promotes client self-management, enhances efficiency of care, and reduces hospital readmissions for a wide range of conditions.
- Ethical issues may arise in telehealth, including consent to treat, privacy and confidentiality, and adhering to professional standards.
- Telehealth should not be used solely for the convenience of the occupational therapy practitioner.

Introduction

The American Occupational Therapy Association (AOTA; 2018) defines *telehealth* as "the application of evaluative, consultative, preventive, and therapeutic services delivered through information and communication technology" (p. 1). The World Health Organization (WHO) and the International Telecommunication Union determined, "Telehealth contributes to achieving universal health coverage in countries by improving access to quality and cost-effective health services for clients regardless of their setting" (WHO, 2022, p. vii). Telehealth in occupational therapy practice increased substantially throughout the COVID-19 pandemic, and as a result, telehealth has become a more common means of delivery of occupational therapy services (AOTA, n.d.-a, n.d.-b, 2021).

Telehealth has helped clients to save time and money, especially for those who live in rural areas with limited transportation or in areas of inclement weather, thus facilitating easy access to health care services and managing barriers to independent living (AOTA, 2018; Cason, 2014; Dirnberger & Waisbren, 2020; Lindeman, 2011; Powell et al., 2017; Sanders et al., 2012; Wallisch et al., 2019). Occupational therapy services provided through telehealth have included client evaluation, intervention, consultation, education, and training; and monitoring health factors, such as blood pressure and follow-through to support clients' use of assistive technology (Seron et al., 2021). Practitioners typically provide occupational therapy services through telehealth using synchronous videoconferencing, though other technologies such as texting and voice-only phone calls can be used (AOTA, 2018).

Telehealth can improve access to care, reduce hospital admissions and readmissions, prevent secondary complications of chronic diseases, and provide an enhanced sense of security in accessing support to address health-related concerns (AOTA, 2018; Hopp et al., 2007; Morony et al., 2017; Wosik et al., 2020). Occupational therapy practitioners are among the rehabilitation health care providers who may use telehealth technologies for service delivery. Telehealth uses include consultation, client evaluation, client monitoring, supervision, and intervention (AOTA, 2018). Some examples of interventions delivered through telehealth have included wheeled mobility and seating assessments (Bell et al., 2020), poststroke rehabilitation (Ostrowska et al., 2021), ADL assessments (Cason, 2014), pediatric occupational therapy services (Camden & Silva, 2021), care for persons with dementia and education for their caregivers (Boyle et al., 2022), group intervention in mental health (Ferrari et al., 2022), and polytrauma rehabilitation (Bendixen et al., 2008). In addition to services with individuals and groups, occupational therapy services through telehealth contribute directly to population health by facilitating self-management of chronic conditions, providing behavioral health screening, and improving the overall health and wellness of clients (Dahl-Popolizio et al., 2020).

As a result of using telehealth, the Veterans Administration has reported a significant decrease in hospital stays and admissions, travel reduction savings, increased client satisfaction, and improved independence (Darkins, 2014). Additionally, clients who opted to use telehealth were satisfied with the services providing clear communication, prompt decision making for their care, and online access to records (Mueller et al., 2020).

To practice ethically, occupational therapy practitioners must consider the unique features of telehealth service delivery for both its advantages and disadvantages. Advantages include providing education to encourage clients' self management, and improving the transfer of clients' information and electronic records (Wootton, 2012). Possible ethical issues with occupational therapy services through telehealth include inequality of client access, especially for those with cognitive impairment; low socioeconomic status making technology not affordable; or living in geographically remote areas where internet services are not available. Furthermore, client autonomy, dignity, and right to refuse treatment might be perceived as compromised with the use of telehealth (Kidholm et al., 2012). The presence of care extenders (e.g., family members, support staff), sometimes referred to as *e-helpers,* may cause privacy and confidentiality ethical issues, especially if the same third party would not necessarily be present during in-person treatment sessions. For example, a practitioner may need to discuss issues of bathing or toileting during a telehealth session, possibly creating a sense of discomfort or feelings of intrusiveness for the client if a care extender is present. In addition, clients or care extenders must be comfortable with and competent in using the technology (Torsney, 2003). For clients, technology competence often can be problematic due to sequela of the condition for which they require rehabilitation services. Sensory loss due to normal aging (e.g., diminished hearing and vision) or cognitive, motor, language, or vocal impairments can impede clients' ability to operate the technology or benefit from services delivered from a distance (Richmond et al., 2017).

Occupational therapy practitioners providing services through telehealth technology must develop and maintain competency in several areas. Following the client's consent to use telehealth, the practitioner must select the appropriate telehealth technology; provide the appropriate training to the client and their caregiver, if appropriate; review and monitor all the clinical data; and provide active care as well as case management by communication with the client's physician (Darkins et al., 2008). Beyond competency in administering typical occupational therapy assessments and interventions, practitioners must be knowledgeable about the implications of providing these services using technology as opposed to in person, as modifications in materials, techniques, or instructions may be required (Richmond et al., 2017).

Three ethical issues in regard to telehealth warrant further exploration: informed consent, privacy and confidentiality, and quality care.

INFORMED CONSENT

Occupational therapy practitioners must fully disclose information about the specific services (e.g., benefits, risks, potential outcomes, providers of services, reasonable alternatives) and implications of the use of technology during intervention. Clients should be informed of the risks and benefits, their rights and responsibilities (including the right to refuse treatment), and organizational policies for the retention and storage of audio and video recordings and electronic medical records (American Psychological Association [APA], 2023).

Some risks related to providing services through telehealth include the potential for loss of client privacy or confidentiality, lack of knowledge and skills of the care recipient or care extender when needed to assist with equipment, the possibility for equipment malfunction, potential costs associated with the use of technology (e.g., internet subscription, cellular data), potential for client feelings of less-personalized care, or modifications to assessment administration and scoring procedures (APA, 2023; Bauer, 2001; van Wynsberghe & Gastmans, 2009). Occupational therapy practitioners should consider all these risks as well as benefits when determining whether to provide occupational therapy services through telehealth.

Occupational therapy practitioners should document the informed consent process and content in compliance with applicable state laws and regulations (Health Resources and Services Administration, 2022). Initially and throughout the duration of intervention, clients should be given opportunities to ask questions to ensure comprehension and ongoing affirmative consent. Lastly, practitioners must respect clients' right to refuse service provision using telehealth.

PRIVACY AND CONFIDENTIALITY

Occupational therapy practitioners must maintain confidentiality throughout all electronic communications. Providers should ensure that clear policies related to service provision; documentation; and transmission, retention, and storage of audio, video, and electronic recordings and records are in place and follow Health Insurance Portability and Accountability Act of 1996 (HIPAA; P. L. 104-191) privacy rules to protect the privacy and confidentiality of clients' protected health information. To maximize privacy and confidentiality, organizations and practitioners should use authentication or encryption technology (Richmond et al., 2017). Strategies include ensuring that equipment and connections are secure and taking steps to make certain unauthorized third parties do not accidentally enter the room during a video conferencing session (APA, 2023; Hyler & Gangure, 2004). Practitioners should inform clients of the possibility of any third-party presence (e.g., technology assistant) and obtain client permission for the same (APA, 2023). Clients have the right to know that, despite efforts to protect their privacy and confidentiality, breaches may occur. In these instances, practitioners should understand and adhere to appropriate procedures addressing the compromise of the client's privacy and confidentiality of protected health information (AOTA, 2018).

QUALITY CARE AND ADHERENCE TO STANDARDS

Occupational therapy practitioners delivering services using a telehealth service delivery model must consider the impact of the technology on the services delivered to ensure they provide the best care possible and adhere to all professional and legal standards. Determining the appropriateness of occupational therapy using telehealth technology should be made on a case-by-case basis according to sound clinical reasoning and should be consistent with published professional standards (Richmond et al., 2017). The decision to use a telehealth service delivery model should be client-centered and based on advocating for recipients to attain needed services rather than on factors related to convenience or administrative directives. In addition, when using telehealth, practitioners must be aware of the potential impact of technology on the communication process (e.g., distorted or delayed audio or video transmission) and take steps to minimize disruption. Finally, practitioners should be knowledgeable as to how technology could affect the reliability of assessments when performing client evaluations using telehealth. Practitioners should remain abreast of the current evidence related to conducting evaluations using telehealth technology (AOTA, 2018).

Occupational therapy practitioners must be aware of state licensure laws (of each state where involved parties reside or are receiving services) and of each state's regulations related to telehealth (AOTA, n.d.-a, n.d.-b, 2018, 2021, 2023).

Relation to the AOTA Code of Ethics

Occupational therapists and occupational therapy assistants who provide services through telehealth face unique ethical considerations. The AOTA Code of Ethics (the Code), in conjunction with other AOTA official documents, offers guidance for these considerations. See Exhibit 20.1 for specific ethical standards related to telehealth.

EXHIBIT 20.1.
ETHICAL STANDARDS RELATED TO TELEHEALTH

- Comply with current federal and state laws, state scope of practice guidelines, and AOTA policies and Official Documents that apply to the profession of occupational therapy.
- Respect and honor the expressed wishes of recipients of service.
- Establish a collaborative relationship with recipients of service and relevant stakeholders to promote shared decision making.
- Do not engage in actions or inactions that jeopardize the safety or well-being of others or team effectiveness.
- Obtain informed consent (written, verbal, electronic, or implied) after disclosing appropriate information and answering any questions posed by the recipient of service, qualified family member or caregiver, or research participant to ensure voluntary participation.
- Fully disclose the benefits, risks, and potential outcomes of any intervention; the occupational therapy personnel who will be providing the intervention; and any reasonable alternatives to the proposed intervention.
- Respect the client's right to refuse occupational therapy services temporarily or permanently, even when that refusal has potential to result in poor outcomes.
- Provide information and resources to address barriers to access for persons in need of occupational therapy services.
- Maintain the confidentiality of all verbal, written, electronic, augmentative, and nonverbal communications in compliance with applicable laws, including all aspects of privacy laws and exceptions thereto (e.g., HIPAA, Family Educational Rights and Privacy Act).
- Maintain privacy and truthfulness in delivery of occupational therapy services, whether in person or virtually.

Note. From the Standards of Conduct from the AOTA Code of Ethics.

Reference to Other AOTA Documents

AOTA (2018) has examined current issues important to telehealth practice in the Telehealth and Occupational Therapy position paper. Some practice and ethical considerations outlined in this document include informed consent/consent to treat, privacy/confidentiality, effectiveness of this service delivery model, competency, compliance with licensure laws and regulations, and ensuring compliance with current standards of practice. AOTA has also provided resources for telehealth use, including a decision-tree guide for deciding whether telehealth is appropriate for a client (AOTA, n.d.-b).

For school and early intervention occupational therapy practitioners, AOTA has additional resources related to evaluation, monitoring progress, documentation, and interprofessional collaboration through telehealth (AOTA, 2020).

Knowledge of and adherence to billing and reimbursement regulations are also important considerations when providing occupational therapy services (AOTA, 2018). AOTA provides up-to-date guidance on insurance coverage for occupational therapy services provided through telehealth (AOTA, n.d.-b).

Occupational therapy practitioners are obligated to take responsibility for maintaining high standards and continuing competence in practice (see the Standards of Practice for Occupational Therapy and Standards for Continuing Competence in Occupational Therapy official documents at https://www.aota.org/practice/practice-essentials/aota-official-documents). Practitioners should take steps to ensure their own competence and weigh benefits of service provision with the potential for client harm.

Standards for supervision of occupational therapy personnel, including occupational therapy assistants, apply to services provided. State licensure boards should be consulted to determine state-specific supervision requirements for occupational therapy assistants and whether supervision can occur through telehealth (see the Guidelines for Supervision, Roles, and Responsibilities During the Delivery of Occupational Therapy Services official document).

Reference to Other Standards

Practitioners should refer to licensure laws in all states in which they provide occupational therapy services through telehealth to ensure they are adhering to the guidelines for telehealth for each state (AOTA, 2022).

Tips

- Use best practices for telehealth with each client.
- Consider both client and practitioner competence for technology use when delivering services through telehealth.
- Protect privacy and confidentiality of health information.
- Review state laws regarding telehealth for occupational therapy to ensure compliance.
- Review third-party payor requirements for telehealth.

Summary

Occupational therapists and occupational therapy assistants are using technology to provide interventions and services to people who may not otherwise have access to them. Practitioners should be aware of ethical considerations that accompany telehealth and the use of emerging technology in practice. First, practitioners must exercise clinical reasoning when deciding whether providing services through telehealth technology is an appropriate option. Practitioners should fully disclose to clients the risks, benefits, and nature of service delivery using technology. In addition, the client, their family, or service extenders may need to develop knowledge and skills in operating technology. The technology used must be of sufficient quality to provide dependable services and include protective measures to meet HIPAA privacy standards. Informed consent must be obtained. Practitioners must protect clients' privacy and confidentiality. Practitioners must ensure their own competency and optimize interventions for delivery through telehealth. Further, they must adhere to local, state, and federal laws, standards, and regulations. Practicing according to standards and guidelines published in several AOTA official documents can promote the safe and effective delivery of occupational therapy services through telehealth. By adhering to the highest level of ethical standards, occupational therapy practitioners can join other health care providers in using telehealth to better serve their clients.

CASE EXAMPLE 20.1. TELEHEALTH AND INFORMED CONSENT

Serena, an occupational therapist working at a Children's Hospital in one state asked **Nell,** an occupational therapy mobility specialist in another state, to consult with a client. **Becky** is a 13-year-old girl with cerebral palsy who has multiple impairments and a recent growth spurt, which has rendered her seating system obsolete. Nell agreed to consult with Becky and her caregiver using a HIPAA-compliant, real-time videoconferencing platform. Before setting up the videoconference, both occupational therapists checked their state licensure to be sure they would be compliant with telehealth services provided.

Serena explained to Becky and her mother how the teleconferencing session with Nell would work. During the session Nell would ask them all questions and instruct Serena to do specific physical assessments. Becky and her mom enthusiastically agreed to participate, because traveling to the other state would have been very difficult and costly for them, and they were anxious for a seating system that would improve Becky's ease of functioning.

The session proceeded as planned. However, after the standard, initial questions were answered, Nell wanted more information about Becky's pelvic mobility to determine the best seating options. If the session were in person, Nell would be able to use light touch to manipulate Becky's pelvis to obtain this information. Because that was not possible, Nell asked Serena to pull down Becky's pants and lift her shirt so she could better observe Becky's mobility. Upon hearing this, Becky started to cry, and Serena decided to end the session.

Questions
1. Despite having followed all anticipated issues during telehealth, situations may arise that change the outcome and cause a dilemma related to ethics. What ethical standards were met or not met during this session?
2. How could this telehealth session have been better planned so a successful outcome would have been obtained?

CASE EXAMPLE 20.2. SUPERVISION AND TELEHEALTH

Chris is a certified and licensed occupational therapy assistant who has 10 years of experience working at a rural skilled nursing facility (SNF) but has no experience in telehealth. The supervisor is **Jamie,** a licensed and registered occupational therapist who works at two SNFs about 60 miles from the SNF where Chris works. During Jamie's Level II fieldwork, approximately 50% of the caseload was through telehealth. To meet professional and state supervisory standards and regulations, Jamie and Chris meet weekly through a business communication platform with chat and video conferencing where they typically discuss the clients on caseload, as well as complete professional development for both of them.

Chris has one client who is discharging from the SNF in 2 days. Jamie and Chris have discussed plans to see this client biweekly through telehealth after the client is home. Jamie completed the initial evaluation more than a month ago when the client was admitted to the SNF and has been monitoring the progress through Chris' progress notes. Chris and Jamie have discussed plans for the telehealth visits to include the client's follow-through with adaptive equipment and development of a routine for a home exercise program.

Jamie and Chris both participated in the first telehealth visit so the evaluation could be completed, and the treatment plan written. Although consent for the visit was obtained, Jamie did not fully explain the purpose of the evaluation nor the reason for the occupational therapy services. During the ensuing telehealth visits Chris was able to determine and recommend adaptive equipment for the client and, with client's approval, help to obtain the needed equipment. Chris also helped the client with routine cues for the active assistive range of motion exercises assigned while at the SNF. Because this was Chris' first experience using telehealth with a client, Jamie would enter the virtual room discreetly for several minutes once a week to check on Chris's approaches.

Approximately 1 week prior to the anticipated discharge from telehealth, Jamie had an unexpected medical leave and was not able to continue providing supervision for Chris' caseload. Chris continued the treatment for two more sessions, then discharged the client, identifying that the goals were met.

Questions
1. According to the Code, what ethical issues were created in the above scenario?
2. Apply an ethical decision-making framework. How could the ethical issues in this scenario have been avoided?

CASE EXAMPLE 20.3. SAFETY IN TELEHEALTH

Terry is a licensed occupational therapist who is working for the Veterans Health Administration (VHA) and has completed all education related to telehealth as assigned by the organization. Terry's first telehealth visit was an evaluation of a **veteran** living 60 miles away from the nearest VA facility. The veteran's primary care physician had recommended occupational therapy to improve his function and independence in his home because he lived alone. Terry initiated the telehealth visit by introducing the veteran to occupational therapy and obtaining the veteran's personal identification. Terry had the veteran complete several standardized assessments prior to assessing the home itself for adaptive

(Continued)

CASE EXAMPLE 20.3. SAFETY IN TELEHEALTH *(Cont.)*

equipment. After an initial interview to determine areas of difficulty, Terry had the veteran complete several standardized assessments that included range of motion, functional reach, and static and dynamic balance. Because the veteran had not identified balance issues during the interview, Terry had the veteran complete the 4-stage balance test. During the tandem stance, the veteran lost his balance and was unable to catch himself. When the veteran reported he was unable to get up from the floor, Terry began looking for an emergency contact number in the veteran's chart and home county. He was finally able to call emergency medical services for the veteran and remained in the telehealth visit with the veteran until they arrived.

Questions
1. What are some of the ethical concerns identified in this scenario?
2. What could Terry have done differently prior to this telehealth evaluation?
3. What could Terry have done differently during this telehealth evaluation?

Acknowledgment

Joanne Estes, MS, OTR/L, authored an earlier edition of this Advisory Opinion.

REFERENCES

American Occupational Therapy Association. (n.d.-a). *Advocacy issues: Expanding telehealth.* https://www.aota.org/advocacy/issues/telehealth-advocacy

American Occupational Therapy Association. (n.d.-b). *Practice essentials: Telehealth resources.* https://www.aota.org/practice/practice-essentials/telehealth-resources

American Occupational Therapy Association. (2018). Telehealth in occupational therapy. *American Journal of Occupational Therapy, 72*(Suppl. 2), 7212410059. https://doi.org/10.5014/ajot.2018.72S219

American Occupational Therapy Association. (2020). *Evaluation considerations for delivering virtual school-based OT services via telehealth.* https://www.aota.org/-/media/corporate/files/practice/covid-19/evaluation-considerations-delivering-virtual-school-based-telehealth.pdf

American Occupational Therapy Association. (2021). *COVID-19 state updates: Summary of telehealth, insurance, and licensure developments; and comprehensive state-by-state chart.* https://www.aota.org/advocacy/advocacy-news/state/state-news/covid-19-summary-telehealth-insurance-licensure

American Occupational Therapy Association. (2022). *Occupational therapy and telehealth: State statutes, regulations, and regulatory board statements.* https://www.aota.org/-/media/corporate/files/advocacy/state/telehealth/telehealth-state-statutes-regulations-regulatory-board-statements.pdf

American Psychological Association. (2023). *Guidelines for the practice of telepsychology.* https://www.apa.org/practice/guidelines/telepsychology

Bauer, K. A. (2001). Home-based telemedicine: A survey of ethical issues. *Cambridge Quarterly of Healthcare Ethics, 10*(2), 137–146. https://doi.org/10.1017/S0963180101002043

Bell, M., Schein, R. M., Straatmann, J., Dicianno, B. E., & Schmeler, M. R. (2020). Functional mobility outcomes in telehealth and in-person assessments for wheeled mobility devices. *International Journal of Telerehabilitation, 12*(2), 27. https://doi.org/10.5195%2Fijt.2020.6335

Bendixen, R. M., Levy, C., Lutz, B. J., Horn, K. R., Chronister, K., & Mann, W. C. (2008). A telerehabilitation model for victims of polytrauma. *Rehabilitation Nursing, 33*(5), 215–220. https://doi.org/10.1002/j.2048-7940.2008.tb00230.x

Boyle, L. D., Husebo, B. S., & Vislapuu, M. (2022). Promoters and barriers to the implementation and adoption of assistive technology and telecare for people with dementia and their caregivers: A systematic review of the literature. *BMC Health Services Research, 22*(1), Article 1573, 1–19. https://doi.org/10.1186/s12913-022-08968-2

Camden, C., & Silva, M. (2021). Pediatric telehealth: Opportunities created by the COVID-19 and suggestions to sustain its use to support families of children with disabilities. *Physical & Occupational Therapy in Pediatrics, 41*(1), 1–17. https://doi.org/10.1080/01942638.2020.1825032

Cason, J. (2014). Telehealth: A rapidly developing service delivery model for occupational therapy. *International Journal of Telerehabilitation, 6*(1), 29–35. https://doi.org/10.5195%2Fijt.2014.6148

Dahl-Popolizio, S., Carpenter, H., Coronado, M., Popolizio, N. J., & Swanson, C. (2020). Telehealth for the provision of occupational therapy: Reflections on experiences during the COVID-19 pandemic. *International Journal of Telerehabilitation, 12*(2), 77–92. https://doi.org/10.5195%2Fijt.2020.6328

Darkins, A. (2014). The growth of telehealth services in the Veterans Health Administration between 1994 and 2014: A study in the diffusion of innovation. *Telemedicine and e-Health, 20*, 761–768. https://doi.org/10.1089/tmj.2014.0143

Darkins, A., Ryan, P., Kobb, R., Foster, L., Edmonson, E., Wakefield, B., & Lancaster, A. E. (2008). Care coordination/home telehealth: The systematic implementation of health informatics, home telehealth, and disease management to support the care of veteran patients with chronic conditions. *Telemedicine and e-Health, 14*, 1118–1126. https://doi.org/10.1089/tmj.2008.0021

Dirnberger, J., & Waisbren, S. (2020). Efficacy of telehealth visits for postoperative care at the Minneapolis VA. *American Journal of Surgery, 220*, 721–724. https://doi.org/10.1016/j.amjsurg.2020.01.015

Family Educational Rights and Privacy Act of 1974, Pub. L. 93-380, 20 U.S.C. § 1232g; 34 CFR Part 99.

Ferrari, S. M. L., Pywell, S. D., da Costa, A. L. B., & Marcolino, T. Q. (2022). Occupational therapy telehealth groups in Covid-19 pandemic: Perspectives from a mental health day hospital. *Cadernos Brasileiros de Terapia Ocupacional, 30*, e3019. https://doi.org/10.1590/2526-8910.ctoRE22883019

Health Insurance Portability and Accountability Act of 1996, Pub. L. 104-191, 42 U.S.C. § 300gg, 29 U.S.C §§ 1181–1183, and 42 U.S.C. §§ 1320d–1320d9.

Health Resources and Services Administration. (2022). *Obtaining informed consent.* https://telehealth.hhs.gov/providers/preparing-patients-for-telehealth/obtaining-informed-consent

Hopp, F. P., Hogan, M. M., Woodbridge, P. A., & Lowery, J. C. (2007). The use of telehealth for diabetes management: A qualitative study of telehealth provider perceptions. *Implementation Science, 2*(1), 1–8. https://doi.org/10.1186/1748-5908-2-14

Hyler, S. E., & Gangure, D. P. (2004). Legal and ethical challenges in telepsychiatry. *Journal of Psychiatric Practice, 10*, 272–276. https://doi.org/10.1097/00131746-200407000-00011

Kidholm, K., Ekeland, A. G., Jensen, L. K., Rasmussen, J., Pedersen, C. D., Bowes, A., . . . Bech, M. (2012). A model for assessment of telemedicine applications: MAST. *International Journal of Technology Assessment in Health Care, 28*(1), 44–51. https://doi.org/10.1017/S0266462311000638

Lindeman, D. (2011). Interview: Lessons from a leader in telehealth diffusion: A conversation with Adam Darkins of the Veterans Health Administration. *Ageing International, 36*(1), 146–154. https://doi.org/10.1007/s12126-010-9079-7

Morony, S., Weir, K., Duncan, G., Biggs, J., Nutbeam, D., & McCaffery, K. (2017). Experiences of teach-back in a telephone health service. *HLRP: Health Literacy Research and Practice, 1*(4), e173–e181. https://doi.org/10.3928/24748307-20170724-01

Mueller, M., Knop, M., Niehaves, B., & Adarkwah, C. C. (2020). Investigating the acceptance of video consultation by patients in rural primary care: Empirical comparison of preusers and actual users. *JMIR Medical Informatics, 8*(10), e20813. https://doi.org/10.2196/20813

Ostrowska, P. M., Śliwiński, M., Studnicki, R., & Hansdorfer-Korzon, R. (2021, May). Telerehabilitation of post-stroke patients as a therapeutic solution in the era of the Covid-19 pandemic. *Healthcare, 9*(6), 654. https://doi.org/10.3390/healthcare9060654

Powell, R. E., Henstenburg, J. M., Cooper, G., Hollander, J. E., & Rising, K. L. (2017). Patient perceptions of telehealth primary care video visits. *Annals of Family Medicine, 15*, 225–229. https://doi.org/10.1370/afm.2095

Richmond, T., Peterson, C., Cason, J., Billings, M., Terrell, E. A., Lee, A. C. W., . . . Brennan, D. (2017). American Telemedicine Association's principles for delivering telerehabilitation services. *International Journal of Telerehabilitation, 9*(2), 63–68. https://doi.org/10.5195/ijt.2017.6232

Sanders, C., Rogers, A., Bowen, R., Bower, P., Hirani, S., Cartwright, M., . . . Newman, S. P. (2012). Exploring barriers to participation and adoption of telehealth and telecare within the Whole System Demonstrator trial: A qualitative study. *BMC Health Services Research, 12*, Article 220. https://doi.org/10.1186/1472-6963-12-220

Seron, P., Oliveros, M., Gutierrez-Arias, R., Fuentes-Aspe, R., Torres-Castro, R., Merino-Osorio, C., . . . Sanchez, P. (2021). Effectiveness of telerehabilitation in physical therapy: A rapid overview. *Physical Therapy, 101*(6), pzab053. https://doi.org/10.1093/ptj/pzab053

Torsney, K. (2003). Advantages and disadvantages of telerehabilitation for persons with neurological disabilities. *NeuroRehabilitation, 18*(2), 183–185. https://doi.org/10.3233/NRE-2003-18211

van Wynsberghe, A., & Gastmans, C. (2009). Telepsychiatry and the meaning of in-person contact: A preliminary ethical appraisal. *Medicine, Health Care, and Philosophy, 12*, 469–476. https://doi.org/10.1007/s11019-009-9214-y

Wallisch, A., Little, L., Pope, E., & Dunn, W. (2019). Parent perspectives of an occupational therapy telehealth intervention. *International Journal of Telerehabilitation, 11*(1), 15. https://doi.org/10.5195%2Fijt.2019.6274

Wootton, R. (2012). Twenty years of telemedicine in chronic disease management: An evidence synthesis. *Journal of Telemedicine and Telecare, 18*(4), 211–220. https://doi.org/10.1258/jtt.2012.120219

World Health Organization. (2022). *WHO–ITU global standard for accessibility of telehealth services.* https://www.who.int/publications/i/item/9789240050464

Wosik, J., Fudim, M., Cameron, B., Gellad, Z. F., Cho, A., Phinney, D., . . . Tcheng, J. (2020). Telehealth transformation: COVID-19 and the rise of virtual care. *Journal of the American Medical Informatics Association, 27*, 957–962. https://doi.org/10.1093/jamia/ocaa067

Ethical Considerations in Private Practice

BRENDA S. HOWARD, DHSc, OTR, FAOTA, and
BRIANNE M. KURCSAK, MS, OTR/L

Key Points

- Ethical issues in private practice include the dual agency of the occupational therapy practitioner as business owner and client advocate. Billing, third-party payer reimbursement, referrals, direct access, and continuity of care can give rise to ethical issues.
- Professional issues, including professional autonomy, ensuring intervention effectiveness, accountability, competition, and professional conduct, can precipitate ethical issues in private practice.
- The private practice business owner must take care to ensure that clients' rights and welfare are protected, especially in cases of power asymmetries and client vulnerability. Client autonomy and safety must be paramount.

Introduction

Private practice can provide a venue in which occupational therapy practitioners with an entrepreneurial spirit can reap the benefits of their work and provide services consistent with their interests. However, practitioners who own a private practice are generally more directly involved with and affected by ethical issues related to business practices than those who work for others. As a private practice owner, the burden is on the practitioner to ensure that they make clinical decisions that are in compliance with core ethical principles related to benefiting the client. Ethical issues in private practice can be categorized into three domains: Business and economic issues, professional issues, and clients' rights and welfare (Hudon et al., 2015).

BUSINESS AND ECONOMIC ISSUES

Business and economic issues become ethical concerns in private practice when financial needs come into conflict with client needs. The occupational therapy practitioner may experience role conflicts when they have a duty to the client, the third-party payer, and the business (Babic, 2015; Hudon et al., 2015; Praestegaard et al., 2013; Wilhelm & Wilhelm, 2021). These role conflicts may begin with client referrals. Conflicts can occur when the referral to the practitioner's business is initiated by the client or one of their family members. If the practitioner is not able to provide the most appropriate care for the client's needs, the practitioner must decide whether to keep the client's business and honor their autonomy of choice, or refer the client elsewhere to provide the most beneficial care (Hudon et al., 2015). Prospective clients have a right to know practice ownership or potential financial gain for either the occupational therapy practitioner or the referring physician. Practitioners have an obligation to be certain that economic gain or a desire to satisfy referral sources do not unduly influence the type and amount of therapy provided. Rather, services provided must carefully reflect the status of the client, collaborative goals, and potential for realistic and meaningful outcomes. If the client's status changes and they are no longer receiving any benefit from skilled occupational therapy, the practitioner should consider options such as providing instruction in a home program, training caregivers, or planning subsequent screening and reevaluation.

Ethical issues may arise when private practice owners sell items to clients at a profit. Such sales may result in conflicts of interest for the business owner when making a profit conflicts with beneficence to the client (Bell, 2021; Hudon et al., 2015). A separate Advisory Opinion addresses this issue (see Chapter 11, "Engaging in Business Transactions With Clients"). The occupational therapy practitioner must be aware of any laws governing sales of products to clients in their geographic area (Bell, 2021).

Although private practice business owners have options for payment for services (fee for service, contracts with insurance companies, billing as an out-of-network provider, or pursuing grants), ethical issues related to billing and payers can still arise (Bell, 2021). The occupational therapy practitioner needs to be aware of and be prepared to address potential issues of undue influence on the duration, type, and frequency of therapy being provided, no matter the payer source or in/out of network benefits. Conflicts of interest may also arise when owners' financial interests are being weighed against evidence-based care (Hudon et al., 2015).

Practice owners need to ensure that they do not set up productivity targets and service delivery models geared to maximize reimbursement without fully considering the impact on individualized and evidence-based care. Designing programs or approaches to therapy provision with the intention only to increase profitability is not consistent with the client-centered philosophy of the profession of occupational therapy or with ethical practice.

Professional Issues

Professional issues that may prompt ethical problems include professional autonomy, ensuring intervention effectiveness, informed consent, accountability, competition, and professional conduct. Private practice affords the occupational therapy practitioner with professional autonomy when making clinical decisions. However, that autonomy should not override providing evidence-based practice that has demonstrated effectiveness in the literature (Hudon et al., 2015). Further, practitioners should always ensure their competence to provide specialized services (Praestegaard et al., 2013) and give clients information about their qualifications (Hazlett, 2019). Accountability includes building intentional structures for transparency and honesty with all stakeholders. Examples include transparency in marketing, such as listing credentials and specialty areas correctly on the business website for each practitioner (Praestegaard et al., 2013); building networks of private practices in order to foster collaboration for clients outside one's areas of competence (Hudon et al., 2015); and using HIPAA-compliant documentation and payment systems. In the case of consulting or non-reimbursable businesses (e.g., health and wellness services, prevention programs, educational services), the practitioner must consider how to set and collect fees for services (Bell, 2021).

Documentation can present additional ethical concerns. Every occupational therapy practitioner has a personal responsibility to be accurate and timely in compliance with documentation and billing standards and regulations. Private practice owners have an additional responsibility to ensure that policies and procedures are in place for enforcing applicable regulations and standards with their employees, because they are also responsible for the business elements of the organization (Bell, 2021). Policies and procedures may include regular medical record review or peer review, an in-service on appropriate documentation, timelines for completing documentation, and continuing education on current coding and billing requirements.

Proper supervision is particularly critical to prevent situations in which an employee leaves the practice and client documentation is incomplete or missing. Without documentation, treatment sessions cannot be billed and reimbursed, and other occupational therapy practitioners who have not treated those clients cannot "fill in" the missing portions of the record. The record is a legal document, and the information it contains must be accurate. The private practice owner has the responsibility for ensuring that employees follow this practice.

If the occupational therapy practitioner practices in a state that allows direct access to occupational therapy without a physician's referral, the practitioner should carefully consider the client's needs and whether or not there is a good fit with occupational therapy to meet those needs. The occupational therapy practitioner has a duty to practice within their scope of practice and specialized knowledge and skills. The occupational therapy practitioner must be qualified to provide the services that the client needs, and should disclose those qualifications to potential clients. One should consider whether they could cause the client harm by attempting interventions for which they have not been trained rather than referring the client to a practitioner who better fits their needs (Hazlett, 2019). In this way, the practitioner can uphold the ethical principle of *nonmaleficence* (avoiding actions that cause harm) at the forefront of the evaluation and treatment process (Beauchamp & Childress, 2019).

Competition between private practice business owners may lead to "siloing," in which practitioners are unwilling to share information between clinics in an attempt to preserve income. This lack of collaboration may harm the client, as important information may be lost from one setting to the next. This harm can be overcome if the business owner has the moral courage to be honest with the client about their capabilities and limitations, and if they exercise fairness with the client, families, and other private practices (Hazlett, 2019). Finally, in the dual roles of business owner and practitioner, occupational therapy practitioners have a responsibility to act in accordance with professional conduct, including all applicable laws, ethical codes, and standards of practice pertaining to the profession (Bell, 2021).

Clients' Rights and Welfare

Ethical issues regarding clients' rights and welfare include power asymmetry, client vulnerability, client autonomy, and informed consent (Hudon et al., 2015). Clients are, by nature of the therapeutic relationship, considered vulnerable and in an asymmetrical power dynamic with the practitioner (Hudon et al., 2015; Praestegaard et al., 2013). It is up to the practitioner to provide the client with their due right to care and respect and to consider their welfare as the utmost priority. To that end, private practice practitioners must respect the principles of *autonomy* and *confidentiality* (Babic, 2015; Hudon et al., 2015). The occupational therapy plan of care should be based on individual evaluation and the client's needs, which identifies their desires and supports autonomy to maximize outcomes. *Autonomy* includes allowing clients a choice in providers when they are referred for therapy (Hazlett, 2019; Therapy Today, 2022). Autonomy also involves carefully weighing the client's right to self-determination against other ethical issues. For example, if a client wishes to continue driving, and the practitioner assesses their driving as not safe, the practitioner must weigh their duty to public safety against the client's right to autonomy (Drolet et al., 2017).

The occupational therapy practitioner must observe privacy and confidentiality regarding both their own social media and the accounts of clients and their families. Deciding whether or not to allow photography or video recording of sessions should include consideration that anything that is recorded can be displayed on the internet. The practitioner runs the risk of losing control of intellectual property, and of others inappropriately using intervention techniques that are posted on social media. Further, family members or caregivers who attend sessions with the client may violate client privacy by posting photos or videos on social media without the client's consent, for which they may hold the practitioner accountable (Therapy Today, 2022).

Occupational therapy practitioners must provide informed consent for clients, including informing the client of the options they have for intervention and what the practitioner can provide (Babic, 2015; Hudon et al., 2015; Praestegaard et al., 2013; Wilhelm & Wilhelm, 2021). When cost, scarcity of resources, and allocation of resources are issues, the practitioner must weigh the evidence in the literature and the benefit of services and technologies versus the potential risks and high costs before engaging in decision making with the client (Babic, 2015). In regard to access to care, practitioners must consider whether the client has access to the most appropriate occupational therapy services for their needs. Limited access in rural areas, insurance restrictions, and other issues out of the practitioner's control can affect access to care. Private practice owners can safeguard client access to appropriate, qualified providers by providing a limited amount of pro bono services, maintaining a list of available community services, and seeking grant funding. Further, the practitioner can consider providing telehealth services to those whose only access to occupational therapy services may be remote (AOTA, 2018).

Lastly, the private practice owner may experience the blurring of personal and professional boundaries. The occupational therapy practitioner must manage their own biases when dealing with cultural, political, or religious values and beliefs of clients that are different from their own. The practitioner has a duty to provide care to all persons, regardless of differences. Practitioners, like any other individuals, may have their own biases or preconceived notions that can influence their interactions with clients. To effectively address this challenge, the practitioner must be self-aware and recognize their own biases. They need to constantly evaluate their attitudes, beliefs, and values to ensure they do not interfere with the delivery of unbiased and culturally sensitive care. This self-reflection process enables them to provide equitable treatment to clients and respect their individuality, regardless of differences. By acknowledging and managing their biases, practitioners uphold their ethical duty to provide care to all persons, regardless of their cultural, political, or religious backgrounds. They should approach each client with an open mind, respect their unique perspectives, and tailor their interventions to suit the individual's needs and preferences (AOTA, 2020a, 2021).

When practicing in private settings, there is a risk of forming more intimate friendships or business alliances with clients (Hudon et al., 2015). Occupational therapy practitioners must carefully consider that these intimate or business associations violate ethical standards and can cause considerable harm to the client. Intimate relationships with current clients can result in sanctions or legal action for sexual misconduct (Babic, 2015), and entering into business relationships with current clients can result in a conflict of interest that violates the AOTA Code of Ethics (the Code).

Relation to the AOTA Code of Ethics

Exhibit 21.1 lists standards from the Code that are applicable to private practice.

Reference to Other AOTA Documents

The American Occupational Therapy Association (AOTA) provides a variety of tools and information for private practice business owners on its website in the Payment policy: Private practice essentials for Reimbursement section. AOTA documents on specific practice areas can provide further guidance for private practice owners (AOTA, 2017a, 2017b, 2020b). AOTA's Standards of Practice for Occupational Therapy and Standards for Continuing in Occupational Therapy Competence official documents apply in private practice as well as all other settings.

EXHIBIT 21.1.
ETHICAL STANDARDS RELATED TO PRIVATE PRACTICE

- Ensure transparency when participating in a business arrangement as owner, stockholder, partner, or employee.
- Do not exploit human, financial, or material resources of employers for personal gain.
- Do not exploit any relationship established as an occupational therapy practitioner, educator, or researcher to further one's own physical, emotional, financial, political, or business interests.
- Do not engage in dual relationships or situations in which an occupational therapy professional or student is unable to maintain clear professional boundaries or objectivity.
- Do not engage in any undue influences that may impair practice or compromise the ability to safely and competently provide occupational therapy services, education, or research.
- Refer to other providers when indicated by the needs of the client.
- Provide information and resources to address barriers to access for persons in need of occupational therapy services.
- Maintain the confidentiality of all verbal, written, electronic, augmentative, and nonverbal communications in compliance with applicable laws, including all aspects of privacy laws and exceptions thereto (e.g., Health Insurance Portability and Accountability Act, Family Educational Rights and Privacy Act).
- Maintain privacy and truthfulness in delivery of occupational therapy services, whether in person or virtually.

Note. From the Standards of Conduct from the AOTA Code of Ethics.

Reference to Other Standards

Private practice owners must keep in mind certain applicable state and federal laws related to private practice and potential referral sources. First, occupational therapy practitioners must be familiar with their state regulatory board's occupational therapy practice act to maintain compliance with scope of practice, licensure, and supervision requirements for all practitioners employed by the practice (AOTA, 2023). Second, the practice owner must comply with all local, state, and federal laws pertaining to health care business ownership. These laws include the federal physician self-referral ("Stark") and anti-kickback laws. The term *Stark Law* commonly refers to Section 1877 of the Social Security Act Amendments of 1965 (P. L. 89-97), which prohibits physicians from referring clients to health care entities from which they (or their immediate family) stand to gain financially from payments from Medicare, Medicaid, or other federal funds. It is recommended that private practice owners use legal assistance to ensure compliance with applicable regulations when setting up a business.

Tips

- Stay updated in knowledge and skills for practice as well as laws and policy through consistent engagement in continuing education (Praestegaard et al., 2013).
- Set practice values in advance of ethical conflicts, in order to provide guidelines for meeting the needs of clients, payers, and the business (Drolet et al., 2017).
- Be transparent and honest when communicating with clients, their families, payers, and other stakeholders regarding business ownership, fees and payment for services, evidence-based practice, and the practitioner's knowledge and skills (Hazlett, 2019).
- Create built-in systems of internal and external accountability to avoid ethical pitfalls (DuBois et al., 2019).
- When in doubt, pause for further investigation of ethical issues by reviewing the Code; state practice acts; and other pertinent laws, policies, and regulations before proceeding (Wilhelm & Wilhelm, 2021).

CASE EXAMPLE 21.1. MULTIPLE REFERRALS WITHIN THE SAME FAMILY UNIT REQUIRING PROFESSIONAL COLLABORATION

A **family with three children** is requesting occupational therapy services from a **private practice owner** who employs other occupational therapy practitioners. Only two of the three children qualify for services. The parent is requesting to have all three children seen, so the child without a therapy need is not left out. On evaluation, the parent reports that one of the children who qualified for services had failed a recent swallow study. The clinic does not have a practitioner who specializes in swallowing, but the parent has requested that the private practice see them anyway because it will be most convenient for their schedule. A **practitioner** who has minimal training in swallowing is persuaded to "learn techniques" to avoid a referral to another clinic with a practitioner who is fully trained and competent in feeding and swallowing. When checking their in-network benefits, the practice owner realizes the reimbursement rate is very high for this insurance company, and considers reviewing the evaluation of the child who did not initially qualify to see if there are, in fact, deficits warranting therapy allowing all three to attend.

Questions
1. What are the ethical issues in this scenario?
2. What are the ethical principles and standards that apply?
3. Apply an ethical decision-making framework. What are the next steps the practitioner should take?

Next Steps

Recommendations from the literature for preventing and mitigating ethical issues in private practice include increasing entry-level training and continuing education that target ethical issues encountered in private practice, ethics mentorships (Hudon et al., 2015),

CASE EXAMPLE 21.2. HIPAA VIOLATION WITH ONLINE PAYMENT SERVICE

A **child** is referred for an occupational therapy evaluation to a clinic where the parent knows the business owner on a personal level. Because this clinic offers direct payment for services, the parent requests to pay for the services using a commonly available online payment platform through an app on their phone. The parent was unaware their privacy settings allowed for public visibility to see the transactions made. A mutual friend sees the transaction and inquires of the business owner what the child was evaluated for and why the visit was so costly.

Questions
1. What are the ethical issues in this scenario?
2. What are the ethical principles and standards that apply?
3. Apply an ethical decision-making framework. What are the next steps a practitioner should take?

equipping practitioners to advocate for clients with third-party payers (Bell, 2021), and creating networks of practice to treat more complex clients (Hudon et al., 2015). To remain ethical, private practice owners need to seek out ways to be accountable to self and others (Babic, 2015; DuBois et al., 2019; Hazlett, 2019; Praestegaard et al., 2013). Recommended changes in laws and policies include regulating the sale of products, better external oversight for private practices, and strengthening legislative requirements for self-referrals (Hudon et al., 2015).

Summary

Regardless of the type of services being provided, occupational therapy practitioners must keep the best interests of the client at the forefront when providing private practice services. To ensure that they meet their ethical obligations and professional standards, practitioners must maintain open communication and collaboration among all parties, transparency, and full disclosure of relevant information. Further, they must comply with all applicable laws and ethical principles. With careful consideration of ethical issues, private practice owners can successfully manage their client-centered practice.

Acknowledgment

Deborah Yarett Slater, MS, OT/L, FAOTA, authored an earlier version of this Advisory Opinion.

REFERENCES

American Occupational Therapy Association. (2017a). Guidelines for occupational therapy services in early intervention and schools. *American Journal of Occupational Therapy, 71*(Suppl. 2), 7112410010. https://doi.org/10.5014/ajot.2017.716S01

American Occupational Therapy Association. (2017b). Occupational therapy services in facilitating work participation and performance. *American Journal of Occupational Therapy, 71*(Suppl. 2), 7112410040. https://doi.org/10.5014/ajot.2017.716S05

American Occupational Therapy Association. (2018). Telehealth in occupational therapy. *American Journal of Occupational Therapy, 72*(Suppl. 2), 7212410059. https://doi.org/10.5014/ajot.2018.72S219

American Occupational Therapy Association. (2020a). Occupational therapy's commitment to diversity, equity, and inclusion. *American Journal of Occupational Therapy, 74*(Suppl. 3), 7413410030p1–7413410030p6. https://doi.org/10.5014/ajot.2020.74S3002

American Occupational Therapy Association. (2020b). Role of occupational therapy in primary care. *American Journal of Occupational Therapy, 74*(Suppl. 3), 7413410040p1–7413410040p16. https://doi.org/10.5014/ajot.2020.74S3001

American Occupational Therapy Association. (2021). *AOTA's guide to addressing the impact of racial discrimination, stigma, and implicit bias on provision of services.* https://www.aota.org/-/media/corporate/files/aboutot/dei/guide-racial-discrimination.pdf

American Occupational Therapy Association. (2023). *Payment Policy: Private practice essentials for reimbursement.* https://www.aota.org/practice/practice-essentials/payment-policy/pay1

Babic, A. (2015). *Ethical dilemmas experienced by occupational therapists working in private practice.* (Unpublished master's thesis). University of Sydney.

Beauchamp, T. L., & Childress, J. F. (2019). *Principles of biomedical ethics* (8th ed.). Oxford University Press.

Bell, A. (2021, August). Cash-based practice: It's complicated. *APTA Magazine,* 16–19. https://www.apta.org/apta-magazine/2021/08/01/apta-magazine-august-2021/cash-based-practice-its-complicated

Drolet, M., Gaudet, R., & Pinard, C. (2017). Preparing students for the ethical issues involved in occupational therapy private practice with an ethics typology. *Occupational Therapy Now, 19*(2), 9–10.

DuBois, J., Anderson, E., Chibnall, J., Mozersky, J., & Walsh, H. (2019). Serious ethical violations in medicine: A statistical and ethical analysis of 280 cases in the United States from 2008–2016. *The American Journal of Bioethics, 19*(1), 16–34. https://doi.org/10.1080/15265161.2018.1544305

Family Educational Rights and Privacy Act of 1974, Pub. L. 93-380, 20 U.S.C. § 1232g; 34 CFR Part 99.

Hazlett, N. (2019). Consent, collaboration, siloes, and scope: Ethics in private pediatric practice. *Occupational Therapy Now, 21*(2), 17–18.

Health Insurance Portability and Accountability Act of 1996, Pub. L. 104-191, 42 U.S.C. §300gg, 29 U.S.C §§ 1181–1183, and 42 U.S.C. §§ 1320d–1320d9.

Hudon, A., Drolet, M., & Williams-Jones, B. (2015). Ethical issues raised by private practice physiotherapy are more diverse than first meets the eye: Recommendations from a literature review. *Physiotherapy Canada, 67*(2), 124–132. https://utpjournals.press/doi/10.3138/ptc.2014-10

Praestegaard, J., Gard, G., & Glasdam, S. (2013, August). Practicing physiotherapy in Danish private practice: An ethical perspective. *Medical Health Care and Philosophy, 16,* 555–564. https://doi.org/10.1007/s11019-012-9446-0

Social Security Act Amendments of 1965, Pub. L. 89-97, 42 U.S.C. §§ 1395–1395kkk1 (Medicare) and 42 U.S.C. §§ 1396–1396w5 (Medicaid).

Therapy Today. (2022, September 22). Our ethics team and Therapy Today readers consider this month's dilemma: Should I agree to my client recording our online sessions? *Therapy Today, 33*(7), 50–53.

Wilhelm, K., & Wilhelm, L. (2021). Ethical issues in private practice: A phenomenological investigation of music therapy business owners. *Journal of Music Therapy, 58,* 345–371. https://doi.org/10.1093/jmt/thaa025

22

The Role of the Occupational Therapy Practitioner as an Expert Witness

BRENDA KORNBLIT KENNELL, MA, OTR/L, FAOTA, and
BARBARA L. KORNBLAU, JD, OTR/L, FAOTA, DAAPM, CCM, CDMS

Key Points

- It is the ethical duty of the expert witness to possess current experience and advanced knowledge in the area for which they are asked to testify (Ronquillo et al., 2023).
- Often the role of an expert witness is to determine whether a "deviation from the standard of care has occurred" and whether that possibly could have contributed to a client's injury or death (Ronquillo et al., 2023).
- An occupational therapy practitioner serving as an expert witness can uphold the ethical principles of *justice* and *veracity*.

Introduction

An *expert witness* is defined as "a person with specialized knowledge, skills, education, or experience in a particular field who is called upon to provide their expertise in legal proceedings to assist the court with understanding complex technical or scientific issues. . . . A person who is designated as an expert witness must be qualified on the subject of their testimony" (Robinson, 2023). Because of their expertise, an expert witness can

> clarify, explain, and provide an expert opinion on complex and complicated matters that the average person cannot understand . . . Thanks in part to Federal Rule of Evidence 702, an expert witness can help shed light on what occurred and the point of the incident, even if they were not physically present when it happened. Their testimony and professional opinion can help . . . lead to a sounder, more resolute case outcome. (Cloudlex, 2023)

An occupational therapy practitioner may serve as an expert witness as a function of their employment role or as an independent contractor. Sometimes the expert witness is the treating practitioner who must verify the facts that gave rise to the litigation. Other times, the expert witness is an independent contractor who may be asked to analyze the pertinent medical documents, and possibly never meet the parties involved. An expert witness may be engaged to evaluate a claim in order to determine if legal action will be initiated. The expert witness may also review pertinent medical records, provide a written opinion, and possibly answer questions under oath from attorneys on both sides during a deposition or an actual court hearing, although the majority of cases settle before progressing to that point (Ronquillo et al., 2023). Regardless of the context, the primary role of the expert witness is always to render an opinion about whether there was a deviation from the standard of care.

Some examples of situations in which an occupational therapy practitioner may be called on to provide professional opinions as an expert include the following:

- results of a functional capacity evaluation in disability determination or personal injury litigation
- results of an environmental assessment in a dispute about an organization's alleged failure to provide reasonable accommodations for a worker with a disability
- challenge by parents related to the appropriate provision of school-based services for their child who has exceptional educational needs
- supervisory responsibility (e.g., when the application of a physical agent modality performed by an occupational therapy practitioner resulted in harm to a client)
- a dispute between an insurer and a client regarding rehabilitation potential and denial of authorization for coverage of occupational therapy services
- a certified hand therapist reviewing medical records to analyze the appropriateness of a treatment plan and outcome for upper-extremity rehabilitation provided by another practitioner
- determining the appropriateness of disciplinary action against an occupational therapy practitioner related to failure to appropriately supervise another practitioner or a student.

Regardless of the reason for which an occupational therapy practitioner serves as an expert witness, they must uphold ethical principles and standards in this role.

Relation to the AOTA Code of Ethics

Several core values and ethics principles in the AOTA Code of Ethics (the Code) have relevance to an occupational therapy practitioner who is serving as an expert witness. Some are directly applicable to the requirements of that role, while others may be relevant to the testimony provided by the occupational therapy expert witness. The core values of altruism, justice, and truth, and the principles of *justice* and *veracity*, address the need for competence, adherence to rules and policies, and honesty in documentation and billing. An expert witness is utilized when there is a significant complaint or dispute about the services provided by a practitioner. Depending on the resolution, a practitioner may incur disciplinary sanctions on their license, lose their job, have to pay fines, or even serve time in prison. Therefore, it is critical that occupational therapy practitioners serving as expert witnesses follow ethical guidelines and standards of conduct.

Just as occupational therapy practitioners must be competent to provide services to clients, an expert witness must be highly knowledgeable about the area of practice for which they are testifying. The court will base the credibility of the practitioner's professional opinion on their knowledge of current, evidence-based practice and standards, or on customary and usual care applicable to the practice setting. This includes knowing about assessment tools and intervention techniques that are appropriate and those that are contraindicated or outdated. The expert witness must also consider applicable regulations and policies, as the scope of occupational therapy practice differs from state to state. Expert witnesses must be truthful in their testimony and must ensure that all of their billing and documentation is accurate, appropriate, and reasonable. Exhibit 22.1 contains ethical standards from the Code related to serving as an expert witness.

EXHIBIT 22.1.
ETHICAL STANDARDS RELATED TO SERVING AS AN EXPERT WITNESS

- Comply with current federal and state laws, state scope of practice guidelines, and AOTA policies and official documents that apply to the profession of occupational therapy.
- Do not engage in conflicts of interest or conflicts of commitment in employment, volunteer roles, or research.
- Bill and collect fees justly and legally in a manner that is fair, reasonable, and commensurate with services delivered.
- Ensure that documentation for reimbursement purposes is done in accordance with applicable laws, guidelines, and regulations.
- Use, to the extent possible, evaluation, planning, intervention techniques, assessments, and therapeutic equipment that are evidence based, current, and within the recognized scope of occupational therapy practice.
- Provide occupational therapy services, including education and training, that are within each practitioner's level of competence and scope of practice.
- Hold requisite credentials for the occupational therapy services one provides in academic, research, physical, or virtual work settings.
- Represent credentials, qualification, education, experience, training, roles, duties, competence, contributions, and findings accurately in all forms of communication.
- Ensure that all duties delegated to other occupational therapy personnel are congruent with their credentials, qualifications, experience, competencies, and scope of practice with respect to service delivery, supervision, fieldwork education, and research.
- Maintain the confidentiality of all verbal, written, electronic, augmentative, and nonverbal communications in compliance with applicable laws, including all aspects of privacy laws and exceptions thereto.

Note. From the Standards of Conduct from the AOTA Code of Ethics.

Reference to Other AOTA Documents

- The Standards of Practice for Occupational Therapy state that an occupational therapy practitioner must be knowledgeable about evidence-based assessment and intervention, use professional reasoning, and document according to standards and regulations. The standards are helpful to practitioners serving as expert witnesses as well as serving clients or students.
- The American Occupational Therapy Association (AOTA) website houses many other valuable documents for practitioners wanting to serve as expert witnesses. These include the AOTA official documents as well as articles, handouts, and tips regarding assessment, intervention, and documentation in a variety of practice settings (AOTA, n.d.).

Tips

- The expert witness must be competent to identify critical pieces of information, analyze them, and provide an objective opinion or recommendation on the basis of the material they are asked to review. They will typically be asked to provide documentation of their competency to render an opinion. This could include education and employment history (settings and roles), publications, and professional activities and positions (especially those that may represent a potential conflict of interest). Expert witnesses must remember that their primary duty is to the court, not to the party that hired them. They should provide Independent, objective, and unbiased evidence; a written report and oral evidence that is truthful and thorough in professional reasoning; and an honest opinion, even if it doesn't support their client's case (Hadley-Piggin, 2016).
- An expert witness should clearly state when a question or issue is outside their area of expertise or knowledge (O'Neil, 2017).
- Being an expert witness requires the practitioner to be highly accurate, attend to detail, write detailed reports, and demonstrate excellent verbal skills. The occupational therapy practitioner must also be available and have the stamina to provide a well-reasoned opinion throughout the duration of the case, which could last months to years (Franks, 2022).

Next Steps

When an occupational therapy practitioner is called to serve as an expert witness, ethical behavior is as important as competence and expertise. The expert witness must

- ensure the currency, validity, and reliability of resources and tools used to adequately evaluate the case material;
- ensure knowledge and adherence to clinical practice guidelines, professional standards, and research evidence;

- protect patient confidentiality;
- stay within the boundaries of the scope of the profession and personal knowledge and expertise;
- maintain objectivity and avoid the appearance of impropriety (e.g., conflicts of interest and exaggeration); and
- maintain awareness of what must be disclosed (Rule 26, Federal Rules of Civil Procedure; knowledge of the Daubert Test: Evidence 702). A 1923 legal case, *Frye v. United States*, lists factors to determine the reliability of expert witnesses, rules of evidence, and what can be admitted as evidence. Similarly, *Daubert v. Merrill* (1993) expanded *Frye v. United States*. The *Daubert test* is "a method that federal district courts use to determine whether expert testimony is admissible under Federal Rule of Evidence 702, which generally requires that expert testimony consist of scientific, technical, or other specialized knowledge that will assist the fact-finder in understanding the evidence or determining a fact in issue. In its role as 'gatekeeper' of the evidence, the trial court must decide whether the proposed expert testimony meets the requirements of relevance and reliability" (Garner, 2009, p. 453). Even though the Daubert test governs an evaluation of the expert witness testimony, that testimony should be based on scientific evidence and the quality of that evidence. These points are used by courts to determine reliability.
- Maintain records of resources, references, and standards that were used, and keep records of what was done and when it was done.

The amount of competence and expertise that the expert witness needs may vary depending on the case. Typically, attorneys will want an occupational therapy practitioner with evidence of experience and competence in areas relevant to the case. Being conscientious and transparent is a professional and ethical imperative, as is the ability to remain calm and answer questions clearly and confidently.

Expert witnesses are entitled to reasonable compensation. It is important that the occupational therapy practitioner establish fees at the outset of an expert witness engagement. Some employers have established policies and preset expert witness rates depending on employees' levels of experience. It is not acceptable for an occupational therapy practitioner to work as an expert witness on a contingency basis (i.e., fees to be paid based on the outcome of the case), because this establishes the most fundamental type of bias—financial interest in the outcome of the case. Fair compensation is typically based on hourly rates, with one rate for research, preparation, and analysis, and potentially a higher daily rate for testimony. Credibility is at risk when there is a large discrepancy between the rate being charged and the usual and customary rate for an expert witness (i.e., was this expert "bought" to express a particular opinion?; Bergman & Moore, 2010).

In establishing expert witness fees, occupational therapy practitioners acting as independent contractors should consider the following:

- their typical hourly wage for their services in clinical situations
- the relative loss of revenue if they are unable to treat (and charge) patients during the time they are serving as an expert witness
- the amount of time needed for preparation

- the range of fees charged by other occupational therapy practitioners who serve as expert witnesses
- their unique qualifications and the relative value of their accumulated expertise (likely the most important and variable factor influencing the rate).

Following these steps will ensure the occupational therapy practitioner is billing for services in an appropriate manner, as required by the Code.

CASE EXAMPLE 22.1. ACTING AS AN EXPERT WITNESS

Charley, an occupational therapist, came to work one day at Valley Pediatric Clinic and told **Tonya,** another therapist, that a parent had lodged a complaint and lawyers were involved. Charley said, "I'm really scared I could lose my license. The child was referred for severe feeding issues. I'm not certified for feeding therapy, but **Janine** (the occupational therapy manager) showed me some techniques she learned at her Level II fieldwork 6 years ago. It's been going okay, but the child does cough and gag a lot. The parents are in the middle of an acrimonious divorce and now Parent A is claiming that Parent B is getting therapy for the child that is harmful and out of our scope of practice. The attorney for Parent B just sent us a letter saying they are going to look for an occupational therapy expert witness to back us up." Tonya thought for a few minutes and then told Charley, "I have 10 years of experience in pediatrics, I've been to several workshops at the national conference about pediatric feeding, I treated three feeding clients a few years ago, and I was at the top of my class in school. I could be an expert witness for Parent B." Charley felt hopeful and agreed to pass Tonya's contact information along to Parent B's attorney.

Parent B's attorney agreed to hire Tonya as an expert witness, after seeing her CV which stated that she was certified in pediatric feeding techniques and had 10 years of experience in pediatric feeding. When reviewing all the records provided by the attorney, Tonya noticed that Charley's documentation did not include any parent education on swallowing precautions. There was also no evidence to show that Janine supervised or taught Charley, or that Charley demonstrated competence in the feeding techniques. Tonya did not mention this to Parent B's attorney or put it in her report, as they were paying her, and she wanted to help them and Charley.

Tonya was scheduled for a deposition with the attorneys for both parents. Parent A's attorney questioned Tonya's qualifications and asked for proof of her feeding certification. Tonya was unable to provide it and was disqualified as an expert witness. During the deposition of Parent A's expert witness, the witness testified that there was no evidence to show that Charley was competent, especially because the techniques Charley used were outdated. Evidence was presented that showed the techniques had frequently led to aspiration in the past with other clients and did not meet current standards of practice. Parent B and the attorney were blindsided, as Tonya had not mentioned any of this in her report or deposition. Parent B lost the case, and Charley and Janine incurred disciplinary action by their state regulatory board. In turn, the regulatory board reported Tonya to the AOTA Ethics Commission.

Questions
1. At different times, Tonya violated various standards of conduct from the Code. Which standards were violated and when?
2. It appears that Tonya recognized some issues when reviewing the medical records. What should she have done at that point?
3. After the Ethics Commission receives the complaint, what should the next steps be? (See the Enforcement Procedures for the process the Ethics Commission must follow.)

Summary

Serving as an expert witness can be an important role for an occupational therapy practitioner. Legal and ethical considerations, as well as specific competencies, must be considered. The occupational therapy practitioner serving as an expert witness has an ethical duty to possess advanced knowledge and skills in the subject area for which they are testifying and to uphold any laws and regulations related to their practice and their role as expert witness.

Acknowledgments

Wayne L. Winistorfer, MPA, OTR; and **Deborah Yarett Slater, MS, OT/L, FAOTA**, authored an earlier edition of this Advisory Opinion.

REFERENCES

American Occupational Therapy Association. (n.d.). *AOTA official documents*. https://www.aota.org/practice/practice-essentials/aota-official-documents

Bergman, P., & Moore, A. (2010). *NOLO's deposition handbook* (5th ed.). NOLO.

Cloudlex. (2023). *What is an expert witness?* https://www.cloudlex.com/glossary/what-is-an-expert-witness/

Daubert v. Merrell Dow Pharmaceuticals, Inc., (1993) No. 92-102.

Federal Rules of Civil Procedure for the United States District Courts: Title V. Disclosures and Discovery Rule 26. Duty to Disclose; General Provisions Governing Discovery Effective September 16, 1938, as amended to December 1, 2014. https://www.uscourts.gov/sites/default/files/federal_rules_of_civil_procedure_december_1_2022_0.pdf

Federal Rules of Evidence: Opinions and Expert Testimony: Article VII, Rule 703. Effective July 1, 1975, as amended to December 1, 2014. https://www.google.com/url?q=https://www.uscourts.gov/sites/default/files/federal_rules_of_evidence_-_december_2020_0.pdf&sa=D&source=docs&ust=1698947911419116&usg=AOvVaw0zMEND9_55BCNzrTSm4rT6

Franks, B. (2022). *The role of an occupational therapist as an expert witness*. https://nrtimes.co.uk/the-role-of-an-occupational-therapist-as-an-expert-witness-somek/

Frye v. United States. 293 F. 1013 (D.C. Cir. 1923).

Garner, B. A. (Ed). (2009). *Black's law dictionary* (9th ed.). West.

Hadley-Piggin, J. (2016). Expert evidence: The roles and responsibilities of the expert witness. *Keystone Law*. https://www.keystonelaw.com/keynotes/expert-evidence-the-roles-and-responsibilities-of-the-expert-witness

O'Neil, C. (2017). *The duties and responsibilities of expert witnesses*. https://www.lexology.com/firms/jams/charles_o_neil_

Robinson, J. (2023). Legal information institute. *Cornell Law School*. https://www.law.cornell.edu/wex/expert_witness

Ronquillo, Y., Robinson, K. J., & Nouhan, P. P. (2023). *Expert witness*. StatPearls Publishing. https://www.ncbi.nlm.nih.gov/books/NBK43600

Client Abandonment

ASHLEY WAGNER, OTD, OTR/L

Key Points

- Client abandonment results when an occupational therapy practitioner withdraws from necessary client treatment without giving reasonable notice or providing a competent replacement.
- Legally—An occupational therapy practitioner must be aware of the state and organizational policies regarding client abandonment where they work.
- Ethically—An occupational therapy practitioner must find a balance between client needs and practitioner rights and responsibilities to ensure that the process of stepping away from the ongoing care needs of a client upholds the ethical standards of the profession.

Introduction

Although the legal definition of *client abandonment* varies in specifics across states, most definitions state that occupational therapy practitioners stepping away from the care of a client with ongoing service needs must provide sufficient notice to facilitate an appropriate transition of care and limit any foreseeable harm to the client (Indest, 2012). Additionally, some state laws speak to client autonomy or collaboration surrounding the discontinuation or transition of care and to the practitioner's role in establishing an interim plan of care for a client when a gap in skilled services is anticipated (Weissberg, 2019). While all occupational therapy practitioners are expected to adhere to the legal guidelines relevant to their practice and license, practitioners are also expected to consider their ethical responsibilities when terminating the therapeutic relationship with a client who continues to benefit from skilled occupational therapy services.

Assuming that the occupational therapy practitioner is stepping away from the client for appropriate or involuntary reasons (e.g., employment change, client relocation, identified conflict of interest), the ethical responsibility of the practitioner then focuses on ensuring a timely transition plan (as defined by legal or organizational policy) is established that limits client harm while promoting client autonomy. Outgoing providers should provide appropriate referrals and complete any relevant paperwork to assist in this transition.

They should collaborate with their supervisor and other practitioners as appropriate to avoid unnecessary gaps in care. They should also avoid creating hostile environments in or during the termination of their therapeutic relationship that would make it harder for the client to establish a healthy therapeutic relationship with any future practitioner who assumes their care (Weissberg, 2019). While such a responsibility may initially seem straightforward, contextual circumstances may contribute to ethical tension for the practitioner as they work to balance continuity of client care with available resources and practitioner rights.

Ethical tensions may arise, for example, if a client is no longer able to pay for services after an occupational therapy practitioner has assumed their care; or if a barrier to ensuring necessary services can continue is created by geography, change in client medical status, or transportation issues. Grajo and Rushanan (2022) speak to the possible ethical tension surrounding termination of services that results from limitations of financial or staffing resources. The authors propose that knowing and assisting the client in accessing resources available within the community is ethically necessary to mitigate the harm caused by terminating the therapeutic relationship. Another suggestion to mitigate such harm can be the transparent collaboration with clients as soon as possible after the practitioner knows that termination of the therapeutic relationship is imminent.

Allowing clients to prepare for the upcoming transition and empowering them to participate in transition planning will help them prepare for the loss of the therapeutic relationship and any negative emotions or sense of abandonment that they may experience as a result (Govender, 2015). While harm stemming from the relational loss to the client is never the intended or even predicted outcome of terminating client care, the potential for such harm should be considered in how an occupational therapy practitioner approaches the transition. Acknowledging the potential of such emotional harm should reinforce the ethical importance of prompt notification of any anticipated disruption to the relationship. This ethical responsibility even holds true for situations involving temporary service provision, such as with research or clinical fieldwork students. Therefore, it is the ethical responsibility of all practitioners involved in client care and project supervision to consider whether the beneficence of temporary services outweighs the potential harm of feelings of abandonment in situations where continuity of care cannot be ensured and to mitigate such harm through advanced notice and open collaboration with the client (Govender, 2015).

Occupational therapy practitioners, students, researchers, and therapy managers alike may feel ethical distress when contextual aspects limit their ability to provide ongoing care for a client in need of services. However, it should be emphasized that the ethical responsibility of occupational therapy providers encompasses ensuring timely notification (as defined by legal or organizational policy) and appropriate transition planning to mitigate harm that may arise from termination of care. Before terminating the therapeutic relationship, all applicable documentation should be completed, all necessary referrals should be made, and care should be taken to collaborate with the client and future service providers, as feasible. It is not the ethical responsibility of the occupational therapy practitioner to continue client care indefinitely until a comparable service provider can take over care or until the client no longer needs skilled therapeutic services (Weissburg, 2019).

Relation to the AOTA Code of Ethics

The ethical standards that relate to client abandonment are outlined in Exhibit 23.1.

EXHIBIT 23.1.
ETHICAL STANDARDS RELATED TO CLIENT ABANDONMENT

- Do not abandon the service recipient, and attempt to facilitate appropriate transitions when unable to provide services for any reason.
- Refer to other providers when indicated by the needs of the client.

Note. From the Standards of Conduct from the AOTA Code of Ethics.

Reference to Other Standards

The following sources may be useful references when considering ethical practice regarding client abandonment:

- applicable legal guidelines on client/patient abandonment, transition planning, and termination of services
- transition planning and documentation guidelines set by payment sources (e.g., Medicare, Medicaid and other third-party payers; see Centers for Medicare & Medicaid Services, n.d.)
- employer policies and procedures relevant to this topic.

Tips

If the therapeutic relationship must be terminated while there is an ongoing need for client care, ethical occupational therapy practitioners will, within their ability and given the context of termination, work to ensure that the following occur:

- legal and organizational policies related to termination or transition of client services are followed
- the employer and client are given sufficient notice of the upcoming transition
- a transitional plan of care is established in collaboration with the client
- all remaining documentation, billing, and paperwork are completed in a timely manner, in accordance with legal or organizational policies
- continuity of care is established via communication of client needs and priorities to future occupational therapy providers assuming care of the client
- referrals to other service providers and community resources are offered as appropriate.

As always, to the extent possible, client well-being should be prioritized throughout the transition to avoid the occurrence or perception of client abandonment.

CASE EXAMPLE 23.1. LEAVING IN THE MIDDLE OF THE SCHOOL YEAR

An **occupational therapy practitioner** is working in a small school district where they share the district caseload with two other practitioners. Near the middle of November, the practitioner gets an offer from a different organization where they have always wanted to work. They are sad to leave their colleagues and the students with whom they have been working during this school year, but they know that this new employment opportunity is best for them and their family. They arrange to start with the new organization in January.

The occupational therapy practitioner goes to their supervisor with the news about a week after they accept the position. They deliver a letter of resignation, discuss their plans to complete documentation before transitioning, and offer to help with the hiring and orientation of a new practitioner to replace them. The supervisor accepts the letter, but seems offended and questions the practitioner's ethics in "abandoning their clients" in the middle of the school year. The clinician is shaken by this response and seeks guidance from their colleagues, who remind them that they didn't sign a contract binding them to complete the school year. Still, the clinician worries that perhaps the supervisor is correct and they have acted unethically.

Questions
1. Does leaving a school district in the middle of a school year constitute client abandonment?
2. What steps can the practitioner take to address the ethical uncertainty they are experiencing?

CASE EXAMPLE 23.2. RESEARCH IN A RURAL COMMUNITY

An occupational therapy **faculty member** is conducting research on telehealth services for the rural community. As part of the study, short-term, virtual occupational therapy intervention will be provided to older adults who are returning home to a rural community without access to occupational therapy services after an acute hospital stay.

Question
1. Knowing that some clients will need services beyond what is offered during the research intervention, what ethical responsibilities must the researcher fulfill to avoid client abandonment?

Summary

Although in an ideal world all clients would receive the skilled services they deserve without disruption, realistically, there will be times when disruption is unavoidable. In such times, the occupational therapy practitioner should ensure that all applicable legal requirements are met to avoid client abandonment. They should also act to promptly notify their supervisor and client. Before terminating the therapeutic relationship, all applicable documentation should be completed, all necessary referrals should be made, and care should be taken to collaborate with the client and future service providers, as feasible. The ethical focus in such cases should be on mitigating harm to the client and ensuring continuity of care and client autonomy to as great an extent as possible.

Acknowledgment

John F. Morris, PhD, authored an earlier edition of this Advisory Opinion.

REFERENCES

Centers for Medicare & Medicaid Services. (n.d.). *Regulations and guidance.* https://www.cms.gov/Regulations-and-Guidance/Regulations-and-Guidance

Govender, P. (2015). An ethical dilemma: A case of student training, intermittent service and impact on service delivery. *African Journal of Health Professions Education, 7*(1), 8–9. https://doi.org/10.7196/AJHPE.405

Grajo, L. C., & Rushanan, S. G. (2022). Ethical decision making in occupational therapy practice. In J. Clifford O'Brien, & J. Welch Solomon (Eds.), *Occupational analysis and group process* (2nd ed., pp. 174–184). Elsevier.

Indest, G. F. (2012). *Patient abandonment.* https://www.thehealthlawfirm.com/resources/health-law-articles-and-documents/Patient-Abandonment.html

Weissberg, K. D. (2019). *Client abandonment and potential ethical concerns.* https://www.physical-therapy.com/ask-the-experts/client-abandonment-and-potential-ethical-4271

24

Responding to Public Health Crises

BRENDA S. HOWARD, DHSc, OTR, FAOTA

Key Points

- Public health crises require a macro approach to health management.
- Occupational therapy practitioners have a role in public health crises.
- Roles in health crises can include leadership on ethics committees, team management to evacuate disaster survivors with disabilities, modifying environments, infection control, monitoring and providing support for the physical and mental health of the interprofessional team, and educating caregivers of survivors.

Introduction

Occupational therapy practitioners are no strangers to a crisis. Birthed in the aftermath of World War I and seasoned by the Great Depression and World War II (Peters & Reed, 2006), in the United States the profession has survived and thrived while helping others live meaningfully. The years have brought increasingly complex health care challenges, and occupational therapy practitioners have consistently met those challenges. However, the ethical challenges arising with public health crises, such as the COVID-19 pandemic, caused a rise in the moral distress experienced by practitioners resulting from competing duties and obligations. Practitioners had to balance issues surrounding personnel and supply allocation, a duty to provide care versus duty to self and their loved ones' safety, and concerns regarding equitable resource allocation and shifting scope of practice.

Responding to a public health crisis requires a different mindset than responding to a personal health crisis. Personal health crisis responses take place on a micro, or individual, level, as does much of occupational therapy service provision. Public health crises take place on a macro level, such as on a community, regional, national, or world level, and require a system-wide response. Occupational therapy practitioners must be aware of how to contribute to an ethical response to a public health crisis, and how to find resources available to support practitioners during a time of crisis.

Ethical Responses During Disasters in Health Care

HEALTH CARE TEAM RESPONSE

On a global front, health care practitioners are increasingly faced with emerging and re-emerging disease threats resulting from a wake of natural disasters, wars, terror attacks, and pandemics. On the heels of the 9/11 terrorist attacks, the Ebola crisis, the severe acute respiratory syndrome (SARS) epidemic, and health crises post–Hurricane Katrina, among others, questions arose regarding the preparedness of the health industry to adequately respond to these threats (Holt, 2008; World Health Organization [WHO], 2007). Moreover, health care practitioners have experienced an increase in moral distress while trying to negotiate the growing ethical concerns related to responding to these threats. *Moral distress* has been defined as, "when a moral agent (e.g., a practitioner) is unsure of the best course of action to take or encounters a barrier that prohibits doing what he or she knows to be right" (Erler, 2017, p. 15). Practitioners' duty to care for their clients has come into direct conflict with their duties to safeguard the health of themselves and their families (Iserson, et al., 2008; Ulrich, 2020). Globally, there is a need to develop ethical guidelines and standards of care that will address the crisis practitioners face amid these growing threats.

A new specialty of medicine has emerged to address these particular needs. *Disaster medicine* focuses on changing current standards of care to meet the unique challenges faced during these unusual times (Holt, 2008). Additionally, in 2007, WHO released specific guidelines for preventing infection and controlling disease during epidemic and pandemic outbreaks. These guidelines focused on continuous and sustainable improvements in safety in health care, specifically for acute respiratory diseases. The *Journal of Clinical Ethics* dedicated an entire volume to addressing medical practice during disasters and pandemics (Howe, 2010). This volume examined issues surrounding standards of care, resource allocation, and preparedness.

However, despite these discussions, few efforts have been made to apply consistent disaster management strategies on a macro or global level (Civaner et al., 2017; Leider et al., 2017). It is no wonder that health care workers have experienced moral distress; the systems could not be in place to support ethical decision making on a micro level when adequate disaster management planning has not been in place on a macro level. Compounding this lack of macro strategies is the problem of pressure on health care workers. During the COVID-19 crisis, health care workers were challenged by the twofold issues of lacking clear direction from administrators and managing the daily overwhelming burden on the health care system that the crisis precipitated. The workers also had to juggle the adverse effects, physically, mentally, and economically, that the health crisis perpetrated on the workers themselves and their families (Adams & Walls, 2020). Additional issues raised for medical personnel include HIPAA compliance vs. public health need to know (U.S. Department of Health and Human Services Office for Civil Rights, 2020); and health disparities regarding resource allocation and illness recovery related to culture, race, ethnicity, disability, coexisting conditions, and age (Biddison et al., 2018; Leider et al., 2017; McCullough, 2010; Parente et al., 2017). During this time, practitioners reported experiencing increased moral distress (Ulrich, 2020).

Often in times of crisis, decision making turns away from altruism and duty to utilitarian considerations of outcomes (Berger, 2010). Practitioners have reported feeling powerless while emotionally and physically worn out (Ulrich, 2020). Health care practitioners routinely accept the inherent risks of their jobs on a daily basis; however, the rising risks during public health crises call for clearer, evidence-based, and practical standards and protections. Practitioners have balanced competing duties to provide care, duties to society as a whole, and duties to themselves and their families. Thus, guidelines on how to prioritize care, protect clients, and protect the health care practitioners have become of the utmost priority (Ulrich, 2020).

Berlinger and colleagues (2020) provided specific guidelines and standards to address health care needs during times of crisis. With an emphasis on fairness, duty to care, duty to steward resources, transparency, and accountability, these guidelines focus on preparation, resource allocation concerns, and adapting to the situation. Keys to help mitigate the distress experienced by practitioners must also include adequate education, staff training, organizational transparency, and communication (Ulrich, 2020). With appropriate standards in place, health care practitioners can have a greater sense of control along with opportunities to safely meet their professional obligations while also feeling protected (Iserson et al., 2008).

The rising emergence of epidemics and pandemics is a global concern. It is clear efforts are emerging to address the rising concerns faced by health care practitioners worldwide. However, these efforts are small, and efforts on a larger, coordinated scale need to occur to secure optimal response during these times. Berlinger and colleagues (2020) indicated that global efforts must focus on three primary duties: duty to plan, including adequate triage measures; duty to safeguard health care practitioners; and duty to guide practice. As part of this planning, health care practitioners need to balance care for those who fall ill and care for themselves. It is up to health care practitioners to advocate and take action to help ensure that sufficient standards and guidelines are in place to protect all those affected, including themselves.

OCCUPATIONAL THERAPY'S RESPONSE

The role of occupational therapy practitioners in public health crisis response is supported in the literature through professional statements and recommendations. Examples of occupational therapy practitioners as part of interprofessional public health crisis teams include responding to hurricanes, earthquakes, and displacement as a result of armed conflict (Parente et al., 2017). The World Federation of Occupational Therapists (WFOT) and the American Occupational Therapy Association (AOTA) have supported occupational therapy practitioners' involvement at all levels of disaster response planning, from local to national and international, and from preparation to post-disaster and long-term rehabilitation efforts (AOTA, 2017; WFOT, 2014). Practitioners are well prepared to support the health care team and community in such times, by assuming leadership roles on ethics committees and in team management to plan for moving and evacuating disaster survivors with disabilities, modifying environments to accommodate persons with disabilities and address infection control, monitoring physical and mental health barriers to functioning, and considering caregivers of survivors as indirect survivors of disaster (AOTA, 2017; Parente et al., 2017; WFOT, 2014).

Following a disaster, displaced persons need to re-establish routines, occupations, and livelihoods; occupational therapy practitioners can focus on these concerns as well as the mental health and well-being of all disaster survivors (WFOT, 2014). Occupational therapy practitioners are distinctly positioned to monitor and intervene for the health and well-being of the health care team responding to disasters. Practitioners in planning and response roles can ensure that health care workers have scheduled shifts and breaks, housing, food and water supply, and alternative child care so the team can continue to provide needed care to survivors (Adams & Walls, 2020; Hick et al., 2020; Koh & Hoenig, 2020). Occupational therapy practitioners can help alleviate anxiety in the health care team by taking an educative role in infection control and self-care, and maintaining a sense of control and building trust within the team during a crisis (Adams & Walls, 2020).

Inevitably in a health care crisis, resources become a concern. Occupational therapy practitioners can practice and educate others in strategies from the Crisis Standards of Care (Hick et al., 2020), including preparing, conserving, substituting, adapting, reusing, and re-allocating resources. The role of occupational therapy practitioners in disaster preparedness and response directly relates to alleviating ethical challenges: "It is only by making great efforts before disasters, that ethical challenges can be minimized in disaster responses" (Ozge Karadag & Kerim Hakan, 2012, p. 602).

Employers may ask occupational therapy practitioners to operate in nontraditional ways during a time of crisis. Although practitioners may consider some duties outside their scope of practice, they must consider that some duties they perform during crises are in the role of an employee, not the role of a practitioner. For example, during the COVID-19 pandemic, occupational therapy practitioners were given duty reassignments to take temperatures of visitors and monitor traffic flow; act as nursing assistants to bathe, dress, and toilet patients; serve on proning teams; deliver meals and educational packets to students in school systems; and a variety of other roles not directly supported by occupational therapy's scope of practice in the *Occupational Therapy Practice Framework: Domain and Process*. The practitioner may need to consider whether they have the skill set to complete these tasks and whether they can separate their role as an occupational therapy practitioner from their role as an employee. As an example, if a practitioner is performing a particular task that they do not consider to be occupational therapy, and they are not billing or coding the task as occupational therapy, they can perform the task as an employee, just as they would routinely complete such tasks as scheduling, restocking supplies, and cleaning the treatment area. The practitioner may also need to ask themselves if they feel confident and safe in performing these tasks. If the answer is no, then discussions with supervisors may be necessary to determine a path forward.

Relation to the AOTA Code of Ethics

The AOTA Code of Ethics (the Code) contains core values to which occupational therapy practitioners adhere, even in times of crisis. These core values include *altruism*, or demonstrating unselfish concern for the welfare of others; *justice*, which includes uphold-ing moral and legal principles, inclusivity, and equitable resource allocation; *dignity*, or valuing, promoting, and preserving the inherent worth and uniqueness of each person; and *prudence*, using reason to govern oneself, reflect, and temper extremes for ethical reason-ing. Ethical principles of *beneficence*, or demonstrating a concern for the well-being and safety of persons; and *justice*, or promoting equity, inclusion, and objectivity, especially apply in times of public health crisis. Ethical standards from the Code that apply to public health crises include, but are not limited to, those listed in Exhibit 24.1.

Reference to Other AOTA Documents

AOTA has made resources available to address the COVID-19 public health crisis (AOTA, n.d.). These include resources to support practitioner well-being. Staying in touch with how other occupational therapy practitioners have coped during a crisis can help to allevi-ate the moral distress brought about by feeling isolated and overwhelmed.

Reference to Other Standards and Guidance Documents

The WFOT has made resources available for occupational therapists working in areas of disaster, armed conflict, and crisis (WFOT, n.d.). One of the documents provides lists of "do's and don'ts" for rehabilitation service providers during provision of humanitarian aid.

Many professional and interprofessional organizations have issued statements and provided resources for pragmatic and ethical management of a pandemic. The Hastings Center has provided an ethical framework and guidelines for responding to the pandemic (Berlinger et al., 2020). The Centers for Disease Control and Prevention (CDC; 2020) and WHO (2020) have likewise provided resources for disaster management. Other resources are available that were developed during previous health crises and can provide guidance

EXHIBIT 24.1.
ETHICAL STANDARDS RELATED TO RESPONDING TO PUBLIC HEALTH CRISES

- Provide occupational therapy services, including education and training, that are within each practitioner's level of competence and scope of practice.
- Provide professional services within the scope of occupational therapy practice during com-munity-wide public health emergencies as directed by federal, state, and local agencies.
- Treat all stakeholders professionally and equitably through constructive engagement and dialogue that is inclusive, collaborative, and respectful of diversity of thought.

Note. From the Standards of Conduct from the AOTA Code of Ethics.

(Hick et al., 2020; Holt, 2008; McCullough, 2010). Information on how to support health care workers during a crisis is also available (Adams & Walls, 2020; Ulrich, 2020).

Tips

Occupational therapy practice, interventions, services, and information or referral during a health care crisis must reflect the highest standards, duties, ethical principles, and professionalism of practitioners, supervisors, leaders, facilities, organizations, and policymakers. Although health care delivery at such times is not "normal," occupational therapy practitioners strive to do their best work in challenging conditions that are fraught with professional and personal choices that are almost unimaginable in other times.

To accomplish these ends, decisions must meet the following criteria:

- Do no harm.
- Include and actively involve all relevant parties.
- Incorporate current information on the emerging crisis.
- Reinforce informed consent.
- Uphold AOTA core values.
- Be transparent and provide clear communication through documentation.
- Respect patient and client autonomy.
- Be consistent with public health declarations from appropriate government officials.

These criteria are consistent with the core values and principles of the Code.

CASE EXAMPLE 24.1. COMMUNITY-BASED SETTING DURING A PANDEMIC

Brianna was an occupational therapy assistant (OTA) who worked in a community-based early intervention (EI) program in a rural area of the Southwest. She provided occupational therapy services to children from birth to age 5 years, and their families, many of whom struggled with poverty. Brianna served children in various settings, including their homes and day care centers, as well as in community- and school-based preschool programs. She was a single mom with 12-year-old twin boys. She was also the primary caregiver for her mother, who had chronic obstructive pulmonary disease.

As the COVID-19 pandemic began to escalate rapidly around the country, the governor of Brianna's state ordered all educational programs to close. Brianna, her occupational therapy supervisor, and the rest of her work team met virtually to discuss options for continued service provision. The team agreed that services via telehealth were an option to discuss and offer to families. However, the team discovered that most families did not have the technological resources necessary to access such services. The team agreed the next best option was to offer services and support via phone and text consultation, although data collection would be a challenge. Nearly all the families expressed interest in receiving continued support and services in this manner, but many mentioned that they had few educational materials or toys in their homes. The director of the EI program recommended the work

(Continued)

CASE EXAMPLE 24.1. COMMUNITY-BASED SETTING DURING A PANDEMIC *(Cont.)*

team gather in groups of 10 people to assemble individual packets of educational and play materials for delivery to families that needed them.

Brianna expressed concern to both her occupational therapy supervisor and the program director about physically gathering in a group to prepare the materials. Her mother's underlying respiratory concerns caused her significant apprehension regarding this plan. The supervisor responded by stating that if staff members were not experiencing any COVID-19 symptoms, it seemed safe to gather in groups.

The EI program director responded to Brianna's concerns by reinforcing that all staff were expected to participate because, "We are a team, and other people are getting together for essential work." She offered no alternative options for Brianna or other staff members who expressed reluctance to participate, even though Brianna volunteered to assemble all the materials by herself. Brianna also initiated working with her team members to develop a resource document of educational and therapeutic activities using common household materials, negating the need for a work team to gather to prepare physical materials.

As the day to assemble materials approached, Brianna experienced significant moral distress, combined with general anxiety, as diagnosed cases of COVID-19 in her community increased. She remained conflicted on how to balance ethical responsibilities to her employer and clients, and to herself and her family, especially given her role as primary caregiver for her mother. She also believed she had an obligation to the community to minimize the potential spread of the virus.

Questions
1. What are the competing ethical issues Brianna must decide among?
2. How might Brianna use a framework for ethical decision making to help her decide what to do?
3. What resources could Brianna use to help guide her ethical decision making?

Summary

During public health crises, occupational therapy practitioners must focus on making the best possible choices, given the extreme circumstances. Occupational therapy practitioners must weigh the options, confer with colleagues, seek out institutional and professional resources and guidance, follow ethical problem-solving steps, and make the best decisions they can during an extraordinarily difficult time. Furthermore, practitioners can and should step into leadership roles as part of the interprofessional team making decisions regarding disaster preparedness and management. When people look back on public health crises, history will not ask the question, "did they do the right thing?" but rather, "did they do all they could?" (McCullough, 2010). As occupational therapy practitioners focus on the guiding values that strengthen advocacy for clients, the resounding answer will be, "yes."

CASE EXAMPLE 24.2. ACUTE CARE SETTING DURING A PANDEMIC

Lee was an occupational therapist practicing in an acute-care hospital. He had been in this position for 6 years and typically enjoyed the fast-paced, high acuity demands of this setting. Lee's primary responsibilities included providing evaluation and intervention for clients who were admitted to the neurology service; however, since the COVID-19 pandemic had begun to escalate in his state, there had been many iterations of staffing adjustments, and he now covered a combination of intensive care and medical units.

At first, Lee felt confident in his role as an occupational therapist in acute care, but as time passed and the pandemic continued to escalate, he started to question his safety, the safety of others, and whether his services were essential. The constantly changing personal protective equipment (PPE) guidelines, often with multiple as well as evolving reasons for the changes, caused significant moral distress. The changes, paired with strict conservation and reuse of PPE, overwhelmed Lee and his colleagues, who often questioned whether they had followed the correct procedures prior to entering the room of a client who had been diagnosed with COVID-19. Lee had mostly positive experiences with the interprofessional team, who came together to support each other in this time. For example, an ICU nurse helped check Lee's PPE before entering a room so he felt more confident. However, there was one instance when a physician saw him applying PPE prior to entering a client's room and commented that the patient did not need occupational therapy because it was not worth wasting the PPE. This made Lee question his value and role in the care of these clients.

Because of the moral distress and risk he was experiencing, Lee contemplated whether to stop coming to work. He was beginning to think that the benefit to his clients did not outweigh the risks.

Questions
1. Who could Lee turn to for assistance in clarifying options in this situation?
2. What are at least three other options Lee could choose besides not going to work?
3. What ethical principles could Lee use to help select a course of action?
4. To whom could Lee talk to communicate his decision?

Acknowledgments

Brenda S. Howard, DHSc, OTR, FAOTA; **Rebecca E. Argabrite Grove**, MS, OTR/L, FAOTA; **Leslie Bennett**, OTD, OTR/L; **Kimberly Erler**, PhD, OT, HEC-C; **Jan Keith**, BA, COTA/L; **Roger A. Ritvo**, PhD; **Brenda Kennell**, MA, OTR/L, FAOTA; and **Donna Ewy**, MD, FAAFP, MTS, MA, authored an earlier version of this Advisory Opinion.

Mark C. Franco, Ethics Commission Legal Counsel, provided input and review.

REFERENCES

Adams, J., & Walls, R. (2020). Supporting the health care workforce during the COVID-19 global epidemic. *Journal of the American Medical Association, 323,* 1439–1440. https://doi.org/10.1001/jama.2020.3972

American Occupational Therapy Association. (n.d.). *Occupational therapy in the age of Coronavirus (COVID-19)*. https://www.aota.org/practice/clinical-topics/covid-19

American Occupational Therapy Association. (2017). AOTA's societal statement on disaster response and risk reduction. *American Journal of Occupational Therapy, 71*(Suppl. 2), 7112410060. https://doi.org/10.5014/ajot.2017.716S11

Berger, J. (2010). Pandemic preparedness planning: Will provisions for involuntary termination of life support invite active euthanasia? *Journal of Clinical Ethics, 21*, 308–311. https://doi.org/10.1086/JCE201021405

Berlinger, N., Wynia, M., Powell, T., Hester, D. M., Milliken, A., Fabi, R., . . . Piper Jenks, N. (2020). *Ethical framework for health care institutions & guidelines for institutional ethics services responding to the coronavirus pandemic: Managing uncertainty, safeguarding communities, guiding practice*. https://www.thehastingscenter.org/ethicalframeworkcovid19/

Biddison, E., Gown, H., Schoch-Spana, M., Regenberg, A. C., Juliano, C., Faden, R. R., & Toner, E. S. (2018). Scare resource allocation during disasters: A mixed-method community engagement study. *Chest, 153*(1), 187–195. https://doi.org/10.1016/j.chest.2017.08.001

Centers for Disease Control and Prevention. (2020). *Coronavirus disease 2019 (COVID-19)*. https://www.cdc.gov/coronavirus/2019-ncov/index.html

Civaner, M. M., Vatansever, K., & Pala, K. (2017). Ethical problems in an era where disasters have become a part of daily life: A qualitative study of healthcare workers in Turkey. *PLoS ONE, 12*(3), e0174162. https://doi.org/10.1371/journal.pone.0174162

Erler, K. S. (2017). The role of occupational therapy in ethics rounds practice. *OT Practice, 22*(13), 15–18.

Hick, J., Hanfling, D., Wynia, M., & Pavia, A. (2020). Duty to plan: Health care, crisis standards of care, and novel coronavirus SARS-CoV-2. *Perspectives*, 1–13. https://doi.org/10.31478/202003b

Holt, G. R. (2008). Making difficult ethical decisions in patient care during natural disasters and other mass casualty events. *Otolaryngology–Head and Neck Surgery, 139*, 181–186. https://doi.org/10.1016/j.otohns.2008.04.027

Howe, E. G. (2010). A possible application of care-based ethics to people with disabilities during a pandemic. *Journal of Clinical Ethics, 21*, 275–283. https://doi.org/10.1086/JCE201021401

Iserson, K. V., Helne, C. E., Larkin, G. L., Moskop, J. C., Baruch, J., & Aswegan, A. L. (2008). Fight or flight: The ethics of emerging physician disaster response. *Annals of Emergency Medicine, 51*(4). https://doi.org/10.1016/j.annemergmed.2007.07.024

Koh, G. C.-H., & Hoenig, H. (2020). How should the rehabilitation community prepare for 2019-nCoV? *Archives of Physical Medicine and Rehabilitation, 101*, 1068–1071. https://doi.org/10.1016/j.apmr.2020.03.003

Leider, J., DeBruin, D., Reynolds, N., Koch, A., & Seaberg, J. (2017). Ethical guidance for disaster response, specifically around crisis standards of care: A systematic review. *American Journal of Public Health, 107*, e1–e9. https://doi.org/10.2105/AJPH.2017.303882

McCullough, L. (2010). Taking seriously the "what then?" question: An ethical framework for the responsible management of medical disasters. *Journal of Clinical Ethics, 21*, 321–327. https://doi.org/10.1086/JCE201021407

Ozge Karadag, C., & Kerim Hakan, A. (2012). Ethical dilemmas in disaster medicine. *Iran Red Crescent Medical Journal, 14*, 602–612.

Parente, M., Tofani, M., DeSantis, R., Esposito, G., Santilli, V., & Galeoto, G. (2017). The role of the occupational therapist in disaster areas: Systematic review. *Occupational Therapy International*, Article 6474761. https://doi.org/10.1155/2017/6474761

Peters, C., & Reed, K. (2006). Occupational therapy values and beliefs, part II: The great depression and war years. *OT Practice, 11*(18), 17–22.

Ulrich, C. M. (2020). Opinion: How do we protect health care workers from the coronavirus as they protect us? *Boston Globe*. https://www.bostonglobe.com/2020/03/10/opinion/how-do-we-protect- health-care-workers-coronavirus-they-protect-us/

U.S. Department of Health and Human Services, Office for Civil Rights. (2020). *HIPAA privacy and novel coronavirus*. https://www.hhs.gov/sites/default/files/february-2020-hipaa-and-novel-coronavirus.pdf

World Federation of Occupational Therapists. (n.d.). *Occupational therapy and humanitarian response*. https://wfot.org/occupational-therapy-and-humanitarian-response

World Federation of Occupational Therapists. (2014). *Occupational therapy in disaster preparedness and response*. https://wfot.org/resources/occupational-therapy-in-disaster-preparedness-and-response-dp-r

World Health Organization. (2007). *Infection prevention and control of epidemic-and pandemic-prone acute respiratory diseases in healthcare*. https://www.who.int/csr/resources/publications/csrpublications/en/index7.html

World Health Organization. (2020). *Coronavirus disease (COVID-19) outbreak*. https://www.who.int/westernpacific/emergencies/covid-19

Outdated and Obsolete Assessment Tools

BRENDA KORNBLIT KENNELL, MA, OTR/L, FAOTA

Key Points

- Assessment and evaluation materials must be current, evidence based, within the scope of occupational therapy practice, and within the practitioner's expertise.
- Assessment and evaluation materials must be relevant to the client being served.
- Occupational therapy practitioners must not plagiarize or infringe on copyrighted materials.

Introduction

The evaluation process and use of assessment tools in occupational therapy practice benefits the client by accurately reporting the client's capabilities (strengths) and limitations (deficits and weaknesses). According to the *Occupational Therapy Practice Framework: Domain and Process,* the evaluation process includes "assessment tools designed to analyze, measure, and inquire about factors that support or hinder occupational performance." The tools chosen must be tailored to the needs and abilities of each client in order to obtain valid and valuable information that will be used to determine intervention.

The problem of outdated and obsolete assessment tools is not unique to occupational therapy practice. Any discipline or profession that uses standardized assessment tools to gather client data has a similar concern. Normative data that are appropriate for one segment of the population may not necessarily accurately measure another segment. Older assessment tools might have been based on normative data from a sample of the population that does not have the characteristics of the client the occupational therapy practitioner is evaluating. Comparing a person's scores with normative data from a dissimilar group does not accurately indicate that person's capabilities and limitations (Kielhofner & Coster, 2017).

Standardized tests and assessments are copyrighted. It is an ethical and legal responsibility to use only forms or licensed electronic versions as purchased from the publisher, and not to make copies for personal or facility use unless explicitly allowed by the publisher

(Howard, 2014). In addition to violating copyright laws, using old photocopied materials can contribute to the use of tests, assessments, or norms that are obsolete.

Occupational therapy practitioners have an ethical responsibility to select, administer, score, and interpret assessment tools that accurately reflect the client in the context of time and personal factors. Assessment tools that are outdated, obsolete, culturally biased, or address other ages or diagnoses than those of the client may not accurately report a client's capabilities and limitations. Inaccurate measurement, such as errors in administration and scoring, or failure to administer essential components of the instrument, may result in unnecessary or ineffective intervention. If errors in administering and scoring have been observed and reported in published studies, if reliability and validity of the instrument have not been established in the literature, or if the conceptual model of the instrument is missing or discarded, the instrument should not be used (Adams, 2000; Butcher, 2000; Okazaki & Sue, 2000; Silverstein & Nelson, 2000; Strauss et al., 2000). In any of these cases, the client may not receive the full benefit of occupational therapy services because the instrument inaccurately identified limitations or capabilities during the evaluation process. The intervention might have been planned and implemented on the basis of incomplete, inaccurate, or missing facts and data. The occupational therapy practitioner should be knowledgeable about the accuracy and appropriate use of each assessment instrument used to measure client capacities and limitations. Any deficiencies in the application of the test or assessment instrument should be clearly stated in documentation reporting the data or summary.

Occupational therapy practitioners need to use evaluations that are evidence based and within the recognized scope of occupational therapy practice. In addition, occupational therapy practitioners have a responsibility to avoid the use of outdated or obsolete assessment tools, as well as data obtained from such tests, in making intervention decisions or recommendations. Therefore, practitioners also have a responsibility to determine when a test or assessment is considered outdated or obsolete. The Guidelines for Practitioner Use of Test Revisions, Obsolete Tests, and Test Disposal stated,

> Professionals engaged in good testing practices evaluate the potential utility of the test used, select technically sound tests in light of intended standards, recognize the importance of fair testing practices, prepare for the test session, administer tests properly, score and analyze test results accurately, interpret test results properly, communicate the results clearly and accurately, and review the appropriateness of the test and its uses. (Oakland, 2015, p. 1)

Relation to the AOTA Code of Ethics

The ethical use of test and assessment materials is addressed in sections of the AOTA Code of Ethics (the Code) relating to professional integrity, responsibility, and accountability; service delivery; and professional competence, education, supervision, and training. Exhibit 25.1 contains ethical standards from the Code related to outdated and obsolete assessment tools.

EXHIBIT 25.1.
ETHICAL STANDARDS RELATED TO OUTDATED AND OBSOLETE ASSESSMENT TOOLS

- Do not engage in actions that reduce the public's trust in occupational therapy.
- Record and report in an accurate and timely manner and in accordance with applicable regulations all information related to professional or academic documentation and activities.
- Provide appropriate evaluation and a plan of intervention for recipients of occupational therapy specific to their needs.
- Use, to the extent possible, evaluation, planning, intervention techniques, assessments, and therapeutic equipment that are evidence based, current, and within the recognized scope of occupational therapy practice.
- Do not accept gifts that would unduly influence the therapeutic relationship or have the potential to blur professional boundaries, and adhere to employer policies when offered gifts.
- Do not engage in dual relationships or situations in which an occupational therapy professional or student is unable to maintain clear professional boundaries or objectivity.

Note. From the Standards of Conduct from the AOTA Code of Ethics.

Reference to Other Standards

Assessment tools most often become outdated and obsolete because new revisions are published. Occupational therapy practitioners should be aware of revisions and make an effort to determine whether any of the reasons for revision are pertinent to the tests or assessments used in their practice areas. According to the Standards for Educational and Psychological Testing (American Educational Research Association, 2014):

> Tests and their supporting documents (e.g., test manuals, technical manuals, user guides) should be reviewed periodically to determine whether revisions are needed. Revisions or amendments are necessary when new research data, significant changes in the domain, or new conditions of test use and interpretation suggest that the test is no longer optimal or fully appropriate for some of its intended uses. As an example, tests are revised if the test content or language has become outdated and, therefore, may subsequently affect the validity of the test score interpretations. (pp. 83–84)

Tips

Here are some tips to ensure that a tool is appropriate to use:

- If a tool cannot be recalibrated, it should be replaced. Tools like dynamometers and pinch gauges need to be periodically recalibrated in order to provide accurate measurements.

- As assessment tools improve to measure more aspects of client capabilities and limitations, occupational therapy practitioners must be alert to the newer measurement tools and incorporate them into the evaluation process. For example, visual perception tests originally had norms only for children, but many have been re-normed to include adults. Using the newer instruments allows for the accurate assessment of perception in adults while continuing to be effective in assessing children.

- Occupational therapy practitioners should select assessment tools that reflect current occupational performance. Developmental tests may become out of date because of changes in population health, nutrition, and child-rearing practices. For example, the average age of walking has changed from 18 months in the 1940s to 11 months today. A developmental test that was standardized 40 or 50 years ago might not identify a performance deficit that should be addressed to improve the child's function in today's society. Some tests include pictures or models of items that are no longer widely used, such as a rotary telephone or a half-dollar coin. Asking someone to identify these items is not useful in interpreting their ability to use a telephone or make correct change.

- Occupational therapy practitioners should select assessment tools that align with current conceptual models. Tests without an identified conceptual model or theory or with a discarded model or theory may provide accurate measurements, but may be insignificant regarding the client's ability to perform daily tasks. For example, cursive writing is no longer taught in many schools, so testing a child's ability to write in cursive may yield an accurate measurement, but can be interpreted as insignificant to performing daily school tasks. Understanding the conceptual basis of an assessment can increase the chances that the information obtained will be useful in planning and implementing an occupational therapy services program.

- Occupational therapy practitioners should consider whether an assessment tool provides information on occupational performance. For example, assessments such as goniometry and muscle strength testing can indicate client factor impairments. The practitioner should take care to incorporate this information on client factors into its impact on occupational performance when reporting evaluation results.

- Many assessment tools require the client to complete the assessment according to standardized procedures. If the occupational therapy practitioner needs to see how the client participates in occupations using problem solving or demonstrating the process of using an alternate method or adaptation for completing the task, then a different evaluation method should be chosen. For example, if a standardized writing assessment favors placing the task in a way that favors right-handed people, then it may not be the best assessment for a left-handed child.

Next Steps

The occupational therapy practitioner should be knowledgeable about each assessment instrument used to measure client capacities and limitations. Although there is no definitive

CASE EXAMPLE 25.1. USING STANDARDIZED ASSESSMENTS

Pat is a new graduate occupational therapist hired by Happy Kids Clinic and is excited about evaluating 8-year-old **Taylor.** Pat selects and administers the Test of Pragmatic Language–2nd edition (TOPL–2®; Phelps-Terasaki & Phelps-Gunn, 2007) and has the parents fill in the Sensory Processing Measure (SPM®; Parham et al., 2007). Pat also has Taylor do activities that mimic those on the DeGangi-Berk Test of Sensory Integration (TSI®; 1983). Three months later, Taylor's family moves to another city and is referred to New City Clinic, which requests a copy of Taylor's occupational therapy evaluation. The Happy Kids Clinic director receives a call from New City Clinic, expressing concerns that the Happy Kids occupational therapy evaluation violated the AOTA Code of Ethics. When asked to explain the choices for assessment tools, Pat says, "These are what we used at my fieldwork site. Most of the children were assessed with the TSI and the SPM–2" (Parham et al., 2021). "We don't have the TSI, but I had a copy of the form from my fieldwork, so I just did activities like it. I know it's for preschoolers, but I just figured out what the norms would probably be. I couldn't find the SPM–2, but there was an old SPM in the file cabinet, so I used that and called someone from my fieldwork to check norms. I found the TOPL–2 in the speech therapy closet, and I remembered that one as well, so I used it too."

Questions
1. What are areas of concern regarding this occupational therapist's assessment?
2. What standards from the Code have been violated (see Exhibit 25.1)?
3. How would you proceed if you were the clinic director?

CASE EXAMPLE 25.2. USING UPDATED ASSESSMENTS

Ken, an occupational therapist working in an outpatient brain injury program, administers the Cognitive Assessment of Minnesota (CAM; Rustad et al., 1993) to **Mr. Clausen,** age 57 years, who hopes to return to work soon. Ken skips the Money Skills section because he cannot find a 50-cent piece, and he skips the Visual Neglect section because the reproducible form is missing from the test manual. He summarizes the test results he has completed, but his supervisor refuses to allow them to be entered in Mr. Clausen's chart because the results are incomplete. The supervisor suggests that Ken look for the missing pieces of the CAM or retest Mr. Clausen with a similar assessment instrument.

Questions
1. What are areas of concern regarding this occupational therapist's assessment?
2. What standards from the Code could have been violated by submitting these results?

checklist to determine whether a test or an assessment is outdated or obsolete, some general guidelines can be stated. Any test or assessment instrument to be used with clients must meet the following criteria:

- The test or assessment instrument should be the most current edition or version available. If a similar test or assessment has essentially the same content and was published more recently, the occupational therapy practitioner should consider using the newer test or assessment if feasible.

- The content of the test or assessment instrument should be based on a currently accepted theory, frame of reference, or model of practice.
- The content of the test or assessment instrument should be recognized as within the scope of occupational therapy practice.
- The assessment instrument's normative data should be current.
- The sample on which the normative data are based should include participants with the characteristics of the client being assessed (e.g., age, sex, ethnicity, symptoms, diagnosis).
- The assessment instrument should be deemed valid and reliable in the current literature, and there should be current evidence to substantiate use of the assessment tool with the population with whom the occupational therapy practitioner wants to use the tool.
- The language of the test or assessment instrument should be consistent with current usage.
- Printed test forms should be purchased from the publisher and not photocopied, unless copying is explicitly allowed by the publisher.
- The test items should be the same as or similar to those in daily use to measure functional ability, occupational performance, or participation.
- The test instrument should be in good condition (i.e., all parts available and in working order). Materials should not be culturally or personally offensive in any way to the client being served.

Summary

Occupational therapy practitioners use assessment tools as a means of gathering data about a client during the evaluation process. The assessment tools should provide accurate and up-to-date data about the client being evaluated. Practitioners must assume responsibility for selecting, administering, scoring, and interpreting assessment tools that are not outdated or obsolete. Although definitive guidelines for determining whether a test or instrument is outdated or obsolete do not exist, practitioners can observe useful guidelines, such as the criteria outlined in this Advisory Opinion.

Acknowledgment

Kathlyn L. Reed, PhD, OTR, FAOTA, MLIS, authored an earlier version of this Advisory Opinion.

REFERENCES

Adams, K. M. (2000). Practical and ethical issues pertaining to test revisions. *Psychological Assessment, 12,* 281–286. https://doi.org/10.1037/1040-3590.12.3.281

American Educational Research Association. (2014). *Standards for educational and psychological testing.* Joint Committee of the American Educational Research Association, American Psychological Association, & National Council on Measurement in Education.

Butcher, J. N. (2000). Revising psychological tests: Lessons learned from the revision of the MMPI. *Psychological Assessment, 12,* 263–271. https://doi.org/10.1037/1040-3590.12.3.263

DeGangi, G., & Berk, R. (1983). *DeGangi-Berk Test of Sensory Integration (TSI).* WPS.

Howard, B. (2014). Clinical plagiarism and copyright violations. *OT Practice,* 11–14. https://www.aota.org/-/media/Corporate/Files/Secure/Publications/OTP/2014/OTP%20Vol%2019%20Issue%2018.pdf

Kielhofner, G., & Coster, W. (2017). Developing and evaluating quantitative data collection instruments. In R. Taylor (Ed.), *Kielhofner's research in occupational therapy: Methods of inquiry for enhancing practice* (2nd ed., pp. 274–295). F. A. Davis.

Oakland, T. (2015). *Guidelines for practitioner use of test revisions, obsolete tests, and test disposal.* https://www.pearsonassessments.com/content/dam/school/global/clinical/us/assets/When-to-Upgrade.pdf

Okazaki, S., & Sue, S. (2000). Implications of test revisions for assessment with Asian Americans. *Psychological Assessment, 12,* 272–280. https://doi.org/10.1037/1040-3590.12.3.272

Parham, L. D., Ecker, C. L., Kuhaneck, H., Henry, D. A., & Glennon, T. J. (2007). *Sensory Processing Measure.* Pearson Clinical.

Parham, L. D., Ecker, C. L., Kuhaneck, H., Henry, D. A., & Glennon, T. J. (2021). SPM™–2: *Sensory Processing Measure* (2nd ed.). WPS.

Phelps-Terasaki, D., & Phelps-Gunn, T. (2007). *TOPL–2: Test of Pragmatic Language* (2nd ed.). WPS.

Rustad, R. A., DeGroot, T. L., Jungkunz, M. L., Freeberg, K. S., Borowick, L. G., & Wanttie, A. M. (1993). *The Cognitive Assessment of Minnesota.* Pearson.

Silverstein, M. L., & Nelson, L. D. (2000). Clinical and research implications of revising psychological tests. *Psychological Assessment, 12,* 298–303. https://doi.org/10.1037/1040-3590.12.3.298

Strauss, E., Spreen, O., & Hunter, M. (2000). Implications of test revisions for research. *Psychological Assessment, 12,* 237–244. https://doi.org/10.1037/1040-3590.12.3.237

Informed Consent

BRENDA S. HOWARD, DHSc, OTR, FAOTA

Key Points

- Informed consent is a client right and the duty of every occupational therapy practitioner.
- Informed consent consists of *disclosure*—taking the time to fully inform the client or participant; and *consent*—the person provides clear, voluntary agreement to participate in occupational therapy or research.
- Occupational therapy practitioners must observe informed consent with every client encounter and with every research endeavor.

Introduction

Informed consent is a fundamental right of every client and every research participant. Informed consent has its roots in the Nuremberg Code (Ghooi, 2011), the Belmont Report (U.S. Department of Health and Human Services, Office for Human Research Protections, 2022), and Declaration of Helsinki (World Medical Association, n.d.). Following the horrific research studies conducted on human subjects in Concentration Camps in Nazi Germany during World War II, worldwide outcry led to the development of principles and standards for preventing such atrocities in the future (Carlson et al., 2004). When, despite these codes and declarations, it was discovered that Black men in the United States had been studied for the effects of syphilis for decades without their knowledge, consent, or the benefit of antibiotic treatment when it became available (Centers for Disease Control and Prevention, 2022), the public protest led multiple professions to develop their own ethical standards, including the AOTA Code of Ethics.

Before interactions with clients, the law requires that health care practitioners obtain informed consent (Doherty & Purtilo, 2016). Informed consent when rendering services consists of two aspects: disclosure and consent. First, the practitioner must explain what will occur in a service delivery session; and second, they must gain agreement from the client for participation. Voluntary consent from the client, or from a representative (e.g., parents of minors under age 18 years, legal guardians or power of attorney for adults with mental incapacitation), must be ensured (Doherty & Purtilo, 2016). Clients and/or their representatives must reasonably understand what is being asked of them and must assure their voluntary participation before the practitioner provides services. Individuals deserve to fully understand what is being asked of them, the risks and benefits, the alternatives to the presented intervention, and the evidence for or against the intervention.

The occupational therapy practitioner must address barriers to communication and ensure the client understands the information provided. This communication process assures that the client shares in the decision-making process, or is making an informed decision to refuse care, if that is their choice (Doherty & Purtilo, 2016). Many times in clinical practice, the occupational therapy practitioner does not have the client sign a form, but rather seeks verbal assent to the session following an explanation of what the practitioner plans to engage them in (College of Occupational Therapists of Ontario, n.d.). In that case, the occupational therapy practitioner should document how they provided information and how the client indicated consent.

In research, the rules of informed consent are clearly laid out. All researchers must submit their study for review by an Institutional Review Board (IRB). The submission must include the protocol for conducting research with human subjects and must demonstrate how the researchers will obtain informed consent (Doherty & Purtilo, 2016). Recruitment materials must clearly identify the request for participants to be part of a research study. An informed consent document (ICD) must clearly lay out the risks and benefits of participation in the study. The document must also provide contact information for the primary investigator and for the IRB so the research participant can ask questions throughout the study (Doherty & Purtilo, 2016). The ICD must also clearly indicate that the participant may stop participating at any time during the study if they so choose. Finally, the ICD must provide clear and explicit proof that the participant is giving consent voluntarily and without coercion (Doherty & Purtilo, 2016). Researchers must take special care in situations when they are working with vulnerable populations (Taylor, 2017).

Relation to the AOTA Code of Ethics

Informed consent in research and practice relates to the American Occupational Therapy Association (AOTA) core values of freedom, justice, dignity, and truth. Observing informed consent not only complies with the law, but it gives participants the freedom and dignity to participate in the decision-making process. Occupational therapy practitioners participate in truthfulness and full disclosure when providing informed consent. The ethical principles of *autonomy,* or self-determination; and *nonmaleficence,* or causing no harm, also apply. The principle of *justice* states that occupational therapy practitioners will follow applicable laws; and veracity states that they will be truthful. Exhibit 26.1 contains ethical standards related to informed consent.

EXHIBIT 26.1.
ETHICAL STANDARDS RELATED TO INFORMED CONSENT

- Conduct and disseminate research in accordance with currently accepted ethical guidelines and standards for the protection of research participants, including informed consent and disclosure of potential risks and benefits.
- Obtain informed consent (written, verbal, electronic, or implied) after disclosing appropriate information and answering any questions posed by the recipient of service, qualified family member or caregiver, or research participant to ensure voluntary participation.
- Fully disclose the benefits, risks, and potential outcomes of any intervention; the occupational therapy personnel who will be providing the intervention; and any reasonable alternatives to the proposed intervention.
- Describe the type and duration of occupational therapy services accurately in professional contracts, including the duties and responsibilities of all involved parties.
- Maintain privacy and truthfulness in delivery of occupational therapy services, whether in person or virtually.
- Facilitate comprehension and address barriers to communication.

Note. From the Standards of Conduct from the AOTA Code of Ethics.

Reference to Other AOTA Documents

Policy E.18 (AOTA, 2023), AOTA's official document on Interventions to Support Occupations, indicates that occupational therapy practitioners will obtain informed consent, especially in the case of new and emerging techniques, technology, and other interventions without strong supporting evidence, and will disclose the potential risks and benefits of participation.

Reference to Other Standards

- Laws associated with the Health Insurance Portability and Accountability Act of 1996 (HIPAA; P. L. 104-191) require that written client consent be given before disclosing or sharing any of their protected health information (U.S. Department of Health and Human Services, Office for Civil Rights, 2020).
- *Red rules*, while not directly related to informed consent, require occupational therapy practitioners to take a "timeout" prior to initiating any evaluation or intervention to make sure the practitioner has identified the client as being the person who should receive services, using two forms of identification (e.g., name and birth date). Red rules are followed in many hospital settings (Jones & O'Connor, 2016). Taking the time to identify the client and verify that all proper procedures are being followed allows the practitioner to include the informed consent process.

Tips

Using an acronym such as AIDET (Huron Consulting Group, n.d.) can assist an occupational therapy practitioner in remembering to ask for verbal informed consent. The AIDET acronym stands for:

- *Announce:* The practitioner announces themselves and identifies the client as the correct person to participate in occupational therapy.
- *Introduce:* The practitioner introduces themselves and explains the role of occupational therapy and the plan for the session.
- *Duration:* The practitioner states the expected duration of the session.
- *Explanation:* The practitioner explains what they are doing and why, providing evidence as needed prior to and during the session. The practitioner requests client verbal assent or signed consent for the session.
- *Thank:* The practitioner thanks the client at the end of the session

The acronym AIDET has improved client satisfaction and has facilitated education in the health professions (Huron Consulting Group, n.d.).

CASE EXAMPLE 26.1. INFORMED CONSENT IN PRACTICE: WHOOPS!

Alex was an occupational therapy practitioner in an acute care hospital. Alex went to see **Jan,** a 78-year-old female in room 218 who was recovering from a stroke, for ADL intervention. Alex walked into the room, threw the curtains open, and called loudly, "Good morning, Jan! It's time for occupational therapy! Let's get you up on the side of the bed and have you brush your teeth." "No, no, no," moaned the woman in the bed, "I hurt all over and I just can't." "You'll feel better once you are up," chirped Alex. Alex pulled back the covers, swung the woman's feet over the side of the bed, and helped her to sit. The woman turned pale and began breathing rapidly. Alex checked her pulse, and it was fast and faint.

Alex pressed the call button, and on arrival, the nurse asked, "What are you doing? She's on complete bedrest!"

Alex asked, "Isn't this Jan Smythe, 2 days post CVA?"

"No," said the nurse, "Jan was moved to room 220. This is Alice Cooper, and she has a GI bleed and is scheduled for surgery later today." "Whoops!" cried Alex. "Let's help you back to bed, Alice. I'm in the wrong room!"

Questions
1. What informed consent procedures did Alex omit?
2. How could have Alex prevented this from happening?
3. What should Alex do after this happened?

CASE EXAMPLE 26.2. INFORMED CONSENT IN RESEARCH: VULNERABLE POPULATION

Charlie was an occupational therapist in a large, urban middle school where they worked with students with physical and intellectual disabilities in two alternative classrooms. When meeting with their supervisor, Charlie related an idea for a research study. Charlie wanted to create a sensory-friendly environment in one classroom, leave the other classroom in its typical layout, and compare students' ability to attend to educational activities after 1 month. The supervisor asked Charlie whether they needed to inform the parents about the research study. "I don't think so," responded Charlie, "because I won't be touching any of the students. They will just be in different environments. In fact, I don't think I need to go through the Institutional Review Board, because it isn't really human subjects research if I'm not doing anything physically to the students." Charlie wanted to report their findings at an upcoming regional conference and perhaps publish the results in a quarterly newsletter.

Questions
1. Was Charlie correct that they did not have to inform parents or go through an IRB?
2. What consequences would Charlie face if they proceeded with this research?
3. What procedures would Charlie need to follow to adhere to informed consent processes?

Summary

Informed consent is a right for clients and a responsibility for occupational therapy practitioners. Whether in a clinical, community-based, or other practice setting, or in a research environment, informed consent procedures must be followed to support the rights of all persons receiving services legally and ethically. Occupational therapy practitioners must seek to obtain informed consent with every encounter involving persons receiving services or participating in research.

REFERENCES

American Occupational Therapy Association. (2023). *Policy E.18: Interventions to support occupations.* https://www.aota.org/-/media/corporate/files/aboutaota/officialdocs/policies/policy-e18-20230419.pdf

Carlson, R. V., Boyd, K. M., & Webb, D. J. (2004). The revision of the Declaration of Helsinki: Past, present and future. *British Journal of Pharmacology, 57,* 695–713. https://doi.org/10.1111%2Fj.1365-2125.2004.02103.x

Centers for Disease Control and Prevention. (2022). *U.S. Public Health Service untreated syphilis study at Tuskegee timeline.* http://www.cdc.gov/tuskegee/timeline.htm

College of Occupational Therapists of Ontario. (n.d.). *Understanding consent.* https://www.coto.org/clientsandthepublic/working-with-an-occupational-therapist/understanding-consent#:~:text=The%20responsibility%20is%20on%20the,signing%20a%20form

Doherty, R. F., & Purtilo, R. B. (2016). *Ethical dimensions in the health professions* (6th ed.). Elsevier/Saunders.

Ghooi, R. B. (2011). The Nuremberg Code: A critique. *Perspectives in Clinical Research, 2*(2), 72–76. https://doi.org/10.4103%2F2229-3485.80371

Health Insurance Portability and Accountability Act of 1996 (HIPAA), Pub. L. 104-191, 42 U.S.C. § 300gg, 29 U.S.C §§ 1181–1183, and 42 U.S.C. §§ 1320d–1320d9.

Huron Consulting Group. (n.d.). *The AIDET® communication framework.* https://www.huroncon-sultinggroup.com/insights/aidet-communication-framework

Jones, L., & O'Connor, S. (2016). The use of Red Rules in patient safety culture. *Universal Journal of Management, 4*(3), 130–139. https://doi.org/10.13189/ujm.2016.040306

Taylor, R. (Ed.). (2017). *Kielhofner's research in occupational therapy: Methods of inquiry for enhancing practice* (2nd ed.). F.A. Davis.

U.S. Department of Health and Human Services, Office for Civil Rights. (2020). *HIPAA privacy and novel coronavirus.* https://www.hhs.gov/sites/default/files/february-2020-hipaa-and-novel-coronavirus.pdf

U.S. Department of Health and Human Services, Office for Human Research Protections. (2022). *The Belmont Report.* https://www.hhs.gov/ohrp/regulations-and-policy/belmont-report/#xethical

World Medical Association. (n.d.). *WMA Declaration of Helsinki—Ethical principles for medical research involving human subjects.* https://www.wma.net/policies-post/wma-declaration-of-hel-sinki-ethical-principles-for-medical-research-involving-human-subjects/#:~:text=The%20World%20Medical%20Association%20

Section 5. Professional Competence, Education, Supervision, and Training

State Licensure and Ethics

BARBARA ELLEMAN, OTD, MHS, OTR/L

Key Points

- All occupational therapy practitioners must hold a license to practice in the state or territory where occupational therapy services are provided.
- The occupational therapy practitioner is responsible for knowing when their license expires, for completing all requirements for renewal, and for staying up to date on changes to regulations.
- Occupational therapy practitioners who fail to comply with state licensure regulations are subject to legal and disciplinary action from the state licensure board and may be subject to disciplinary actions from the AOTA Ethics Commission, the National Board for Certification in Occupational Therapy (NBCOT®), or other regulatory agencies.

Introduction

Throughout the United States, the District of Columbia, Guam, and Puerto Rico, occupational therapists and occupational therapy assistants are required to hold an occupational license to practice (American Occupational Therapy Association [AOTA], n.d.). An occupational license is issued by a state regulatory board (SRB) and signifies that the person has met the requirements and has the legal authority to work in a specific occupation in that state (Cunningham, 2019). Licensure is a common requirement for many health care professions and ensures that a person possesses a defined skill or specific knowledge to perform a job (Cunningham, 2019). State regulatory boards governing licensure of occupational therapy practitioners aim to protect the safety of the public by regulating the practice of occupational therapy in their state. Licensure protects the integrity of the profession by ensuring that practitioners who provide occupational therapy services have the qualifications to do so (Bloom, 2017).

All occupational therapy practitioners are required to hold a license to practice occupational therapy in each state or territory in which they provide services, though not necessarily in their state of residence. Licensure requirements and regulations governing practice can vary among states and territories, and the occupational therapy practitioner is ultimately responsible for complying with the laws and any changes to those laws that are outlined in each state's practice act (Hall et al., 2016).

Each state's practice act outlines specific regulations governing practice that often include

- terms of licensure,
- documentation of services,
- billing for services,
- scope of occupational therapy practice,
- supervision of licensed and/or unlicensed personnel,
- competency and continuing education requirements, and
- ethical conduct.

All occupational therapy practitioners are ethically bound to be aware of, understand, and adhere to the requirements in the state, territory, or district where they are licensed. Failure to comply with the requirements and regulations of an SRB is unlawful and unethical, and is a direct violation of the AOTA Code of Ethics (the Code) and could result in legal prosecution and/or disciplinary actions, including loss of licensure (Bloom, 2017). Lack of awareness, or misunderstanding, will not prevent or mitigate these actions. Occupational therapy practitioners are responsible for staying informed of their licensure status, updating their SRB when their name or address changes, and renewing their state licensure in a timely manner. Occupational therapy practitioners are also responsible for notifying their employer of any changes in licensure status or requirements. When licensed to practice in different states, occupational therapy practitioners are responsible for understanding and complying with the regulations specific to each state in which they are practicing. For example, state practice acts may indicate how to represent one's credential (e.g., OT/L, OTR/L, OTA/L, or COTA/L). Some states require additional credentialing in order to administer certain interventions (e.g., physical agent modalities). State licensure laws often include standards that must be followed in relation to billing and documentation for occupational therapy services.

Rules and regulations regarding obtaining and maintaining licensure vary and occupational therapy practitioners are ethically responsible for securing, reading, and understanding licensure rules and requirements for their state, territory, or district. If an occupational therapy practitioner provides occupational therapy services without obtaining or renewing their license for any reason, they are breaking the law (state regulation) and acting unethically. In such cases, not only will the occupational therapy practitioner be subject to legal repercussions from the SRB, but the practitioner and employer may be subject to disciplinary and financial repercussions from governing agencies and third-party payers.

Licensure renewal regulations often require evidence of ongoing competence or a specified amount of continuing education. These requirements vary from state to state in terms of what activities qualify, how many hours or points are needed, how often (yearly or every 2 years), and whether ethics or other topics are required. Occupational therapy practitioners must be truthful and not misrepresent the education or professional development activities they participated in to meet renewal criteria. They must be prepared to provide evidence of continued competence according to criteria outlined in their state practice act. Occupational therapists who serve in a supervisory relationship with an occupational therapy assistant are responsible for ensuring that the occupational therapy assistant has met all state requirements for licensure and maintains an active license. Likewise, occupational therapy assistants must ensure that the supervising occupational therapist maintains an active license in the state in which they are practicing.

Relation to the AOTA Code of Ethics

The AOTA Code of Ethics (the Code) provides standards of conduct that guide occupational therapy practitioners and support regulatory measures to protect consumers, the practitioner, and the profession of occupational therapy. When a practitioner violates a law established by their SRB, they simultaneously violate the Code and may be subject to disciplinary action. The ethical standards that relate to state licensure are outlined in Exhibit 27.1.

EXHIBIT 27.1.
ETHICAL STANDARDS RELATED TO STATE LICENSURE

- Comply with current federal and state laws, state scope of practice guidelines, and AOTA policies and official documents that apply to the profession of occupational therapy.
- Inform employers, employees, colleagues, students, and researchers of applicable policies, laws, and official documents.
- Do not engage in illegal actions, whether directly or indirectly harming stakeholders in occupational therapy practice.
- Bill and collect fees justly and legally in a manner that is fair, reasonable, and commensurate with services delivered.
- Ensure that documentation for reimbursement purposes is done in accordance with applicable laws, guidelines, and regulations.
- Hold requisite credentials for the occupational therapy services one provides in academic, research, physical, or virtual work settings.
- Represent credentials, qualifications, education, experience, training, roles, duties, competence, contributions, and findings accurately in all forms of communication.
- Provide appropriate supervision in accordance with AOTA official documents and relevant laws, regulations, policies, procedures, standards, and guidelines.

Note. From the Standards of Conduct from the AOTA Code of Ethics.

Reference to Other AOTA Documents

- AOTA (n.d.) offers numerous resources and answers to common questions related to state licensure.

- Guidelines for Supervision, Roles, and Responsibilities During the Delivery of Occupational Therapy Services outline the parameters of effective supervision between an occupational therapy assistant and an occupational therapist.
- Standards of Practice for Occupational Therapy identify the minimal standards for the delivery of occupational therapy services.
- Standards for Continuing Competence in Occupational Therapy describes the standards to assess, maintain, and document continuing competence in occupational therapy practice.

Reference to Other Standards

- SRBs in individual states and territories detail licensure requirements. The links to each SRB are available through AOTA's Licensure page (AOTA, n.d.).
- National Board for Certification in Occupational Therapy (NBCOT®) Practice Standards (2023) provide standards to which all certified occupational therapy practitioners must adhere.

Tips

- Take steps to ensure that contact information is current with applicable SRBs to ensure receipt of timely notifications and announcements.
- Subscribe to applicable SRB's newsletters, notifications, or social media accounts (where available) to stay up to date.
- Be aware of and complete (at a minimum) the required continuing education and professional development activities needed to maintain state licensure.
- Collect and maintain a record of all continuing education activities.

CASE EXAMPLE 27.1. PRACTICING WITHOUT A LICENSE

An **occupational therapy practitioner** has been licensed to practice occupational therapy in the state where they reside. The practitioner has received reminders that their state license is due for renewal by the end of the month. Despite these notifications, the practitioner finds it hard to carve out the time to complete the renewal process between their full-time job and active home life. They tell themselves they will complete it before the deadline. Unfortunately, the practitioner has to take an unexpected leave of absence from work to care for an ill family member out of state. During the process, the practitioner fails to renew their license. When they return to work 6 weeks later, they continue to work for a full 2 weeks before they are approached by their employer who states that they received notification that the practitioner's license has expired. The practitioner has been practicing for the past 2 weeks on an expired license.

Questions
1. What are the ethical implications of this scenario?
2. What actions should the practitioner take?

CASE EXAMPLE 27.2. CONTINUING EDUCATION AND LICENSE RENEWAL

Over the past year, the employer of a licensed **occupational therapy practitioner** had to cut funding for allotted continuing education in half, and the practitioner was not able to attend the AOTA INSPIRE Annual Conference as they had in previous years. When it is time to renew their license, they realize they are 4 hours short of the total continuing education hours required by the state regulations to renew their license, and there is no longer time to fulfill continuing education requirements before their license is due for renewal.

Questions
1. What are the ethical implications of this scenario?
2. What actions should the practitioner take?

Next Steps

The Occupational Therapy Licensure Compact (OT Compact) is a joint initiative by AOTA and NBCOT (Occupational Therapy Licensure Compact, n.d.). The OT Compact is a formal agreement between multiple states that, once enacted, will offer practitioners the opportunity to provide occupational therapy services across those states through a compact privilege instead of attaining an individual license in each state. Occupational therapy practitioners who hold state licensure in the states that have adopted the OT Compact legislation should stay abreast of changes and updates through their SRB and the OT Compact website (https://otcompact.org). Occupational therapy practitioners should be aware that although many states have adopted the OT Compact legislation, there are additional steps, including an application, that will need to be taken in order for an individual to attain compact privileges to provide occupational therapy services in a compact state after the compact is enacted (Occupational Therapy Licensure Compact, n.d.).

Summary

Any individual providing occupational therapy services in the United States and specified territories must attain and maintain an active license from their SRB to practice occupational therapy. State licensure protects the safety of consumers by ensuring that they are receiving care from qualified individuals. Occupational therapy practitioners are legally bound by state regulations and are ethically responsible to comply with them. Failure to adhere to state regulations could result in legal and/or disciplinary actions with long-term professional or personal ramifications. Practitioners who are vigilant to stay up-to-date and adhere to requirements and maintain timely renewal practices will avoid these devastating outcomes.

Acknowledgments

Melba J. Arnold, MS, OTR/L, and **Diane Hill, COTA/L, AP, ROH,** authored an earlier version of this Advisory Opinion.

REFERENCES

American Occupational Therapy Association. (n.d.). *Licensure.* https://www.aota.org/career/state-licensure

Bloom, G. M. (2017). Ethics and its application to occupational therapy practice. In K. Jacobs & N. MacRae (Eds.), *Occupational therapy essentials for clinical competence* (3rd ed., pp. 715–731). Slack.

Cunningham, E. (2019). Professional certifications and occupational licenses: Evidence from the current population survey. *Monthly Labor Review.* https://doi.org/10.21916/mlr.2019.15

Hall, S. R., Crifasi, K. A., Marinelli, C. M., & Yuen, H. K. (2016). Continuing education requirements among state occupational therapy regulatory boards in the United States of America. *Journal of Educational Evaluation for Health Professions, 13*, 37. https://doi.org/10.3352/jeehp.2016.13.37

National Board for Certification in Occupational Therapy. (2023). *NBCOT® practice standards.* https://www.nbcot.org/professional-conduct/practice-standards

Occupational Therapy Licensure Compact. (n.d.). *About.* https://otcompact.org/about/

28

Promoting Ethically Sound Practices in Occupational Therapy Fieldwork Education

LESLIE E. BENNETT, OTD, OTR/L; MARGOT ELACQUA, OTD, MBA, OTR/L; and SARAH BROCKWAY, EdD, OTR/L

Key Points

- Fieldwork education is a dynamic process that requires collaboration between the academic institutions, fieldwork sites, fieldwork educators, and students.
- Ethical challenges arise when individuals do not maintain high standards of ethical and professional conduct.
- Clear, transparent, and honest communication is essential for managing conflicts that arise in fieldwork education.

Introduction

Occupational therapy fieldwork education is essential in shaping and ensuring the future of the profession. The dynamic nature of today's health care environments and the emergence of the COVID-19 pandemic added challenges to fieldwork education. Despite these challenges, it is important that faculty, academic fieldwork coordinators (AFWCs), fieldwork educators (FWEs), and students (the dynamic triad) work collaboratively to provide a rich fieldwork experience where students can develop and demonstrate the entry-level skills required to become competent practitioners (Estes & Bennett, 2019). Throughout the education process, faculty, AFWCs, FWEs, and students are responsible for maintaining high standards of ethical conduct.

Faculty and AFWC Responsibilities

Academic fieldwork coordinators and faculty are responsible for meeting Accreditation Council for Occupational Therapy Education (ACOTE®) standards, which guide fieldwork education and the development of fieldwork programs. These standards are intended to ensure the following:

- Settings meet curricular goals and provide educational experiences that align with the academic institution's goals.
- Fieldwork experiences promote ethically sound practice and promote the development of entry-level professionals.
- The supervision process protects clients and their families and provides for appropriate role modeling.

AFWCs are increasingly challenged to meet these expectations. Growing demands on the FWEs' time and resources are resulting in a decreased number of FWEs taking on these professional responsibilities (Estes & Bennett, 2019). Diminishing availability of fieldwork sites requires AFWCs to be creative with placements.

Ethical dilemmas can arise when AFWCs are tempted to place students in suboptimal settings to ensure that there are enough sites for every student in each cohort. Applying sound critical reasoning and professional judgment helps determine whether a clinical site can provide appropriate fieldwork experiences that meet current ACOTE standards. When a fieldwork site does not meet the current ACOTE standards, AFWCs must demonstrate moral courage by refraining from placing students at that site or by removing the student when it becomes evident that the site no longer is providing appropriate educational experiences or meeting students' learning needs.

Another area of ethical concern relates to Family Educational Rights and Privacy Act of 1974 (FERPA; P. L. 93-380) guidelines, which govern access to student education information and confidential records. An AFWC may legally share information on how to support a student's performance in the clinic with those at the fieldwork site who have legitimate educational interests, based on the student's time in the classroom. This sharing of information includes those under contractual agreement with a college or university. However, the AFWC must balance the legal boundaries afforded by FERPA with their ethical responsibilities to protect student information. They need to determine whether sharing the information supports a student's success in fieldwork. It is unethical to share information that is not relevant to the student's fieldwork experience and could negatively bias relevant parties toward that student.

Ethically, the AFWC may share only information that is relevant to promoting a student's successful completion of their fieldwork experience. This information could include developing strategies to support the student with multiple demands of a fast-paced environment in a timely manner. However, an AFWC should not be sharing information about the student's struggles or accommodations in the classroom without consent from the student. If an AFWC is unsure whether sharing a student's academic information is within established legal and ethical boundaries, they should seek assistance from the educational institution.

Fieldwork Educator Responsibilities

Fieldwork educators are professionally and ethically obligated to provide appropriate levels of supervision, despite challenges created by current practice demands, including increased productivity rates and staffing shortages (American Occupational Therapy Association [AOTA], 2022; Estes & Bennett, 2019). Fieldwork educators have a primary duty to ensure the safety and well-being of their clients; and they must simultaneously balance their own daily clinical work demands with responsibilities for adequate student supervision. Doing so requires FWEs to honestly appraise students' capabilities to be certain the students are competent to provide safe and effective interventions.

Honest appraisal of a student's capabilities may lead to the determination that a student is not meeting competency standards and thus should fail their fieldwork rotation. Fieldwork educators may struggle with this decision if they believe that students who have successfully completed all the academic requirements for competency should pass fieldwork. They may question whether their supervisory methods were too harsh and caused a student to fail. Conversely, FWEs who are new to supervision will struggle to fail a student as they may blame themselves for the student's failure. Supervisory methods are not always at fault, and a student may struggle to demonstrate clinical competency in a real-life practice setting. When this occurs, FWEs have an ethical obligation to accurately and objectively appraise a student's abilities and draw on their own moral courage to determine whether the student should pass or fail the fieldwork rotation (AOTA, 2018; Estes & Bennett, 2019; Estes & Brandt, 2011).

Ethical fieldwork supervision requires transparent, clear, and open communication, whether written, verbal, or electronic. Fieldwork educators need to provide ongoing objective feedback to students to keep them informed of their progress or areas that require improvement. In addition, precise documentation related to supervisory activities enables the supervisor to more fairly evaluate student performance and ultimately support the final evaluation. These strategies may prevent misunderstanding between the student and FWEs (Estes & Bennett, 2019; Estes & Brandt, 2011).

FWEs are also responsible for ensuring that students are provided with appropriate and effective educational experiences. Fieldwork educators should serve as exemplary role models by adhering to high standards of ethical and professional conduct. They must ensure that students function according to their role expectations. For example, students should not be expected to perform as if they are substitutes for regular employees, to address staff shortages or demands for high productivity. Doing so denies the occupational therapy student their right to an appropriate fieldwork education experience and may violate their state occupational therapy practice act (Estes & Bennett, 2019; Estes & Brandt, 2011).

Concerns related to billing and reimbursement are additional areas of ethical concern. FWEs are responsible for ensuring that billing for services meets local, state, federal, and payer standards and regulations. Furthermore, billing for services provided by the fieldwork students must accurately reflect who provided the services and the actual services provided. Doing otherwise may constitute insurance fraud (Estes & Bennett, 2019; Estes & Brandt, 2011).

Student Responsibilities

Students are a critical component of the dynamic triad in fieldwork education and must adhere to the same legal and ethical standards expected of occupational therapy practitioners to meet client intervention duties and other responsibilities while on fieldwork. Students should be knowledgeable about relevant ethical codes and other policies and procedures for handling concerns about situations or issues that may challenge those standards. Students have a primary duty to protect the safety and well-being of their clients and clients' family members. Doing so requires students to be transparent in communicating with their clients and supervisors. In particular, students have a duty to divulge their status as students to their clients.

Students have a responsibility to be open and transparent about their concerns regarding their own levels of competence and confidence with different treatment interventions to their supervisors. This is especially important for students who are asked to provide interventions for which they may not feel adequately prepared or competent to provide. Encouraging students to incorporate evidence-based practice resources into their interventions can help promote student competence and promote client well-being (AOTA, 2018; Estes & Bennett, 2019; Estes & Brandt, 2011).

Students also need to protect clients' privacy and confidentiality (Estes & Brandt, 2011). They may find themselves in a position of sharing their fieldwork experiences with faculty or classmates in the context of teaching-learning environments. This sharing could be in the form of classroom discussions, written assignments, or virtual discussion boards. In each situation students must discern what, if any, information they can communicate about the clients in a manner that maintains compliance with current HIPAA regulations (Health Insurance Portability and Accountability Act of 1996 [P. L. 104-191]; Centers for Disease Control and Prevention, 2022). Students must not share information related to their fieldwork experiences through online social networking sites.

Like occupational therapy practitioners, students are expected to report any acts they see in practice that are illegal or unethical. Students who find themselves in difficult situations should reach out to their academic institution and the AFWC to minimize the chance of unpleasant consequences later in the fieldwork rotation. The AFWC can assist the student by helping them to analyze the situation, define the issues, explore potential strategies, and determine the most appropriate course of action. The AFWC and the student should maintain ongoing lines of communication throughout the fieldwork rotation so the AFWC can continue to advise and support the student. Students must communicate all concerns in an honest, fair, objective, and respectful manner at all times.

Meeting these ethical responsibilities may not be easy for students. Fieldwork can be a stressful experience for many students as they transition from the academic learning environment to real-life clinical settings. Students may struggle with current systemic constraints (e.g., productivity or infection control standards), conflicting values between themselves and the practitioner or client, or the presence of questionable ethical and professional behaviors they observe from their supervisors and other practitioners (Grenier, 2015). Due to the power differentials, students may have difficulty speaking up. They may fear any repercussions they experience from reporting concerns, including not being taken seriously or facing retribution, which could result in a failure (Holder & Schenthal, 2007).

A final ethical issue facing students is whether to disclose a disability or any accommodations to the AFWC or FWEs. The Americans with Disabilities Act of 1990 (P. L. 101-336) and FERPA and HIPAA laws protect students' confidentiality, leaving students to decide whether to share their status (AOTA, 2023). Students who would like to receive accommodations for qualified disabilities are responsible for initiating requests to receive them and for providing supporting documentation. Students who choose not to share this information must understand that they will not receive those accommodations for which they otherwise have qualified. Most importantly, students who choose not to share their disabilities must ensure that they are able to provide safe and effective client interventions without accommodations (AOTA, 2023; Estes & Brandt, 2011).

Relation to the AOTA Code of Ethics

Applicable standards from the AOTA Code (the Code) may be found in Exhibit 28.1. Local, state, and federal laws that impact practice can help students and occupational therapy practitioners stay up to date with the most current practice standards.

EXHIBIT 28.1.
ETHICAL STANDARDS RELATED TO FIELDWORK EDUCATION

- Ensure that documentation for reimbursement purposes is done in accordance with applicable laws, guidelines, and regulations.
- Record and report in an accurate and timely manner and in accordance with applicable regulations all information related to professional or academic documentation and activities.
- Do not follow arbitrary directives that compromise the rights or well-being of others, including unrealistic productivity expectations, fabrication, falsification, plagiarism of documentation, or inaccurate coding.
- Provide occupational therapy services, including education and training, that are within each practitioner's level of competence and scope of practice.
- Represent credentials, qualifications, education, experience, training, roles, duties, competence, contributions, and findings, accurately in all forms of communication.
- Ensure that all duties delegated to other occupational therapy personnel are congruent with their credentials, qualifications, experience, competencies, and scope of practice with respect to service delivery, supervision, fieldwork education, and research.
- Provide appropriate supervision in accordance with AOTA official documents and relevant laws, regulations, policies, procedures, standards, and guidelines.
- Be honest, fair, accurate, respectful, and timely in gathering and reporting fact-based information regarding employee job performance and student performance.

Note. From the Standards of Conduct from the AOTA Code of Ethics.

Reference to Other AOTA Documents

AOTA has several resources to help educators, clinicians, and students navigate fieldwork education (n.d.-b). The AOTA (2018) Fieldwork Level II and Occupational Therapy Students position statement also provides guidance for FWEs and students.

Tips

- When examining whether their organization can establish an effective fieldwork program, FWEs can start by conducting an analysis of *s*trengths, *w*eaknesses, *o*pportunities, and *t*hreats (SWOT analysis) to establish ethically sound standards for fieldwork.
- Both new and veteran FWEs should complete the Fieldwork Educator Certificate program offered through AOTA (n.d.-a), which addresses conflicts that arise in fieldwork education, including potential ethical violations.
- It is important that all members of the dynamic triad maintain open, transparent, and honest lines of communication at all times.
- Students and FWEs need to demonstrate the moral courage to take action and speak up when confronting ethical issues in practice.

CASE EXAMPLE 28.1. ABSENT FIELDWORK EDUCATOR

Sam is nearing the end of their second Level II fieldwork rotation at a large, university-based hospital. Sam did so well at their first rotation that they were offered a position following completion of their degree. Sam is doing well at their current rotation, receiving a glowing midterm evaluation from **Alex,** their FWE. Sam, however, does not share the same positive assessment about the supervision they are receiving from Alex.

It seems that Alex is rarely around when Sam has questions about their clients, and Sam has noticed that Alex frequently leaves early, especially on Fridays. On a particularly busy Friday afternoon, Alex approached Sam, asking them to pick up three additional clients that Alex could not treat that day. Alex shared that they were headed out of town for the weekend with their partner and wanted to leave early to get ready. On their way out the door, Alex added, "And can you please document treatment notes in the charts of the clients I saw this morning? I jotted down what I did with each one; just write them as if you did the treatments, sign your name, and I will cosign on Monday when I return. Have a great weekend!" Sam is shocked by what Alex has requested.

Questions
1. What ethical standards from the Code have been violated?
2. What should Sam do next?
3. What are the appropriate actions to take at this point in the fieldwork rotation?

CASE EXAMPLE 28.2. CURRENT AREAS OF ETHICAL CONCERN

An **AFWC** was tallying up the ethical issues encountered by occupational therapy students in the academic institution's program within the previous year. The list included the following:

1. Accessing medical records of family, friends, or others not on caseload
2. Social media posting of pictures or identifying client information
3. FWEs not thoroughly vetting the competency of a student prior to the start of hands-on care
4. Crossing professional boundaries of relationships with student, clients, and FWEs, including having inappropriate sexual relationships
5. Student failing to disclose any conflict of interest prior to the start of fieldwork
6. Dishonesty in documentation and billing practices
7. Failure to maintain confidentiality and privacy of student and client information
8. Failure to provide adequate supervision
9. Impaired practice
10. Incompetent practice
11. Inappropriately accepting gifts from clients and others
12. Professional incivility, including bullying in the workplace.

Unethical behavior had been committed by students, by FWEs, and by clients. The AFWC was deeply concerned about the apparent rise in unethical behavior in the profession and wanted to take action.

Questions

1. For each of the identified ethical issues, what sections in the Code have been violated?
2. What potential laws may have been broken?
3. Using an ethical decision-making framework, what is one course of action the AFWC could take?

Summary

Fieldwork education is a critical component of developing competent and ethical occupational therapy practitioners. The dynamic triad (AFWC, FWEs, students) must work to ensure the ethical development and implementation of fieldwork education programs that meet professional standards for developing knowledge and skills required for entry-level practice. Fieldwork education must include development of appropriate professional and ethical conduct.

Of primary concern for all stakeholders is protecting the safety and well-being of the clients served. Beyond this, AFWCs and FWEs are responsible for adhering to the guidelines, standards, regulations, and legal statutes related to fieldwork education. They are also responsible for demonstrating high standards of ethical and professional conduct in all communications and actions, and providing positive role modeling for students. Meeting professional and organizational standards may be challenging, given the nature of the current health care environment.

Students must also be held to these ethical standards during their fieldwork experiences. However, an inherent power imbalance in the supervisor relationship may result in student vulnerability and lead to unique ethical challenges for them. In successfully navigating these ethical challenges, AFWCs, FWEs, and students must work together to generate competent and caring occupational therapy practitioners of the future.

REFERENCES

American Occupational Therapy Association. (n.d.-a). *Fieldwork educators certificate workshop.* https://www.aota.org/education/fieldwork/fieldwork-educators-certification-workshop

American Occupational Therapy Association. (n.d.-b). *Fieldwork management.* https://www.aota.org/education/fieldwork

American Occupational Therapy Association. (2018). Fieldwork level II and occupational therapy students. *American Journal of Occupational Therapy, 72*(Suppl. 2), 7212410020. https://doi.org/10.5014/ajot.2018.72S205

American Occupational Therapy Association. (2022). Occupational therapy fieldwork education: Value and purpose. *American Journal of Occupational Therapy, 76*(Suppl. 3), 7613410240. https://doi.org/10.5014/ajot.2022.76S3006

American Occupational Therapy Association. (2023). *AOTA ethics advisory opinion: Ethical considerations for students and practitioners with disabilities.* https://www.aota.org/practice/practice-essentials/ethics

Americans With Disabilities Act of 1990, Pub L. No. 101-336, 42 U.S.C. pp. 12101–12213 (2008).

Centers for Disease Control and Prevention. (2022). *Health Insurance Portability and Accountability Act of 1996 (HIPAA).* https://www.cdc.gov/phlp/publications/topic/hipaa.html#:~:text=The%20Health%20Insurance%20Portability%20and,the%20patient's%20consent%20or%20knowledge

Estes, J., & Bennett, L. E. (2019). Ethics in fieldwork. In K. Jacobs & G. L. McCormack (Eds.), *The occupational therapy manager* (6th ed., pp. 547–554). AOTA Press.

Estes, J., & Brandt, L. C. (2011, April 25). Navigating fieldwork's ethical challenges. *OT Practice, 16*(7), 7–15.

Family Educational Rights and Privacy Act of 1974, Pub. L. 93-380, 20 U.S.C. § 1232g; 34 CFR Part 99.

Grenier, M.-L. (2015). Facilitators and barriers to learning in occupational therapy fieldwork education: Student perspectives. *American Journal of Occupational Therapy, 69*(Suppl. 2), 6912185070. https://doi.org/10.5014/ajot.2015.015180

Health Insurance Portability and Accountability Act of 1996, Pub. L. 104-191, 110 Stat. 1936.

Holder, K., & Schenthal, S. (2007). Watch your step: Nursing and professional boundaries. *Nursing Management, 38*(2), 29–30. https://journals.lww.com/nursingmanagement/Fulltext/2007/02000/Watch_your_step__Nursing_and_professional.10.aspx

29

Supervision and Collaboration Between Occupational Therapists and Occupational Therapy Assistants

BARBARA ELLEMAN, OTD, MHS, OTR/L; MARITA HENSLEY, COTA/L;
BRENDA KORNBLIT KENNELL, MA, OTR/L, FAOTA; and
LAUREN N. SPONSELLER, PhD, OTD, MSOT, MEd, OTR/L, CLA

Key Points

- Occupational therapy assistants receive *clinical supervision* from occupational therapists.
- Occupational therapy assistants can provide *administrative supervision* to occupational therapists.
- Occupational therapists and occupational therapy assistants should work collaboratively to deliver optimal care.

Introduction

Successful occupational therapy practitioners in an evolving health care delivery system must be familiar with and consider professional ethical standards as they confront potential new challenges of health care reform. Occupational therapy assistants are typically employed in positions in which they work collaboratively with occupational therapists who supervise them and delegate clinical work. Occupational therapy assistants need to be supervised appropriately according to state practice acts, regulations, and organizational policies. In most settings, occupational therapy assistants receive *clinical supervision* for client-related interventions as delegated by an occupational therapist. The official documents of the American Occupational Therapy Association (AOTA), such as the AOTA Code of Ethics (the Code) and the Guidelines for Supervision, Roles, and Responsibilities During the Delivery of Occupational Therapy Services, describe and support the framework for supervisory relationships in the delivery of occupational therapy services.

However, in some settings, occupational therapy assistants assume dual roles. They may be "rehab directors, regional managers, recruiters, and entrepreneurs (business owners)" (Jacobs, 2016, p. 95), providing managerial and administrative oversight of occupational therapists and other professionals while also implementing all or part of the plan of care delegated by the supervising occupational therapist. This is no different than having a manager who is a physical therapist, speech-language pathologist, or nurse. All occupational therapy practitioners begin training to be managers in school as they learn about breaking down tasks, assessing needs, educating others, finding resources, evaluating performance, managing time, and documenting results (Smoot, 2019). When working as occupational therapy managers, they also plan for daily staffing issues, coordinate with other disciplines, monitor use of resources, review measurable outcomes, and ensure compliance with facility policies. This is called *managerial* and/ or *administrative supervision* and can also include monitoring productivity and attendance, safety and quality management, and caseload assignment. Any practitioner who is trained in these areas can assume these roles. This role is different from *clinical supervision* that the occupational therapist provides to the occupational therapy assistant, and that addresses the appropriateness, quality, and competence of occupational therapy intervention.

Relation to the AOTA Code of Ethics

Occupational therapists and occupational therapy assistants both have college degrees and state licenses, and have demonstrated entry-level competence through fieldwork experience and a national certification exam. Both are qualified professionals who should have a collaborative relationship. To facilitate that partnership it is important to recognize that both make valuable contributions. Although the occupational therapist has ultimate responsibility for the evaluation and plan of care, occupational therapy assistants can contribute to the assessment process and work collaboratively with the occupational therapist to develop goals and an intervention plan. In some settings where the occupational therapists are PRN or cover multiple sites, it is the occupational therapy assistant who does the majority of the treatment and therefore has the most knowledge about the client's progress, barriers, preferences, and potential. Having scheduled and unscheduled communication and sharing between the occupational therapist and occupational therapy assistant leads to best client outcomes.

It is important to consider the unique issues that may arise from these collaborative and administrative roles and relationships. The Code addresses these issues in terms of clinical supervision, assignment of duties, collaboration, representation of qualifications, professional competence, and communication.

STANDARDS AND IMPLICATIONS

See Exhibit 29.1 for standards of conduct from the Code that apply to occupational therapist–occupational therapy assistant relationships.

Occupational therapists and occupational therapy assistants comply with current laws, follow protocols under their organization/employer, ensure transparency, and respect the

EXHIBIT 29.1.

ETHICAL STANDARDS RELATED TO COLLABORATION AND SUPERVISION BETWEEN OCCUPATIONAL THERAPISTS AND OCCUPATIONAL THERAPY ASSISTANTS

- Provide occupational therapy services, including education and training, that are within each practitioner's level of competence and scope of practice.
- Terminate occupational therapy services in collaboration with the service recipient or responsible party when the services are no longer beneficial.
- Hold requisite credentials for the occupational therapy services one provides in academic, research, physical, or virtual work settings.
- Ensure that all duties delegated to other occupational therapy personnel are congruent with their credentials, qualifications, experience, competencies, and scope of practice with respect to service delivery, supervision, fieldwork education, and research.
- Provide appropriate supervision in accordance with AOTA official documents and relevant laws, regulations, policies, procedures, standards, and guidelines.
- Engage in collaborative actions and communication as a member of interprofessional teams to facilitate quality care and safety for clients.
- Demonstrate courtesy, civility, value, and respect to persons, groups, organizations, and populations when engaging in personal, professional, or electronic communications, including all forms of social media or networking, especially when that discourse involves disagreement of opinion, disparate points of view, or differing values.

Note. From the Standards of Conduct from the AOTA Code of Ethics.

responsibilities of their own and other professions to develop a collaborative environment. Occupational therapists and occupational therapy assistants are also responsible for engaging in actions that encourage the public's trust in the profession, reporting either known or potential suspicions of inappropriate practice, and ensuring there is no engagement in any conflicts of interest.

Occupational therapists and occupational therapy assistants are responsible for respecting the wishes of recipients of service, establishing a collaborative partnership to promote shared decision making, and maintaining appropriate boundaries with clients. This responsibility also includes prioritizing the safety and well-being of others.

The occupational therapist can complete, document, and synthesize the results of an evaluation, while an occupational therapy assistant may contribute to the documentation of evaluation results. All occupational therapy practitioners are to ensure that documentation for reimbursement purposes is consistent with laws and regulations, and to bill and collect fees legally in a manner that is sensible. Documentation should also be accurate and recorded in a punctual manner.

Both the occupational therapist and occupational therapy assistant are responsible for ensuring that intervention is provided in a timely manner, is provided for the appropriate duration, and is appropriate for the recipient. This includes choosing intervention activities and modalities based on the service recipient's needs and preferences rather than those of the treating occupational therapy practitioner or facility.

It is the responsibility of both the occupational therapy assistant and the occupational therapist not only to ensure that they are competent and qualified to conduct practice, but also to ensure that their occupational therapist/occupational therapy assistant partner (occupational therapy assistant manager/employee) holds the appropriate credentials and is competent to perform the functions of their job. For example, if the occupational therapy assistant has advanced training and experience in a specialty area, the occupational therapist must possess knowledge and competence in this area to provide adequate supervision.

Both occupational therapists and occupational therapy assistants should ensure that all communication within and outside of the supervisory interactions include confidentiality and respect for each other. When a record of supervisory interactions is required by state licensure or employer, it is the responsibility of both parties to ensure that confidentiality is maintained and security of the information is assured.

In all interactions with each other, the occupational therapist and occupational therapy assistant (occupational therapy assistant manager/employee) should incorporate cultural sensitivity and humility, respecting differing viewpoints and collaborative approaches to resolve differences in the partnership created by the supervision expectation.

Reference to Other AOTA Documents

The Guidelines for Supervision, Roles, and Responsibilities During the Delivery of Occupational Therapy Services delineates roles and responsibilities of occupational therapists and occupational therapy assistants regarding assessment, intervention, documentation, and clinical supervision.

Reference to Other Standards

The following documents may be useful references when considering ethical practice and the occupational therapist–occupational therapy assistant relationship.

- Individual states have specific guidelines for supervision, and practitioners should refer to their state practice acts.
- Practitioners should be aware of specific guidelines related to payment sources in their individual practice area (e.g., Medicare, Medicaid, other third-party payers).
- Practitioners should be knowledgeable about guidelines and policies determined by their employers.

Tips for Successful Occupational Therapist–Occupational Therapy Assistant Partnerships

Rowe (2016) offers the following tips:

- Use AOTA documents as a resource to grow in understanding the relationship.
- Understand your state laws.

- Understand that it is a two-way street.
- Put that ego down.
- Embrace strengths and weaknesses.
- Be honest.
- Always be appreciative.
- Communication is key.
- Don't be possessive.
- Celebrate your love of this amazing profession.

When occupational therapists and occupational therapy assistants engage in an effective collaborative relationship, they utilize open communication and approach the dyad as a partnership, recognizing mutual responsibility and embracing the opportunity to learn from each other and grow together. Each practitioner understands their role. When in doubt, there are resources provided by AOTA and other organizations to help with clarifying and delineating each role. Effective occupational therapist and occupational therapy assistant partnerships reflect mutual respect for the value the other brings to the collaboration. Each person is appreciative of the unique contributions of the other. They have a plan of action that mutually supports the other's needs and preferred mode of collaboration. When challenges or conflicts arise, each seeks to find common ground and solve problems, prioritizing the needs of clients and their mutual desire to advance and protect their chosen profession.

CASE EXAMPLE 29.1. OCCUPATIONAL THERAPY ASSISTANT AS MANAGER

Kelly is an occupational therapy assistant and the Rehabilitation Manager in a skilled nursing facility. The administrative staff has been pressuring Kelly to increase the occupational therapy department's revenue and to mandate that all plans of care include "modalities as needed." One of the occupational therapists on staff has begun adding modalities to all new plans. Kelly recognizes that several of the residents do not require physical agent modalities as part of their intervention. Although the plan of care is written by the evaluating occupational therapist (preferably in collaboration with the occupational therapy assistant), part of Kelly's administrative supervision of the occupational therapy staff includes ensuring that intervention is ethical. During a staff meeting, Kelly reiterates the need for client-centered plans and intervention individually tailored to each client; and she outlines other plans to improve revenue. During the meeting the occupational therapist says, "You don't understand. You're just an occupational therapy assistant. I bet they couldn't even afford ultrasound and e-stim machines at your community college. Leave this decision to the expert—me." That evening, the occupational therapist posts on social media, "Can't believe I have to take orders from a certified occupational therapy assistant. #incompetentmanager #communitycollegeeducation," and tags several other employees on the post. Two other staff members "like" the post. A physical therapist tells Kelly about it, and the next day Kelly arranges a disciplinary meeting with the occupational therapist.

Questions
1. Which ethics standards of conduct are relevant in this case?
2. How should the practitioners proceed?

CASE EXAMPLE 29.2. OCCUPATIONAL THERAPIST–OCCUPATIONAL THERAPY ASSISTANT CLINICAL SUPERVISION

Casey is the supervisor in a pediatric clinic. The updated plan of care for 2-year-old Raj includes goals to increase acceptance of solid food. Raj has been working with the occupational therapy assistant for a few months, but as part of clinical supervision, Casey recognizes that the occupational therapy assistant is not competent in this area. Casey reassigns Raj to another staff member who is skilled in feeding. Casey also sets up a plan with the occupational therapy assistant to develop service competency in pediatric feeding, as this is an area of interest for the occupational therapy assistant's professional development.

Questions
1. Which ethics standards of conduct are relevant in this case?
2. How should the practitioners proceed?

CASE EXAMPLE 29.3. OCCUPATIONAL THERAPIST–OCCUPATIONAL THERAPY ASSISTANT COLLABORATIVE PARTNERSHIP

Avery is a new graduate occupational therapist who accepted a position in a large public school system. She has been assigned to supervise an occupational therapy assistant with 24 years of experience in schools. The occupational therapy assistant regularly assesses her students using a standardized assessment, as the previous occupational therapist requested, when the student demonstrates changes in status. Avery has heard of the assessment but is not competent in its use. Avery explains that she is not comfortable using this assessment and asks the occupational therapy assistant to stop using it. The occupational therapy assistant verbalizes frustration regarding this request, explaining that the assessment is an excellent tool in determining changes in the student's overall response to treatment. The occupational therapy assistant insists on continuing use of the assessment and offers to train Avery. Avery refuses this offer and recommends an alternative assessment that the occupational therapy assistant has experience using but feels it will not show the changes because the other assessment was used during the initial evaluations. Despite ongoing supervisory meetings, at the end of the school year Avery chooses not to continue with this school system, citing discomfort with the occupational therapy assistant working under Avery's license.

Questions
1. Which ethics standards of conduct are relevant in this case?
2. How should the practitioners proceed?

Next Steps

- Occupational therapists and occupational therapy assistants are equally responsible for promoting a collaborative partnership. Practitioners must be knowledgeable of and adhere to relevant organizational, state, and federal guidelines and regulations.
- If an ethical violation occurs, practitioners should report the violation to the appropriate authority (e.g., human resources, organizational leadership, state regulatory board,

federal regulatory agency or specific organizations such as AOTA, National Board for Certification in Occupational Therapy).

- Practitioners can direct questions and inquiries related to ethics to ethics@aota.org.

Summary

"Establishing a partnering relationship between the occupational therapy assistant and the occupational therapist is imperative in order to create an optimal working environment and deliver effective client care" (Scheerer, 2002, p. 193). It is also both acceptable and ethical for qualified occupational therapy assistants to serve in management roles in which they have administrative responsibility for occupational therapists. Occupational therapists and occupational therapy assistants must understand their individual ethical responsibility to engage in collaborative partnerships. The Code, other AOTA official documents, state practice acts, and employer policies should be used to guide supervision and provide direction in the face of ethical dilemmas.

Acknowledgments

Loretta Foster, MOS, COTA/L; and **Rae Ann Smith, OTD, OTR/L** authored an earlier version of this Advisory Opinion.

REFERENCES

Jacobs, K. (Ed.). (2016). *Management and administration for the occupational therapy assistant: Leadership and application skills*. Slack Inc.

Rowe, N. (2016). *10 tips to building a strong OT/OTA relationship*. https://www.aota.org/publications/student-articles/career-advice/ot-ota-relationship

Scheerer, C. R. (2002). The partnering model: Occupational therapy assistant and occupational therapy students working together. *Occupational Therapy in Health Care, 15*(1–2), 193–208. https://doi.org/10.1080/J003v15n01_17

Smoot, M. (2019). Succeeding as a new leader or manager. In K. Jacobs & G. L. McCormack (Eds.), *The occupational therapy manager* (6th ed, pp. 625–631). AOTA Press.

Ethical Considerations for Students and Practitioners With Disabilities

RENA B. PUROHIT, JD, OTR/L, and KATHRYN L. SORENSEN, OTD, OTR/L, ADAC

Key Points

- Reasonable accommodations for students and practitioners with disabilities are a right under law.
- Educational institutions and employers must inform students and employees about policies and procedures related to obtaining and implementing reasonable accommodations.
- The medical and disability status of students and practitioners must remain confidential.

Introduction

As the occupational therapy profession strives to become more inclusive of people from diverse backgrounds, it is essential to be intentional and methodical in creating opportunities for and providing support to students and practitioners with disabilities. It is critical to meet the imperative call to "take bold new steps to become an organization and profession that embraces DEI [diversity, equity, and inclusion] and justice for all members, professionals, students, clients, and underrepresented and/or marginalized individuals or groups" as published in the American Occupational Therapy Association's (AOTA's) Diversity, Equity, and Inclusion Strategic Plan Report (2021a, p. 4). Supporting students and practitioners with disabilities goes far beyond a professional vision. Providing support is mandated by federal law, as written in the Americans with Disabilities Act (ADA) of 1990 and Section 504 of the Rehabilitation Act of 1973 (Disability Rights Education & Defense Fund, n.d.). As a profession that desires to be a leader in inclusion among health care professions, occupational therapy educational programs and places of work must create and implement policies designed to educate and empower students and practitioners with disabilities. While holding this charge, it is also essential to remain ethically responsible to students, practitioners, and future clients, as outlined in the AOTA Code of Ethics (the Code).

Background

Section 504 was the first disability civil rights law to be enacted in the United States. It prohibits discrimination against people with disabilities in programs that receive federal financial assistance and sets the foundation for the ADA of 1990, which extended civil rights in the form of accommodations and accessibility to individuals with disabilities in both public and private entities (Disability Rights Education & Defense Fund, n.d.; U.S. Department of Education [ED], 2020). The intention of the ADA is to protect against discrimination on the basis of a disability. Specifically, the ADA defines a person with a disability as someone who (1) "has a physical or mental impairment that substantially limits one or more major life activities," (2) "has a history or record of such an impairment", or (3) "is perceived by others as having such an impairment" (U.S. Department of Justice, n.d.). Some conditions may warrant medical intervention or result in a deficit but may not rise to the level of impairment as defined by the ADA. Together, these legislative mandates protect people with disabilities in almost all aspects of American life, including housing, education, employment, and recreation. In any situation in which an otherwise qualified person might be prevented from achieving his or her potential because of a disability, Section 504 and the ADA demand that opportunities be available for all.

Implications for Occupational Therapy Students and Practitioners

REASONABLE ACCOMMODATIONS

The ADA and Section 504 are anti-discrimination acts, not entitlement acts. This legislation requires that individuals receive the opportunity to participate in educational and vocational endeavors for which they are otherwise qualified. All educational institutions and workplaces that employ more than 15 people are required to provide reasonable accommodations (appropriate modifications, aids, and services) that enable a qualified student or employee with a disability to have an equal opportunity to participate in the educational program or workplace (ED, 2020; U.S. Equal Employment Opportunity Commission, n.d.). Documentation of a specific disability does not translate directly into specific accommodations. Reasonable accommodations are unique to each person and should be based on the functional impact of the condition and how likely it is that the condition will affect the person's interaction with the environment (e.g., course assignments, essential functions, physical design). The responsibility for initiating accommodation rests with the person with the disability. It is important to note that an equal opportunity to participate does not mean that there will be equal outcomes. Just like their typical peers, some students with disabilities will fail coursework or fieldwork, and some practitioners will not meet the standards of the workplace. The ADA focuses on whether people with disabilities have equal access to an education or employment opportunity for which they are otherwise qualified (U.S. Department of Justice, n.d.). The ADA is not intended to optimize or give an advantage for success: "The intent of the law, again, was to level the playing field, not to tilt it" (Gordon & Keiser, 1998, p. 5).

The process of applying for reasonable accommodations is similar in both academia and the workplace. Students apply for accommodations through an administrative office, such as the Office of Disability Services (ODS), and practitioners apply through the appropriate personnel department designated by their employer. In both instances, it is imperative that the individual with the disability communicate their needs, and that the institution engage in an interactive process by which both parties can work together to determine accommodations that are reasonable and appropriate for the student, employee, site, and clients.

SELF-IDENTIFICATION AND PRIVACY

There is a lot of perceived stigma and misinformation around identification and disclosure as it relates to people with disabilities disclosing to ensure that their civil rights are protected. This disclosure does not mean that their professors, colleagues, or even direct supervisors need to know their disability. Although there are certain people at an institution who do need to see verification of one's disability, federal laws protect the privacy and confidentiality of people with disabilities to allow them to have the accommodations they need with the least amount of disclosure and vulnerability. For example, the Family Educational Rights and Privacy Act of 1974 (FERPA; P. L. 93-380) protects the privacy of all students' educational records. Educational institutions must have written consent from a student before releasing information from their educational records (ED, 2021). The student alone determines whether to share information, decides what information to share, selects which faculty members may receive information, and what information a fieldwork site is given. "The Department of Justice has indicated that a faculty member generally does not need to know what the disability is, only that it has been appropriately verified by the individual (or office) assigned this responsibility on behalf of the institution" (Association on Higher Education and Disability, 1996, p. 1). This also applies to fieldwork settings, as it is often sufficient for a site to know the accommodation but not the exact diagnosis of a student. It is best for all parties that this permission be in writing, so there can be specific and clear details about what educators are and are not permitted to share. For all people with disabilities, protection of confidential information is not only part of FERPA but also the ADA and Section 504. Only the individual(s) involved in making the determination about whether an accommodation is reasonable need to know a specific diagnosis or medical history, and only those individuals involved in implementing the reasonable accommodation need to be made aware of any approved accommodations (U.S. Equal Employment Opportunity Commission, 2002).

A person with a disability may make the decision not to self-identify or apply for accommodations for any reason; however, it is important that people with disabilities are aware that unless they apply for a reasonable accommodation under the ADA and Section 504, and those protections are approved by the educational institution or workplace, no associated privileges are afforded (ED, 2011). This decision is to be respected. Given the skill set of occupational therapy practitioners, one of the inherent challenges that comes with working with students or coworkers with disabilities is the natural desire to provide accommodations that were not asked for or approved. As difficult as it might be, all faculty, clinical educators, supervisors, coworkers, and practitioners must only provide the accommodations that students and coworkers with disabilities have requested and been approved for. Employers cannot force an employee to apply for or accept any accommodations (U.S. Equal Employment Opportunity Commission, n.d.).

Technical Standards and Essential Job Functions

After determining that a person meets the definition of disability under the ADA, the next step in determining reasonable accommodations is to look at the technical standards of an educational program (in the classroom) or essential job functions (at fieldwork or a worksite). Occupational therapy and occupational therapy assistant educational programs are strongly encouraged to include a list of technical standards for prospective and current students to use as a reference to determine what reasonable accommodations might be needed for effective participation in their program. A variety of documents have helped clarify the essential job functions of an occupational therapist or occupational therapy assistant (AOTA, 2020, 2021b; National Center for O*Net Development, 2022a, 2022b). Educational institutions have an ethical obligation to set students up for success with realistic accommodations that will translate to the workplace after graduation. Similarly, places that employ occupational therapy practitioners are strongly encouraged to create a list of essential job functions that practitioners can use to help initiate reasonable accommodations. Students and practitioners with disabilities have an ethical obligation to recognize that they are engaging in a therapeutic relationship with a recipient of occupational therapy services. Moreover, providers (both students and practitioners) are ethically obligated to apply for accommodations that will ensure they do not inflict harm or injury to clients.

ACCESSIBILITY

It is important to ensure that occupational therapy programs and workplaces are accessible for students, practitioners, and clients with disabilities. The ADA lays out guidelines for accessibility of buildings, classrooms, bathrooms, and parking, but many older campus locations and sites where occupational therapy practitioners work are not up to date with these federal standards, making it challenging for people with physical disabilities to access them. When teaching in a classroom, presenting at a conference, or providing an in-service in the workplace, it is important to consider implementing universal design principles where applicable, and ensuring that learning management platforms are inclusive for students and faculty with various learning styles and abilities (Harbour & Greenberg, 2017). It is also important for educational programs to foster partnerships with community organizations representing people with disabilities to make certain that the program and curriculum are reflective of their voices (Harbour & Greenberg, 2017; Scott, 2019).

Beyond accessibility and federal standards, inclusive classrooms and workplaces consist of informed leaders, accepting attitudes, and positive interactions, where participation and contribution to an inclusive environment for people with disabilities are supported (Bonaccio et al., 2020; Scott, 2019). Institutions can improve the learning and work environment by assessing accessibility and disability services through surveys, providing training programs, and providing opportunities for engagement with community disability initiatives (Harbour & Greenberg, 2017). It is imperative that occupational therapy practitioners ensure that people with disabilities are included in the larger conversation about justice, equity, diversity, and inclusion.

AOTA is committed to acting with intention to create an environment where all people within the professional community, including students and practitioners with disabilities, are valued and able to give their best in the communities where they live and work. AOTA strives to recognize and uplift diversity within the profession and is committed to creating opportunities to foster inclusivity, participation, justice, and representation (AOTA, 2021a).

Relation to the AOTA Code of Ethics

The Code is designed to reflect the dynamic nature of the occupational therapy profession, the evolving health care environment, and emerging technologies that can present potential ethical concerns in practice, research, education, and policy. Exhibit 30.1 contains ethical standards from the Code related to ethical considerations for students and practitioners with disabilities.

Tips

To ensure people with disabilities are not being discriminated against in the school or workplace, the following tips are recommended both for people with disabilities and institutions:

PEOPLE WITH DISABILITIES

- Take time to learn your rights and understand the laws.
- Be proactive about asking for your accommodations. Talk to personnel from the appropriate office to learn more about what accommodations you might need.
- Engage in the interactive process, which is a dialogue between an educational institution or employer and an individual with a disability to determine a reasonable accommodation (ED, 2011).
- Maintain your reasonable accommodation request and determination in writing. It is always best to have a written record of your request and determination.

EDUCATION AND WORKPLACE INSTITUTIONS

- Prepare to have people with disabilities in your program/workplace by listing technical standards and essential functions and ensuring that there is a clear plan in place for people with disabilities to apply for reasonable accommodations.
- Inform people with disabilities about how to apply for accommodations early and often during the application process, and then have clear communication and reminders regularly. All faculty, practitioners, staff, and students should know how to apply for an accommodation at any time.
- Engage in the interactive process, which is a dialogue between an educational institution or employer and an individual with a disability to determine a reasonable accommodation (ED, 2011).
- Respect and implement the accommodations that are approved, and do not provide accommodations that are not approved.

EXHIBIT 30.1.

ETHICAL STANDARDS RELATED TO ETHICAL CONSIDERATIONS FOR STUDENTS AND PRACTITIONERS WITH DISABILITIES

- Comply with current federal and state laws, state scope of practice guidelines, and AOTA policies and Official Documents that apply to the profession of occupational therapy.
- Inform employers, employees, colleagues, students, and researchers of applicable policies, laws, and Official Documents.
- Do not inflict harm or injury to recipients of occupational therapy services, students, research participants, or employees.
- Provide students with access to accurate information regarding educational requirements and academic policies and procedures relative to the occupational therapy program or educational institution.
- Maintain the confidentiality of all verbal, written, electronic, augmentative, and nonverbal communications in compliance with applicable laws, including all aspects of privacy laws and exceptions thereto (e.g., Health Insurance Portability and Accountability Act, FERPA).
- Facilitate comprehension and address barriers to communication (e.g., aphasia; differences in language, literacy, health literacy, or culture) with the recipient of service (or responsible party), student, or research participant.
- Demonstrate a level of cultural humility, sensitivity, and agility within professional practice that promotes inclusivity and does not result in harmful actions or inactions with persons, groups, organizations, and populations from diverse backgrounds, including age, gender identity, sexual orientation, race, religion, origin, socioeconomic status, degree of ability, or any other status or attributes.

Note. From the Standards of Conduct from the AOTA Code of Ethics.

CASE EXAMPLE 30.1. STUDENT DISCLOSURE OF DISABILITY

Tanisha is meeting with the **academic fieldwork coordinator** (AFWC) to prepare for her first Level II fieldwork (FWII) experience. Although she has spoken to the AFWC about her diagnosis of anxiety disorder and dyslexia, Tanisha has not formally applied for reasonable accommodations through her university's ODS. She states that some of her instructors just gave her more time for tests and other assignments. She does not understand why the other occupational therapy instructors did not automatically give those accommodations to her, and she thinks those professors are not supportive. The AFWC informs Tanisha that she has the right to apply for accommodations to support her at her fieldwork site and asks her whether she thinks it might benefit her to have extra time for documentation. Tanisha states that she does not see the benefit of accommodations, as she has managed to get good grades in the program. She also does not want to reveal to the fieldwork site that she has a disability because she plans to apply for jobs in this city after graduation. She says she does not want to be discriminated against and wants to prove that she can perform without assistance. After the AFWC explains to Tanisha that she can be approved for an accommodation without the site knowing her specific disabilities (they would just be informed of the accommodations); Tanisha still decides not to disclose or ask for accommodations through the ODS at her FWII placement clinical site.

When the AFWC contacts Tanisha after week 2 to check her progress, Tanisha says things are okay. At a week 4 site visit, Tanisha's fieldwork educator, **Jeremy,** tells the AFWC that he is concerned about Tanisha's difficulty with confidence, time management, and documentation. He says that Tanisha is doing well when she is engaged with clients, but often states she doesn't "feel ready" to do an evaluation or take on more clients, and therefore does not always do what is asked. She also seems to sometimes "shut down" in stressful situations and she is making a lot of mistakes and taking a lot of time with documentation. Jeremy asks whether Tanisha has a learning disability or other disability that he should know about, and he requests advice on how to help her be more successful with confidence and documentation. The AFWC lets Jeremy know that Tanisha does not have any accommodations, and encourages him to document Tanisha's difficulties and to give her frequent and specific feedback. The AFWC says that if these suggestions don't correct the problems, a learning contract or additional site visit could be considered. Before leaving the site visit, the AFWC privately talks to Tanisha and again asks if she thinks accommodations might be helpful and reminds her of the potential risks of not having an accommodation. Tanisha says she is overwhelmed but does not want her site to think less of her, so she is not going to apply for accommodations.

Tanisha's mid-term Fieldwork Performance Evaluation (FWPE) scores show she is struggling with documentation (both time and accuracy) and managing her emotions and anxiety in stressful situations (she has yet to do an evaluation because she does not feel ready). Jeremy states that Tanisha is falling behind and requests to have a learning contract initiated with specific goals she must meet in 1 week to continue her fieldwork at that site. The learning contract is put in place without Tanisha applying for accommodations through the university. At the end of the week with the learning contract in place, Tanisha has not met her goals and is dismissed from her FWII placement by the site. Tanisha reports to the Director of the program that she asked Jeremy for more time to do her notes during the week and he said he could not allow that unless she applied to her university's ODS. She feels that because faculty gave her accommodations without her going through ODS, Jeremy should have given them to her as well. She reports that she has been discriminated against by her site for having a disability and that she should not have been dismissed because she asked for an accommodation.

(Continued)

CASE EXAMPLE 30.1. STUDENT DISCLOSURE OF DISABILITY *(Cont.)*

Questions

1. What would you do if you were the AFWC?
2. What standards from the Code do you think apply to this situation?
3. What laws apply to this scenario?
4. What are the ethical obligations of the fieldwork coordinator?
5. How would you navigate this challenging conversation with Tanisha?
6. To whom would you reach out for additional support and knowledge about this scenario?

CASE EXAMPLE 30.2. ESSENTIAL JOB FUNCTIONS

Adam is a student with spina bifida who uses forearm crutches. He informs the **AFWC** that he wants to do his FWII at an inpatient rehabilitation center for people with spinal cord injuries. The AFWC recommends that he apply for reasonable accommodations at the ODS, and asks for permission to disclose his needs to potential sites (without disclosing identifying information) to see if a site can be found that meets his accommodation needs. Adam agrees, gives written consent, and applies to the ODS for an accommodation to not have to lift more than 10 pounds while on fieldwork. The educational institution's ODS contacts the AFWC with this request and the AFWC then reaches out to potential sites to start the interactive process to determine whether Adam's request is reasonable. Six sites indicate that an essential job function of their site is for therapists to be able to perform transfers and keep people safe independently; therefore, an accommodation to not lift more than 10 pounds would not be reasonable. Finally, one site supervisor states that, while an essential job function at the site is for all therapists to be able to do transfers independently, they would be willing to work with Adam to just require him to explain how to do transfers to his fieldwork educator. The ODS office approves the accommodation at the agreement of the site to waive this essential job function.

The AFWC is glad that Adam has a placement in a setting he wants to be in, but they are also concerned about whether his inability to transfer clients is going to affect his ability to be employed in this setting after graduation. While there are some facilities that do not require occupational therapy practitioners to transfer clients independently, at the very least he will need to ensure he can keep clients and himself physically safe at all times. The AFWC is torn between placing Adam at this site with an accommodation that would not be permitted if he were an employee, and allowing him to learn in the setting he desires. The AFWC decides to have a conversation with Adam about the pros and cons of doing his FWII at this site and to let him know that six sites, in addition to the site that agreed to take him, found that this accommodation would not be reasonable if he were an employee. The AFWC lets Adam know that they will ultimately respect his decision if he wants to do FWII at this site, but also encourages him to consider a setting that will allow him to fully engage in the educational experience and learn skills that will set him up to be employed after graduation. Adam admits he was not fully thinking about what accommodations would or would not be reasonable as an employee, and that staff in all the places he shadowed said he "would make a great therapist." He admits that if a client were to lose their balance, he would not be able to safely catch them. Adam is understandably upset and torn about what to do.

(Continued)

CASE EXAMPLE 30.2. ESSENTIAL JOB FUNCTIONS *(Cont.)*

Questions
1. What would you do if you were the AFWC?
2. What standards from the Code do you think apply to this situation?
3. What laws apply to this scenario?
4. What are your ethical obligations as a fieldwork coordinator?
5. How would you navigate this challenging conversation with Adam?

CASE EXAMPLE 30.3. REASONABLE ACCOMMODATIONS

Alex is an occupational therapy practitioner with 10 years of experience working in inpatient rehabilitation. Over the last 6 months, Alex experienced several personally challenging situations outside of work and ended up taking 6 weeks off through the Family and Medical Leave Act (1993) for personal reasons. Alex returned to work "ready to go," but during the first week back, Alex was frequently tardy to work, made uncharacteristic errors in documentation and reports, and had two safety incidents. Initially, Alex's coworkers and supervisor did not think this was alarming given the personal challenges Alex had going on, but after another week and an additional safety incident, Alex's supervisor, **Sam**, decided to talk to Alex. Sam pointed out that Alex's quality of work had decreased, and that any additional safety incidents would result in probation. Sam reminded Alex about reasonable accommodations and the process of how to apply for them. Alex, afraid of being stigmatized, denied that anything was wrong and chose not to apply for accommodations.

After 2 more weeks, Alex continued to be late, had one more safety incident, and still made an alarming number of documentation errors. As a result, Alex was put on probation. Alex went to the Human Resources office to let them know about being diagnosed with depression and anxiety earlier in the month and explained that this was the reason for the change in work performance. Alex then applied for three accommodations: (1) to have a flexible schedule that allows Alex to come in and leave at any time; (2) for coworkers to proofread all notes, documentation, and reports for errors; and (3) to be granted immunity from previous safety incidents.

Questions
1. Are the accommodations that Alex applied for reasonable? Why or why not (what information is needed to determine if they are reasonable)?
2. What standards from the Code do you think apply to this situation?
3. What federal laws apply to this scenario?
4. Did the workplace meet its ethical obligations to support Alex's disability leading up to this point?

Summary

Educators: Occupational therapy educators must ensure the focus is not just on helping students with disabilities to successfully graduate, but also on empowering students to understand how reasonable accommodations can allow them to be successfully qualified occupational therapy practitioners after completing their educational program. It is imperative to adhere to federal laws and the ethical standards set forth by the profession's governing body and to keep the focus on setting students up for success as practitioners, not just as students.

Employers and practitioners with a disability: In the workplace, it is the responsibility of the employer to have policies and procedures in place and to communicate to employees how they can apply for a reasonable accommodation. It is also important to communicate to employees that any information shared will be kept confidential. There are many reasons why a person with a disability might not apply for reasonable accommodation. The stigma associated with acknowledging a disability can be a very emotionally challenging process for many people. However, applying for reasonable accommodations will not only allow people with disabilities the opportunity to be successful in their institution, but will also provide a first-hand experience that can be a powerful tool for empowering and supporting future clients.

The ultimate obligation and job of educators and employers is to make certain that the professional standards of conduct are being followed as evidenced by (1) educating students and practitioners about their rights and obligations, (2) allowing people with disabilities to make decisions about their accommodation and disclosure choices, and (3) ultimately ensuring client safety in all situations. By allowing federal laws, professional guidelines, and institutional policies to serve as a guide, the legal and ethical requirements for inclusion will be met. It is also imperative that our institutions be welcoming; actively promoting accessibility for all; and fostering an environment inclusive of people with disabilities that reflects the values, principles, and standards of the occupational therapy profession.

REFERENCES

American Occupational Therapy Association. (2020). Guidelines for supervision, roles, and responsibilities during the delivery of occupational therapy services. *American Journal of Occupational Therapy, 74*(Suppl. 3), 7413410020. https://doi.org/10.5014/ajot.2020.74S3004

American Occupational Therapy Association. (2021a). *AOTA diversity, equity, and inclusion strategic plan report.* https://www.aota.org/-/media/corporate/files/aboutaota/dei-strategic-plan-report.pdf

American Occupational Therapy Association. (2021b). Standards of practice for occupational therapy. *American Journal of Occupational Therapy, 75*(Suppl. 3), 7513410030. https://doi.org/10.5014/ajot.2021.75S3004

Americans with Disabilities Act of 1990, Pub. L. 101-336, 42 U.S.C. §§ 12101–12213 (2000).

Association on Higher Education and Disability. (1996). Confidentiality and disability issues in higher education [brochure]. Author.

Bonaccio, S., Connelly, C. E., Gellatly, I. R., Jetha, A., & Martin Ginis, K. A. (2020). The participation of people with disabilities in the workplace across the employment cycle: Employer concerns and research evidence. *Journal of Business and Psychology, 35*(2), 135–158. https://doi.org/10.1007/s10869-018-9602-5

Disability Rights Education & Defense Fund. (n.d.). *Section 504 of the Rehabilitation Act of 1973.* https://dredf.org/legal-advocacy/laws/section-504-of-the-rehabilitation-act-of-1973/

Family and Medical Leave Act of 1993, 29, U.S.C. §§ 2601–2654 (2006).

Family Educational Rights and Privacy Act, of 1974, Pub. L. 93-380, 20 U.S.C., § 1232g, 34CFR Part 99.

Gordon, M., & Keiser, S. (1998). *Accommodations in higher education under the Americans with Disabilities Act (ADA): A no-nonsense guide for clinicians, educators, administrators, and lawyers.* GSI Publications.

Harbour, W. S., & Greenberg, D. (2017). *Campus climate and students with disabilities* [Research brief]. National Center for College Students with Disabilities. https://ici-s.umn.edu/files/h9Fy39M6hQ/nccsd_campus_climate_brief_-_final_pdf_with_tags2

Health Insurance Portability and Accountability Act of 1996, Pub. L. 104-191, 42 U.S.C. § 300gg, 29 U.S.C §§ 1181–1183, and 42 U.S.C. §§ 1320d–1320d9.

National Center for O*NET Development. (2022a). *Occupational therapists.* https://www.onetonline.org/link/summary/29-1122.00

National Center for O*NET Development. (2022b). *Occupational therapy assistants.* https://www.onetonline.org/link/summary/31-2011.00

Rehabilitation Act of 1973, Pub. L. 93–112, 29U.S.C. §§ 701–7961.

Scott, S. (2019). *Access and participation in higher education: Perspectives of college students with disabilities* [Research brief]. National Center for College Students with Disabilities. https://files.eric.ed.gov/fulltext/ED602378.pdf

U.S. Department of Education, Office for Civil Rights. (2011). *Students with disabilities preparing for postsecondary education: Know your rights and responsibilities.* https://www2.ed.gov/about/offices/list/ocr/transition.html

U.S. Department of Education. (2020). *Protecting students with disabilities.* https://www2.ed.gov/about/offices/list/ocr/504faq.html

U.S. Department of Education. (2021). *Family Educational Rights and Privacy Act (FERPA).* https://www2.ed.gov/policy/gen/guid/fpco/ferpa/index.html

U.S. Department of Justice. (n.d.). *Introduction to the Americans with Disabilities Act.* https://www.ada.gov/topics/intro-to-ada/

U.S. Equal Employment Opportunity Commission. (2002). *Enforcement guidance on reasonable accommodation and undue hardship under the ADA.* https://www.eeoc.gov/laws/guidance/enforcement-guidance-reasonable-accommodation-and-undue-hardship-under-ada

U.S. Equal Employment Opportunity Commission. (n.d.). *The ADA: Your responsibilities as an employer.* https://www.eeoc.gov/publications/ada-your-responsibilities-employer

Section 6. Communication

31

Ethical Communication

BRENDA KORNBLIT KENNELL, MA, OTR/L, FAOTA

Key Points

- When people communicate effectively, they can exchange ideas, thoughts, opinions, knowledge, and data. Both the sender and the receiver can feel satisfied that the message was received and understood with clarity and purpose (Coursera, 2023).
- Communication forms include verbal and nonverbal, written, visual, and listening. Venues for communication include social media, websites, and online forums; phone and video chats; through paper mail and email; and in person (Coursera, 2023).
- It is the ethical duty of every occupational therapy practitioner to provide clear, compassionate, and culturally appropriate communication.

Introduction

People communicate with each other every day, whether in writing, in person, or through online platforms, but how much of the communication reaches the audience in the way it was intended? According to Coursera (2023), effective communication must meet the 5 Cs—it must be "clear, correct, complete, concise, and compassionate" (para. 5). Effective communication is how occupational therapy practitioners give and receive information to and from clients, caregivers, colleagues, students, and the public. When communication is confusing, unclear, misleading, disrespectful, intimidating, or harassing, it can affect the trust and relationship between people, the accuracy and quantity of information gathered from clients, training given to a caregiver, instructions to a student or employee, or the perspectives of other disciplines about occupational therapy and its practitioners. It is the ethical duty of every occupational therapy practitioner to provide clear, compassionate, and culturally appropriate communication, and to continually reflect on and improve their communication abilities with colleagues and clients. Practitioners are compelled to refrain from unethical communication behaviors.

Face-to-face communication includes more than the words that are used or not used (verbal communication), but also how the words are said (paraverbal communication). *Paraverbal communication* includes tone, pitch, and cadence of speech. These are the sounds and emotions conveyed when speaking, the volume and range of high to low pitch of the voice, and the speed of speech. These factors can affect how the recipient perceives what is said (Bennett, 2023). People may speak quickly or slowly depending on their regional dialect; familiarity, proficiency, and comfort with the language they are speaking; and emotions felt at the moment. People can misinterpret or misrepresent these emotions based on their own paraverbal style. For example, someone may speak quickly and loudly when excited about a topic or information, but the listener may believe the speaker is angry. Emphasis on specific words can also affect the meaning or interpretation of a message. The words in these four messages from a supervisor to an employee are identical, but the differing emphasis conveys different messages of encouragement, praise, surprise, or criticism:

- *This* report is great.
- This *report* is great.
- This report *is* great.
- This report is *great*.

In addition, the body language, positioning, and proximity of the speaker and the recipient of the message (nonverbal communication) affect how a message is received. These nonverbal communication factors can provide cues that clarify or contradict the verbal message. For example, when someone says, "You're such a pain" to a colleague while smiling broadly, the recipient may ascertain that the speaker is making a joke. When an occupational therapy practitioner stands over a seated client, student, or employee, their physical position can convey a sense of authority and make the recipient feel powerless or overwhelmed, rendering them unable to clearly receive the intent and the words that are spoken. In the United States, failing to make eye contact with the speaker is typically considered disrespectful, but direct eye contact can be uncomfortable for neurodivergent people, and it is considered rude in certain cultures (U.S. Department of Health and Human Services [DHHS] Office of Minority Health, n.d.-a). Written, printed, or texted communication lacks paraverbal and nonverbal cues, which can affect how the recipient perceives the message. In these written modes, people use emojis to convey emotion; and italics, bold print, underlining, and capitalization to express emphasis.

Gestures can also interfere with effective communication among and with people of different cultures. Many gestures common in the United States have different meanings and are actually rude or offensive in other countries. For example, the thumbs-up symbol is the equivalent of extreme disrespect and cursing in Greece, Iran, Russia, and West Africa. Crossed fingers are a symbol for female genitalia in Vietnam. Curling a finger to beckon someone to "come here" is used only for dogs in the Philippines (Teixeira, 2023).

While growing up, everyone is exposed to the beliefs and opinions of those around them. These beliefs, combined with information from a variety of sources, including books, music, film, television, and the news, may lead to the development of stereotypes about other people. Stereotypes can have positive or negative connotations and can lead to implicit or unconscious bias about people based on race, ethnic origin, age, gender identity, or other attributes. Implicit bias can lead to microaggressions—words or actions that communicate bias against certain people (Limbong, 2020). When microaggressions are evident, people are often unaware of what they have communicated or the impact on the recipient. When confronted, the offending individual may become defensive, deny any such intention, or downplay the effect on others

(Limbong, 2020). Intentional or not, microaggressions can derail effective communication, erode trust, and inhibit further interaction. People from majority cultures need to consider the impact of what and how they communicate and be open and responsive to feedback.

Relation to the AOTA Code of Ethics

The AOTA Code of Ethics (the Code) encompasses the core values, ethical principles, and standards of conduct that can guide occupational therapy practitioners toward ethical behavior, both interpersonally and professionally. Occupational therapy practitioners observe the core values of *equality* and *dignity* and the ethical principle of *fidelity* when they treat all persons fairly and with respect and integrity. They exemplify these core values when they engage in communication that is civil, inclusive, and culturally sensitive. The core values of *freedom*, *justice*, and *dignity*; and the ethical principles of *beneficence* and *autonomy*; are demonstrated through respecting the confidentiality and privacy of clients, caregivers, colleagues, employees, and students; and ensuring that communication is collaborative, understandable, and honors choice and diversity of thought. *Truth*, or *veracity*, protects against communication that is deceptive or misleading. See Exhibit 31.1 for standards related to ethical communication in the Code.

Reference to Other AOTA Documents

The American Occupational Therapy Association's (AOTA's) Diversity, Equity, and Inclusion Resource Library (AOTA, n.d.-b) has several valuable resources addressing communication:

- Unconscious Bias Training (Atewologun et al., 2018)
- Implicit Bias Testing (Project Implicit, 2022)
- "What's Your Pronoun? Strategies for Inclusion in the Workplace" (Out & Equal, 2020)
- Diversity, Equity, Inclusion, & Justice Vocabulary (Avarna Group, n.d.)
- Learning Modules on Microaggressions and Facing Difficult Conversations (AOTA, n.d.-a)

Reference to Other Resources

The National Board for Certification in Occupational Therapy (NBCOT®) has resources including the following:

- 13 Simple Ways You Can Have More Meaningful Conversations (Hall, 2013)
- JEDI Reflection Points learning modules (NBCOT, n.d.).

The American Psychological Association (APA) *Publication Manual* (7th ed.; 2019) has an excellent section on bias-free language in professional writing.

EXHIBIT 31.1.
ETHICAL STANDARDS RELATED TO COMMUNICATION

- Maintain the confidentiality of all verbal, written, electronic, augmentative, and nonverbal communication in compliance with applicable laws, including all aspects of privacy laws and exceptions thereto (e.g., Health Insurance Portability and Accountability Act, Family Educational Rights and Privacy Act).
- Preserve, respect, and safeguard private information about employees, colleagues, and students unless otherwise mandated or permitted by relevant laws.
- Demonstrate responsible conduct, respect, and discretion when engaging in digital media and social networking, including, but not limited to, refraining from posting protected health or other identifying information.
- Facilitate comprehension and address barriers to communication (e.g., aphasia; differences in language, literacy, health literacy, or culture) with the recipient of service (or responsible party), student, or research participant.
- Do not use or participate in any form of communication that contains false, fraudulent, deceptive, misleading, or unfair statements or claims.
- Do not engage in verbal, physical, emotional, or sexual harassment of any individual or group.
- Do not engage in communication that is discriminatory, derogatory, biased, intimidating, insensitive, or disrespectful or that unduly discourages others from participating in professional dialogue.
- Engage in collaborative actions and communication as a member of interprofessional teams to facilitate quality care and safety for clients.
- Treat all stakeholders professionally and equitably through constructive engagement and dialogue that is inclusive, collaborative, and respectful of diversity of thought.
- Demonstrate courtesy, civility, value, and respect to persons, groups, organizations, and populations when engaging in personal, professional, or electronic communications, including all forms of social media or networking, especially when that discourse involves disagreement of opinion, disparate points of view, or differing values.

Note. From the Standards of Conduct from the AOTA Code of Ethics.

Tips

Inclusivity: Using inclusive language means avoiding words and phrases that can be offensive or exclusionary to individuals, groups, or populations. This includes written forms, signs, surveys, and so forth.

- Use person-first language instead of identity-first language (e.g., a person who has a disability vs. a disabled person). This is a general guideline, as some people or populations prefer identity-first language, such as many autistic people and members of the Deaf community.

- Use gender-neutral terms. Refer to individuals or groups as "they" or "them" instead of "he" or "she." Address a group as "team" or "folks" instead of "guys."
- Use people's preferred pronouns and names.
- Avoid jargon and acronyms such as ADLs, SCI, or SLP; or idioms such as "break a leg," meaning "good luck."
- Avoid using terms implying that diagnoses equal victimhood, such as "stroke victim" or "suffers from cerebral palsy."
- Don't use mental health diagnoses as metaphors for everyday feelings. For example, don't say "Stop being so OCD about your notes" or "I feel so ADD right now" (Seiter, 2018).
- Don't infantilize older adults. Referring to someone as "cute," calling them "honey" instead of using their name, using a sing-song voice, or directing comments and questions to others in the room undermines the person's competence and autonomy.

Printed communication: Facilitating effective printed communication in the workplace may include changes to forms and signage.

- Forms that ask about gender should include options such as "nonbinary gender," an option to write in "other," and an option for "prefer not to answer."
- When asking about race or ethnicity, a form should contain mixed race or multi-ethnic choices, an option for "other," and an option for "prefer not to answer."
- Translation services and forms in languages frequently spoken in the service area should be available. This includes sign language and telecommunications options for people with hearing impairments.
- Forms should be available in large print. Braille forms may be difficult to obtain, but an alternative is having someone available to read forms to someone who is blind or has low vision.
- Printed communication should be written at a third-grade level. An option for having someone read forms to clients should be available for those with low literacy.
- Signs should show multicultural images and not include images that could be offensive to any individual, group, or population. This could include religious symbols such as a cross or Star of David.
- Signs indicating locations of different offices should include a representative symbol if possible, along with printed names of locations.

Conversation: Hall (2013) offers these suggestions to make face-to-face conversations more meaningful:

- Listen to what someone is saying, instead of thinking ahead about your response.
- Ask questions for clarification or to indicate that you are engaged in the conversation.
- Demonstrate interest in what others are saying.
- Ask how you can help others, instead of assuming you know what they want or need.

Unconscious bias: The JEDI (justice, equity, diversity, inclusion) learning modules from NBCOT offer these suggestions regarding implicit bias (NBCOT, n.d.):

- Pause and think logically before speaking.
- Listen to what others are saying and don't jump to conclusions.
- Be willing to make adjustments in what you are thinking.

Next Steps

To effectively communicate with a wide variety of people, it is important to recognize that communication styles and preferences differ. It is important to tailor communication to the intended audience, whether that be clients, family members, students, physicians, teachers, interdisciplinary colleagues, or third-party payers. Occupational therapy practitioners must be aware of barriers and avoid jargon and multi-meaning terms that can be misunderstood. Language used in both verbal and written communication should be

---

CASE EXAMPLE 31.1. CLIENT INTERACTION

Janelle enjoyed her job working in early intervention. There were two new children on her caseload last week. When she arrived at the first house, the mother answered the door wearing traditional clothing from her home country. Janelle entered the home, immediately went to the family room, and sat on the floor. "Come here cutie," she said as she beckoned to the little boy with her finger. The mother sat quietly with a displeased look on her face. Janelle offered the child several activities to address fine motor skills. They built towers with blocks and when the towers fell down, Janelle said, "Look, the house is falling down." She pointed to herself with one finger, and then pointed to the little boy and said, "Now it's your turn." The mother made a distressed sound. Speaking slowly and enunciating every syllable, Janelle said to the mother, "I need to ask you a few questions about your son." Pointing to the older sibling, she asked, "Will your daughter translate for you?" The mother stood up and said, "I do not need a translator, and I most certainly will not have a child tell me what you are saying. I will answer your questions, and then you may leave." Janelle asked a few questions and then stood to leave. "Thank you, you've been *very helpful*. I'll see you next week", she said as she rolled her eyes.

The next day, the supervisor told Janelle that the boy's mother had asked to be assigned to a different occupational therapy practitioner, due to Janelle's lack of respect and poor communication. When Janelle questioned what the mother complained about, the supervisor replied, "She thought you were condescending and spoke to her like a child. She said you used offensive gestures and said and did things that reminded her of what they went through when their home was attacked during the war. She also saw you roll your eyes and speak to her sarcastically. She said she cannot trust you to provide the best care for her child."

Questions
1. How did Janelle's paraverbal and nonverbal communication impact her interaction with the child's mother?
2. What standards of conduct from the Code did Janelle violate?
3. What action(s) do you think Janelle and the supervisor should take to avoid situations like this in the future?

CASE EXAMPLE 31.2. PROFESSIONAL COMMUNICATION

The faculty of an occupational therapy doctoral program met with the students in their research group midway through the semester to assess professional behavior and progress on the project. The students in the group were nervous about meeting with **Dr. Avery,** as he spoke very fast and loudly. He loved to use acronyms that the class hadn't learned. When meeting with one research group, Dr. Avery referred to Shea, a nonbinary student in the class, as "he." Dr. Avery stood and walked around the office during the meeting, and then stood with arms crossed, looking down at Ling. "I'm pretty impressed with your English comprehension, Ling, but I was surprised that you of all people bombed the quiz on statistical analysis last week." Dr. Avery turned to Marcus, and asked when he was going to turn in his two late assignments. "You are bordering on a C in the course, Marcus. You don't want to fail again, do you? And Carson, your last report was (made gesture of thumbs down). My 11-year-old son could write better than this."

Questions
1. How did Dr. Avery's verbal, paraverbal, and nonverbal communication impact the professional-student relationship?
2. What standards of conduct from the Code did Dr. Avery violate?
3. Using an ethical decision-making framework, what course of action do you think the Program Director should take with the students and with Dr. Avery?

inclusive, clear, and free of bias. Pictures and symbols can enhance written communication. It is important to ask questions if a message is unclear, and encourage others to do the same (DHHS, n.d.-b). When an occupational therapy practitioner hears or sees communication that is disrespectful, derogatory, or offensive, they have an ethical duty to speak up. It is the responsibility of all practitioners to facilitate change if the communication in their workplace is toxic or inappropriate.

Summary

The ability to communicate effectively is critical to the profession of occupational therapy. The *Occupational Therapy Practice Framework: Domain and Process* describes the integral occupational therapy process of *therapeutic use of self,* which includes interpersonal communication skills to "shift the power of the relationship to allow clients more control in decision making and problem solving, which is essential to effective intervention" (AOTA, 2020, p. 20). Appropriate information gathering and assessment is most effective when the occupational therapy practitioner acknowledges and uses the client's preferred style and method of communication. Obtaining referrals and authorization for treatment in different settings requires the ability to effectively and appropriately communicate with other disciplines, families, referral sources, third-party payers, and the public. Respectful, accurate, and culturally responsive verbal and written communication is essential.

REFERENCES

American Occupational Therapy Association. (2020). Occupational therapy practice framework: Domain and process (4th ed.). *American Journal of Occupational Therapy, 74*(Suppl. 2), 7412410010. https://doi.org/10.5014/ajot.2020.74S2001

American Occupational Therapy Association. (n.d.-a). *Diversity, equity, and inclusion learning modules.* https://www.aota.org/practice/practice-essentials/dei/diversity-equity--inclusion-toolkit-learning-modules

American Occupational Therapy Association. (n.d.-b). *Diversity, equity, and inclusion resource library.* https://www.aota.org/practice/practice-essentials/dei/diversity-equity--inclusion-toolkit-resource-library

American Psychological Association. (2019). *Publication manual of the American Psychological Association* (7th ed.).

Atewologun, D., Cornish, T., & Tresh, F. (2018). Unconscious bias training: An assessment of the evidence for effectiveness. *Equality and Human Rights Commission Research Report 113.* https://www.ucd.ie/equality/t4media/ub_an_assessment_of_evidence_for_effectiveness.pdf

Avarna Group. (n.d.) *Diversity, equity, inclusion, & justice vocabulary.* https://theavarnagroup.com/resources/equity-inclusion-diversity-vocabulary/

Bennett, M. (2023). *What is paraverbal communication? A guide for professionals.* Niagara Institute. https://www.niagarainstitute.com/blog/paraverbal-communication

Coursera. (2023). *What is effective communication? Skills for work, school, and life.* https://www.coursera.org/articles/communication-effectiveness

Family Educational Rights and Privacy Act of 1974, Pub. L. 93-380, 20 U.S.C. § 1232g; 34 CFR Part 99.

Hall, J. (2013). 13 Simple ways you can have more meaningful conversation. *Forbes.* https://www.forbes.com/sites/johnhall/2013/08/18/13-simple-ways-you-can-have-more-meaningful-conversations/?sh=f4e69a04fe95

Health Insurance Portability and Accountability Act of 1996, Pub. L. 104-191, 42 U.S.C. § 300gg, 29 U.S.C §§ 1181–1183, and 42 U.S.C. §§ 1320d–1320d9.

Limbong, A. (2020). *Microaggressions are a big deal: How to talk them out and when to walk away.* NPR Life Kit. https://www.npr.org/2020/06/08/872371063/microaggressions-are-a-big-deal-how-to-talk-them-out-and-when-to-walk-away

National Board for Certification in Occupational Therapy. (n.d.). *JEDI reflection points: Justice, equity, diversity, and inclusion tools for self-reflection and growth.* https://jedireflectionpoints.nbcot.org/

Out & Equal. (2020). *What's your pronoun: Strategies for inclusion in the workplace.* https://www.aota.org/practice/practice-essentials/dei/diversity-equity--inclusion-toolkit-resource-library

Project Implicit. (2022). *Implicit association test.* https://implicit.harvard.edu/implicit/selectatest.html

Seiter, C. (2018). *An incomplete guide to inclusive language for startups and tech* [Buffer Blog]. https://buffer.com/resources/inclusive-language-tech/

Teixeira, M. I. (2023). *15 insulting gestures in different cultures.* Lingoda. https://blog.lingoda.com/en/15-insulting-gestures-in-different-cultures/

U.S. Department of Health and Human Services Office of Minority Health. (n.d.-a). *Think cultural health: Communication styles.* https://thinkculturalhealth.hhs.gov/assets/pdfs/resource-library/communication-styles.pdf

U.S. Department of Health and Human Services Office of Minority Health. (n.d.-b). *Think cultural health: Effective cross-cultural communication skills.* https://thinkculturalhealth.hhs.gov/assets/pdfs/resource-library/effective-cross-cultural-communication-skills.pdf

Ethics and Social Media

BRENDA KORNBLIT KENNELL, MA, OTR/L, FAOTA, and
JOYCE E. RIOUX, EdD, OTR/L, SCSS, FAOTA

Key Points

- Practice professionalism across social media outlets, just as one would do for in-person communications.
- Protect clients' privacy and confidentiality.
- When using social media, put practices in place to optimize benefits and minimize pitfalls.

Introduction

In 2005, about 5% of Americans used social media; by 2021, that number had risen to 72% (Pew Research Center, 2021). Social media has become popular and is ever evolving. Today, sites and apps exist for social networking (e.g., Facebook, Twitter), professional networking (e.g., CommunOT, LinkedIn), media sharing (e.g., YouTube), content production (e.g., blogs, microblog platforms such as Instagram and Pinterest), knowledge and information aggregation (e.g., Wikipedia), and virtual reality training spaces (Adobe Express, 2022). On a personal level, people may use social media to stay in touch with friends, keep up to date on news, network with others, share opinions, research products, and be entertained. On a professional or business level, people may use social media to disseminate information; network with colleagues; seek advice; and promote a brand, event, or professional presence (Federation of State Medical Boards, 2019).

When occupational therapy practitioners elect to use social media in their private or professional lives, they need to understand how to navigate these different contexts without inadvertently compromising their professional roles and responsibilities, therapeutic relationships, and depiction of other people and places (e.g., clients, colleagues, workplace, occupational therapy profession). Common ethical dilemmas that may surface when using social media include dilemmas around role, tempo, integrity, speech, and competence (Kvalnes, 2020).

ROLE DILEMMAS

As social media users, occupational therapy practitioners may hold many roles (e.g., private individual, friend, professional, employee, employer; Kvalnes, 2020). As private individuals, practitioners need to know that their personal and professional presence on social media will likely meld. In today's digital age, with overlapping networks, information can be easily leaked, viewed, or shared with others outside one's social circle even when privacy settings are in place (ESET UK, 2022). All interactions (e.g., photographs, comments, likes) intended for family, friends, and acquaintances should always meet the benchmark of being workplace appropriate. Privacy settings should also be routinely checked as updates in social media features can impact visibility. As professionals, practitioners may experience clients attempting to "friend" them on their personal accounts. One must be cautious of accepting friend requests because doing so can blur the boundaries between client and professional. Practitioners must also use caution when considering viewing clients' personal social media presence, as this practice may violate a client's personal boundaries and negatively impact the therapeutic relationship.

TEMPO DILEMMAS

Social media allows users to post information, share links, contribute to discussions, and approve or disapprove of content at the click of a button (Kvalnes, 2020). This fast tempo can result in dilemmas, as users may respond before thinking. Celebrities, politicians, and professional athletes often face backlash after their inappropriate or offensive posts, yet their careers often rebound after a public apology (Ballotpedia, 2023; ESPN, 2019; Yang, 2020). Average citizens (e.g., occupational therapy practitioners) may not be afforded that same grace and could face steep disciplinary actions, including loss of employment or professional licensure (ABC News, 2020). Practitioners need to remember that they are the editors of their own work and need to decide what is appropriate to post and how to respond to posts (Ventola, 2014).

INTEGRITY DILEMMAS

Maintaining professional responsibilities across social media platforms is essential. Sharing or liking posts, either intentionally or inadvertently, that include comments or depictions that disparage persons, groups, organizations, or populations can negatively affect others' perceptions of an occupational therapy practitioner's integrity, lead to uncivil behavior, and result in a rippling effect of consequences. Practitioners also have a legal responsibility to protect clients' private and confidential information in accordance with laws (e.g., Health Insurance Portability and Accountability Act of 1996 [HIPAA], Family Educational Rights and Privacy Act of 1974 [FERPA]) and are not excused from this responsibility in social media platforms (Harvan, 2019). Violations can occur by posting information or photos about clients or their conditions either innocently (e.g., photo of child or parent during a pediatric clinic event) or maliciously (e.g., revealing information about a celebrity client). Responding to a client complaining about or praising a practice or facility may also lead to a HIPAA or FERPA violation when enough detail is present to identify the client. Putting practices in place that do not compromise integrity and legal responsibilities is essential.

SPEECH DILEMMAS

Expressing opinions in social media is commonplace. When expressing opinions or defending a stance, one may believe that they are protected under their constitutional rights, "such as freedom of speech, freedom from search and seizure, and the right to privacy; however, these rights can be successfully challenged" (Ventola, 2014, p. 498). Occupational therapy practitioners should always practice legally responsible and professional communication.

COMPETENCE DILEMMAS

Given that social media content is user generated, the quality of information can vary from being reliable and accurate to being questionable and damaging. When searching for content or asking for advice, one should always apply caution. Taking the time to verify that content is credible by triangulating with reliable sources is a good strategy before implementing anything into practice. When coming across content that is inaccurate, unsafe, or contraindicated, the occupational therapy practitioner should thoughtfully compose a response that refutes the content and directs to credible sources.

Relation to the AOTA Code of Ethics

The AOTA Occupational Therapy Code of Ethics (the Code) requires that occupational therapy practitioners adhere to standards of conduct. Although using social media is not inherently unprofessional or unethical, practitioners need to carefully select what, where, and how much to post and respond to on social media. Exhibit 32.1 contains ethical standards from the Code related to social media use.

Among the core values of the Code are *truth* and *prudence*. *Truth* refers to "being accountable, honest, forthright, accurate, and authentic in attitudes and actions." *Prudence* requires thoughtfulness, discretion, and application of good sense when making decisions. When occupational therapy practitioners exercise truth and prudence in their social media practices, there is greater benefit for all. Practitioners following these guidelines can better maintain their professional integrity, responsibility, and accountability; foster healthy therapeutic relationships with clients; uphold professional and legal standards of confidentiality; and conduct themselves in a civil manner that preserves respect.

EXHIBIT 32.1.
ETHICAL STANDARDS RELATED TO USE OF SOCIAL MEDIA

- Respect the practices, competencies, roles, and responsibilities of one's own and other professions to promote a collaborative environment reflective of interprofessional teams.
- Do not engage in actions that reduce the public's trust in occupational therapy.
- Proactively address workplace conflict that affects or can potentially affect professional relationships and the provision of services.
- Maintain privacy and truthfulness in delivery of occupational therapy services, whether in person or virtually.
- Demonstrate responsible conduct, respect, and discretion when engaging in digital media and social networking, including but not limited to refraining from posting protected health or other identifying information.
- Ensure that all marketing and advertising are truthful, accurate, and carefully presented to avoid misleading recipients of service, research participants, or the public.
- Demonstrate courtesy, civility, value, and respect to persons, groups, organizations, and populations, including all forms of social media or networking, especially when that discourse involves disagreement of opinion, disparate points of view, or differing values.
- Demonstrate a level of cultural humility, sensitivity, and agility within professional practice that promotes inclusivity and does not result in harmful actions or inactions with persons, groups, organizations, and populations from diverse backgrounds, including age, gender identity, sexual orientation, race, religion, origin, socioeconomic status, degree of ability, or any other status or attributes.

Note. From the Standards of Conduct from the AOTA Code of Ethics.

Reference to Other Standards

The American Occupational Therapy Association (AOTA) uses an Event Code of Conduct that pertains to both online and in-person events. This document states that AOTA "will not tolerate any form of incivility, harassment, bullying, or microaggressions at its events, whether in person, online, or hybrid format" (AOTA, n.d.). It further states, "all participants in AOTA events are expected to treat others with respect and consideration, follow event rules, and alert AOTA facilitators and/or staff of any inappropriate behavior." While not directly applying to social media, this document does apply to any social media posting regarding AOTA conferences, Representative Assembly, or other volunteer meetings. Discourse regarding sensitive topics being discussed by AOTA membership must remain civil both in person and in the social media arena.

Tips

- Employers should set social media policies, a training/retraining schedule for all employees, and a review cycle to update policies with social media advances (Harvan, 2019).

- When using social media, occupational therapy practitioners should
  - only share content from credible sources,
  - adhere to privacy and confidentiality laws,
  - keep personal and professional accounts separate,
  - frequently update private security settings, and
  - be respectful and professional in communications (Ventola, 2014).

CASE EXAMPLE 32.1. SHARING CLIENT INFORMATION

Janine loved her new job in pediatrics. On Friday, the clinic hosted a field day event for their clients. They went to a park, served refreshments, and played lots of games designed by the occupational therapy staff. Janine was very proud of the obstacle course she designed for the event and was so happy to see the children enjoying it. That weekend Janine posted pictures of kids smiling and laughing with her on the obstacle course on Instagram and wrote, "Remember when I said I would never work in pediatrics? Well, look at me now!" She linked the post to the company's Facebook page. On Monday when Janine arrived at the clinic, the owner/director told her that three of her families had requested to be moved to another occupational therapy practitioner, and four others had called to say they were transferring to another clinic.

Questions
1. What standards from the Code may Janine have violated?
2. What do you think is the appropriate course of action?
3. Which type(s) of dilemmas do you think were illustrated?

CASE EXAMPLE 32.2. BLURRING WORK AND PERSONAL LIFE

Roger enjoyed his home health job in a large county, which included rural, urban, and suburban areas. He liked his co-workers, and they all followed each other on social media sites. One day after work Roger went to a vigil with a friend following a recent mass shooting at an LBGTQ+ dance. There were protesters across the street with anti-LGBTQ+ signs, some blaming the victims and their lifestyles. The next night Roger saw a post on Instagram of two of his coworkers among the group of protesters. He contacted another coworker who was gay, and they talked long into the night about whether they wanted to continue working with these two people. When they arrived at work on Monday, they saw the two coworkers in the director's office. "Did you hear?" asked one of the nurses. "Those two are being terminated because of an Instagram post. They went to that vigil the other night straight from work, wearing their polo shirts with our company insignia, and were carrying signs with hate messages. Three clients have already called this morning refusing to be treated by them anymore."

Questions
1. What standards from the Code may have been violated?
2. What do you think is the appropriate course of action?
3. Which type(s) of dilemmas do you think were illustrated?

CASE EXAMPLE 32.3. SHARING WORKPLACE FRUSTRATIONS

Sara was an occupational therapy student who had completed half of her second Level II fieldwork placement at Loving Care Skilled Nursing Facility. Her supervisor, **Belinda,** told Sara that she was not on track to successfully complete her fieldwork due to delays in completing documentation, difficulty establishing rapport with the residents, and a lack of consistency in following safety precautions. Throughout the day Sara was impatient with her clients and became frustrated when they couldn't complete her planned activities. That evening Sara relaxed watching some YouTube videos and then decided to post to TikTok. With a glass of wine in her hand, she turned on music and danced suggestively, singing about Belinda the Wicked Bitch of the West, and "Miss I-Don't-Want-To-Do-Therapy Mabel." She finished her video by saying, "If you love your family, don't send them to Loving Care Health Center."

Questions
1. What standards from the Code may have been violated?
2. What do you think is the appropriate course of action?
3. Which type(s) of dilemmas do you think were illustrated?

Summary

This Advisory Opinion is not to convey that occupational therapy practitioners cannot use social media for personal or professional purposes. Instead, it is offered as guidance to better understand possible dilemmas that can present themselves when best practices are not put into place. The proliferation of social media platforms offers millions of people worldwide opportunities to stay connected, gather and share media, produce content, and aggregate information. People may feel that their postings are personal in nature and not subject to review or judgment by others; yet that is not the case. Today, personal and professional boundaries can easily blur. Practitioners need to be mindful of always observing ethical standards when engaging in social media use.

Acknowledgments

Joanne Estes, MS, OTR/L, and **Lea Cheney Brandt, OTD, MA, OTR/L,** authored an earlier edition of this Advisory Opinion.

REFERENCES

ABC News. (2020). *As social media posts surface and cause backlash, businesses rethink policies for employees.* https://abc11.com/durham-nc-social-media-marketing-what-is/6263724/

Adobe Express. (2022). *The eight top social media sites you should prioritize in 2023.* https://www.adobe.com/express/learn/blog/top-social-media-sites

American Occupational Therapy Association. (n.d.). *AOTA event code of conduct.* https://www.aota.org/events/code-of-conduct

Ballotpedia. (2023). *Elected officials suspended or banned from social media platforms.* https://ballot-pedia.org/Elected_officials_suspended_or_banned_from_social_media_platforms

ESET UK. (2022). *Eight reasons to keep your social media set to private.* https://www.eset.com/uk/about/newsroom/blog/8-reasons-to-keep-your-social-media-set-to-private/

ESPN. (2019). *Jermaine Whitehead just the latest in long line of sports figures to run into trouble on social media.* https://www.espn.com/nfl/story/_/id/23660805/jermaine-whitehead-just-latest-long-line-sports-figures-run-trouble-social-media

Family Educational Rights and Privacy Act of 1974, Pub. L. 93-380, 20 U.S.C. § 1232g; 34 CFR Part 99.

Federation of State Medical Boards. (2019). *Social media and electronic communications.* https://www.fsmb.org/siteassets/advocacy/policies/social-media-and-electronic-communications.pdf

Harvan, A. C. (2019). *HIPAA compliance in the social media age: What physicians should know.* Pennsylvania Medical Society. https://www.pamedsoc.org/list/articles/hipaa-social-media

Health Insurance Portability and Accountability Act of 1996, Pub. L. 104-191, 42 U.S.C. § 300gg, 29 U.S.C §§ 1181–1183, and 42 U.S.C. §§ 1320d–1320d9.

Kvalnes, O. (2020). *Digital dilemmas: Exploring social media ethics in organizations.* Palgrave Macmillan. https://doi.org/10.1007/978-3-030-45927-7

Pew Research Center. (2021). *Social media fact sheet.* https://www.pewresearch.org/internet/fact-sheet/social-media/

Yang, R. (2020). The biggest celebrity apologies on social media in 2020. *Entertainment Weekly.* https://ew.com/celebrity/celebrity-apologies-2020/?slide=a62035cc-f8d0-4415-a1b2-a89214ea5ade#a62035cc-f8d0-4415-a1b2-a89214ea5ade

Occupational Therapy Ethics Rounds in Practice

BARBARA ELLEMAN, OTD, MHS, OTR/L; BRENDA S. HOWARD, DHSc, OTR, FAOTA; BRENDA KORNBLIT KENNELL, MA, OTR/L, FAOTA

Key Points

- Occupational therapy practitioners may experience ethical tensions and moral distress regardless of training, experience, or practice setting.
- Ethical issues can often be anticipated and may have the potential to be addressed proactively or prevented through consultation with other practitioners.
- Occupational therapy ethics rounds can be an important medium for cultivating sensitivity toward anticipated and emerging ethical issues and for preparing practitioners to deal with ethical problems in practice.

Introduction

Occupational therapy practitioners play an important role in improving the quality of life for service recipients in a variety of settings. However, in the complex and dynamic landscape of practice settings, practitioners are often confronted with ethical challenges (Durocher et al., 2016; Durocher & Kinsella, 2021). The duty to act ethically extends beyond rote adherence to standards or codes. Practitioners should also embrace systems that promote and prioritize an ethical culture in the workplace. Ethics rounds offer one approach to proactively navigate ethical challenges and promote the highest standard of care by potentially preventing ethical challenges before they arise or addressing them as they occur (Schmitz et al., 2018; Silén et al., 2016; Wocial et al., 2017).

Occupational therapy ethics rounds are a medium for open dialogue and honest reflection, as a means to practice ethically and mitigate moral distress. *Moral distress* was first defined by Jameton (1984) as when, "one knows the right thing to do, but institutional constraints make it nearly impossible to pursue the right course of action" (p. 6). Erler (2017) clarified that "moral distress is tension that arises when a moral agent (e.g., a practitioner) is unsure of the best course of action to take or encounters a barrier that prohibits doing what he or she knows to be right" (p. 15). Ethical issues can lead to moral distress, which can negatively impact the practitioner, client care, and the practice setting. Moral distress among occupational therapy practitioners has been explored in a variety of practice settings with varied clients and has been found to impact quality of care, personal and work life, and staff retention (Higgins et al., 2021; Howard et al., 2023; Mukherjee et al., 2009; Penny et al., 2014; Rivard & Brown, 2019; Slater & Brandt, 2009; Tinkham et al., 2021).

Although referred to as *occupational therapy ethics rounds* in this Advisory Opinion, interprofessional participation is strongly encouraged. The format of occupational therapy ethics rounds may vary across settings; however, the goal of promoting an ethical culture through dialogue remains. Ethics rounds may consist of reviewing ethical principles and codes of conduct, applying ethical decision-making frameworks to a hypothetical case, or discussing ethical issues the interprofessional or occupational therapy team are facing in practice. The team can reflect on various perspectives and collectively share insights in an effort to prepare practitioners to make informed decisions when faced with an ethical problem (Branch & George, 2017). This process incorporates the use of clinical narratives, reflection, debriefing, communication skills, conflict management, and problem solving. Ethics rounds offer several potential benefits to practitioners and organizations, such as increasing practitioners' awareness of ethical challenges; providing an opportunity for open and honest reflection and dialogue without negative consequences; minimizing moral distress; sharing and receiving support from colleagues; developing skills to solve or prevent ethical issues; and promoting a culture that prioritizes ethics in practice. Ethics rounds encompass many components of ethical clinical practice and provide an opportunity for practitioners to consider what shapes and guides their own ethical decision making.

Ethics rounds provide a means for occupational therapy practitioners to remain apprised of current and emerging ethical challenges. Engaging in ongoing discussions with colleagues can alert practitioners to potential conflicts and promote an adaptable and well-informed approach to client care. Increased awareness and understanding of ethical challenges can aid in ethical decision making and may mitigate ethical challenges before they arise. Ethics rounds serve as a training ground to develop and refine ethical reasoning skills. Figure 33.1 depicts sources of guidance practitioners can use to support ethical reasoning.

As occupational therapy practitioners engage in discussions centered on complex cases, they learn to analyze situations from multiple ethical perspectives and refine their familiarity with the AOTA Code of Ethics (the Code) and regulatory standards. This practice helps them develop the ability to weigh the ethical principles involved, consider relevant values, and arrive at well-reasoned ethical decisions. These skills are transferable and valuable in promoting ethical problem solving as an integral part of everyday clinical decision making. Involving colleagues from other disciplines (e.g., physical therapists, classroom teachers, nurses) can widen everyone's perspective of the issues and ethical ramifications involved in the client's care. Collaborative

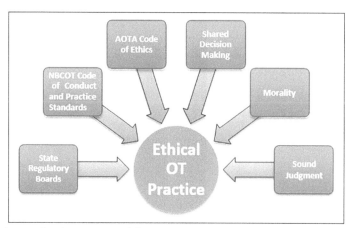

Figure 33.1. Guides to ethical occupational therapy practice.

Note. AOTA = American Occupational Therapy Association; NBCOT = National Board for Certification in Occupational Therapy; OT = occupational therapy.
Source. Erler (2017). Copyright © 2017 by the American Occupational Therapy Association. Used with permission.

discussion with other professionals can be beneficial when the varying disciplines or family members have conflicting priorities or opinions about the value of treatment, and therefore complying, refusing, changing, or ending treatment. Ethics rounds may not always result in a definitive answer to an ethical question, but the process will provide increased clarity and additional perspective on ethical tensions, concerns, or issues.

Relation to the AOTA Code of Ethics

The Code clearly defines standards of conduct and core values to promote ethical actions by occupational therapy practitioners and students. The Code requires that occupational therapy practitioners adhere to standards of conduct and specifically outlines core values of the profession of occupational therapy that should be taken into consideration during interactions and used as a guide toward ethical action. Understanding the Code is a crucial component of fostering an ethical culture in one's area of practice. The incorporation of ethics rounds in practice upholds the long-established core values of altruism, equality, justice, and prudence. Reference to applicable standards of conduct can assist practitioners in evaluating and making decisions about an ethical challenge. Although any core values, ethical principles, or ethical standards may be applicable to a case being discussed by a team during ethics rounds, Exhibit 33.1 contains examples of ethical standards from the Code that are related to and support the incorporation of ethics rounds in occupational therapy.

EXHIBIT 33.1.
ETHICAL STANDARDS RELATED TO ETHICS ROUNDS

- Comply with current federal and state laws, state scope of practice guidelines, and AOTA policies and official documents that apply to the profession of occupational therapy.
- Abide by policies, procedures, and protocols when serving or acting on behalf of a professional organization or employer to fully and accurately represent the organization's official and authorized positions.
- Respect the practices, competencies, roles, and responsibilities of one's own and other professions to promote a collaborative environment reflective of interprofessional teams.
- Establish a collaborative relationship with recipients of service and relevant stakeholders to promote shared decision making.
- Respect the client's right to refuse occupational therapy services temporarily or permanently, even when the refusal has potential to result in poor outcomes.
- Terminate occupational therapy services in collaboration with the service recipient or responsible party when the services are no longer beneficial.
- Report systems and policies that are discriminatory or unfairly limit or prevent access to occupational therapy.
- Engage in collaborative actions and communication as a member of interprofessional teams to facilitate quality care and safety for clients.
- Treat all stakeholders professionally and equitably through constructive engagement and dialogue that is inclusive, collaborative, and respectful of diversity of thought.

Note. From the Standards of Conduct from the AOTA Code of Ethics.

Reference to Other Standards

- The National Board for Certification in Occupational Therapy (NBCOT®; 2022) Code of Conduct outlines professional standards for practitioners.
- State and district regulatory boards often refer to the Code as a resource for ethical practice.
- Codes of ethics from professions other than occupational therapy are important to examine in an interprofessional team setting.

Tips

Organizers who want to implement ethics rounds in their setting should consider the following:

SCHEDULE

- Start small and be realistic when scheduling.

- Schedule during or around already planned meeting times or as an optional continuing education activity during or after work hours.
- Follow a frequency that meets the needs of the facility and individuals (e.g., monthly, quarterly, bi-annually).

FORMAT

A sample structure for a 60-minute ethics rounds could include the following:

- Present the case, topic, article, or scenario (15 minutes)
- Summarize the ethical issues (5 minutes)
- Facilitate a group discussion (30 minutes)
- Summarize the discussion, reiterate major points, and identify next steps (10 minutes)

CONTENT

- Examine a current or retrospective case.
- Analyze a journal article or ethical case in the news.
- Discuss the ethical ramifications of a specific topic (e.g., productivity demands, role of occupational therapy in an emerging population or practice area, barriers to access to occupational therapy services, organizational or insurance barriers, new or emerging interventions).
- Mentor students or early career practitioners in solving ethical dilemmas.

RESOURCES

- Learn what resources (e.g., personnel, library, policies) are available in the setting or facility for supporting ethics rounds. Some hospital systems may have medical ethicists or ethics committees who can provide support.
- Collaborate with the interprofessional team and enter into discussions with those already holding ethics discussions. For example, nursing may incorporate ethics discussions into team huddles (Pavlish et al., 2021).
- Explore current literature or a case or topic relevant to the practice setting.
- AOTA Ethics Advisory Opinions provide a valuable resource related to current topics. Opinions provide an overview of the topic, highlight related standards in the Code, and often include sample ethical scenarios that could be considered for discussion and to save preparation time.

Next Steps

Organizers who want to implement ethics rounds in their setting should rally support from leadership at the facility by sharing important documents and literature to justify the need. A review of the Code and AOTA Ethics Advisories could help identify topic areas

CASE EXAMPLE 33.1. SMOKING AS AN OCCUPATION

John, age 58 years and right-hand dominant, was in an accident that resulted in a left femur fracture, right-hand amputation, and left thumb and index finger amputation. He has been angry and reluctant to participate in any therapy. The **occupational therapy practitioner** working with him in acute rehabilitation was attempting to build rapport and engage him in ADLs. After hearing the role of occupational therapy explained, John finally made eye contact with the practitioner and said that his only goal was to be able to smoke a cigarette without someone else holding it for him. When asked what meaningful occupations he wanted to participate in, he said, "I want to participate in smoking. That's what's meaningful to me." Since admission, despite the medical team's advice not to smoke cigarettes, John had been going outside to smoke cigarettes multiple times a day with the assistance of his family. Although the practitioner wanted to be client centered and help John achieve his stated goals through rehabilitative and compensatory strategies, the thought of helping him smoke has created ethical tension and moral distress.

Questions
1. How do you react to John's goal? Do you think it has the potential to cause ethical tension in the interprofessional team? Why or why not?
2. What ethical principles or standards from the Code are relevant to this case? Do any of the principles or standards conflict with each other?
3. What is the role of interprofessional care in this case?
4. What resources exist to assist the occupational therapy practitioner in confronting this ethical dilemma?
5. What are the practitioner's potential next steps?

CASE EXAMPLE 33.2. PRODUCTIVITY

Participants in an interprofessional team ethics rounds discussion believed that the productivity standards at the skilled nursing facility in which they worked were too high. They reviewed the *Consensus Statement on Clinical Judgment in Health Care Settings* (AOTA et al., 2014). Although this document offered support for their ethical issue, it did not give the team recent information or data on how productivity standards should be set in their setting. The team was left feeling unsure about what to do.

Questions
1. What challenges exist to meeting productivity standards in practice?
2. What other resources should the team seek to provide data and support for challenging existing productivity standards?
3. Using an ethical decision-making framework, what additional steps should the team take in addressing productivity standards?
4. How does the Code apply to the topic of productivity?
5. What are the team's potential next steps? What strategies could the team employ to take their concerns to management?

CASE EXAMPLE 33.3. PEDIATRIC TEAM AND FAMILY WISHES

An **8-year-old child** was admitted to the intensive care unit of a pediatric hospital for the 10th time in 12 months. The child had been diagnosed with a rare form of cancer, and their condition had deteriorated substantially. The medical consensus was that the child's condition was no longer responding to medical intervention and that the child would not survive. However, the child's parents wanted all possible measures to be taken to save the child's life and prevent further decline. Because of their desire, the physician had ordered physical and occupational therapy to begin daily intervention with the child. During the first visit, the **occupational therapist** found that the child was very uncomfortable and unable to participate in basic ADL performance. Upon discussing a plan of care with the parents, including goals for positioning for comfort and decreasing pain, the parents adamantly responded that they wanted the child to be getting out of bed, eating, and getting dressed. The therapist conferred with other team members and found that the parents had made similar statements to them, and that they expected all heroic life-saving measures to be followed.

Questions
1. What are the ethical principles in conflict between the interprofessional team and the child's parents?
2. What resources might the team use in their ethical decision-making process?
3. What additional information does the team need to achieve a plan of action with the child's parents?

for discussion specific to the practice setting. Organizers do not always have to present or feel compelled to have all of the answers. The organizers should determine who will be involved, establish procedures for conducting the meetings, set an initial schedule, and identify discussion leaders and topics for discussion. They should establish a confidential and open forum in which all respectful opinions are welcome.

Summary

Ethics rounds offer the opportunity for discussion and reflection on current laws, rules and policies, and critical incidents that have arisen or may arise in practice. Purposeful reflection and consideration of the most ethical action considering the policies and rules provide the opportunity for the team to identify the most caring response to an ethical issue and avoid conflicts of interest or actions that jeopardize the effectiveness of the team. Occupational therapy practitioners have the obligation to abide by relevant policies, procedures, and regulations, and to inform others of policies that are discriminatory or unfair. The diligence and thoughtfulness that occupational therapy practitioners strive to maintain during all interactions with clients are sometimes challenged by ethical tensions or conflicts. Ethical issues can lead to moral distress, which has a negative impact on practitioners, their ability to provide appropriate care, and the practice setting. Developing a forum for occupational therapy practitioners to reflect on ethical issues openly and honestly can have a powerful impact on fostering an ethical culture, providing an effective strategy to minimize moral distress, maximizing awareness of ethical challenges, and developing skills to effectively problem solve or prevent ethical issues.

Acknowledgment

Kimberly S. Erler, MS, OTR/L, authored an earlier version of this Advisory Opinion.

REFERENCES

American Occupational Therapy Association, American Physical Therapy Association, & American Speech-Language-Hearing Association. (2014). *Consensus statement on clinical judgment in health care settings.* https://www.aota.org/-/media/corporate/files/practice/ethics/apta-aota-asha-concensus-statement.pd

Branch, W. T., Jr., & George, M. (2017). Reflection-based learning for professional ethical formation. *AMA Journal of Ethics, 19*(4), 349–356. https://doi.org/10.1001/journalofethics.2017.19.4.medu1-1704

Durocher, E., Kinsella, E. A., McCorquodale, L., & Phelan, S. (2016). Ethical tensions related to systemic constraints: Occupational alienation in occupational therapy practice. *Occupational Therapy Journal of Research, 36*(4), 216–226. https://doi.org/10.1177/1539449216665117

Durocher, E., & Kinsella, E. A. (2021). Ethical tensions in occupational therapy practice: Conflicts and competing allegiances. *Canadian Journal of Occupational Therapy, 88*, 244–253. https://doi.org/10.1177/00084174211021707

Erler, K. S. (2017). The role of occupational therapy in ethics rounds practice. *OT Practice, 22*(13), 15–18.

Higgins, P., Kellish, A., Fleming, D., Gotthold, S., & Tiziani, M. (2021). The double-edged sword of moral distress and burnout among health science clinical educators. *American Journal of Occupational Therapy, 75*(Suppl. 2), 7512510259p1. https://doi.org/10.5014/ajot.2021.75S2-RP259

Howard, B. S., Beckmann, B., Flynn, D., Haller, J., Pohl, M., Smith, K., & Webb, S. (2023). Moral distress in the time of COVID-19: Occupational therapists' perspectives. *Occupational Therapy in Health Care*, 1–17. https://doi.org/10.1080/07380577.2023.2181625

Jameton, A. (1984). *Nursing practice: The ethical issues.* Prentice Hall.

Mukherjee, D., Brashler, R., Savage, T. A., & Kirschner, K. L. (2009). Moral distress in rehabilitation professionals: Results from a hospital ethics survey. *PM & R: The Journal of Injury, Function, and Rehabilitation, 1*, 450–458. https://doi.org/10.1016/j.pmrj.2009.03.004

National Board for Certification in Occupational Therapy. (2022). Code of Conduct. https://www.nbcot.org/professional-conduct/code-of-conduct

Pavlish, C. L., Brown-Saltzman, K., Robinson, E. M., Henriksen, J., Warda, U. S., Farra, C., . . . Jakel, P. (2021). An ethics early action protocol to promote teamwork and ethics efficacy. *Dimensions of Critical Care Nursing, 40*(4), 226–236. https://doi.org/10.1097/DCC.0000000000000482

Penny, N. H., Ewing, T. L., Hamid, R. C., Shutt, K. A., & Walter, A. S. (2014). An investigation of moral distress experienced by occupational therapists. *Occupational Therapy in Health Care, 28*, 382–393. https://doi.org/10.3109/07380577.2014.933380

Rivard, A. M., & Brown, C. A. (2019). Moral distress and resilience in the occupational therapy workplace. *Safety, 5*(1), 10. https://doi.org/10.3390/safety5010010

Schmitz, D., Groß, D., Frierson, C., Schubert, G. A., Schulze-Steinen, H., & Kersten, A. (2018). Ethics rounds: Affecting ethics quality at all organisational levels. *Journal of Medical Ethics, 44*, 805–809. https://doi.org/10.1136/medethics-2018-104831

Silén, M., Ramklint, M., Hansson, M. G., & Haglund, K. (2016). Ethics rounds: An appreciated form of ethics support. *Nursing Ethics, 23*(2), 203–213. https://doi.org/10.1177/0969733014560930

Slater, D. Y., & Brandt, L. C. (2009). Combating moral distress. *OT Practice, 14*(2), 13–18.

Tinkham, L., Guyton, K., Eddy, E., & Erler, K. (2021). Moral distress among occupational therapy practitioners caring for clients with traumatic brain injury. *Annals of International Occupational Therapy, 4*, 1–7. https://doi.org/10.3928/24761222-20210601-01

Wocial, L., Ackerman, V., Leland, B., Benneyworth, B., Patel, V., . . . Nitu, M. (2017). Pediatric ethics and communication excellence (PEACE) rounds: Decreasing moral distress and patient length of stay in the PICU. *HEC Forum, 29*(1), 75–91. https://doi.org/10.1007/s10730-016-9313-0

Section 7. Professional Civility

34

Professional Civility

BRENDA KORNBLIT KENNELL, MA, OTR/L, FAOTA

Key Points

- "Civility is behavior that shows respect toward another person, makes that person feel valued, and contributes to mutual respect, effective communication, and team collaboration" (Lower, 2012, para. 4).
- "Civility entails honoring one's personal values, while simultaneously listening to disparate points of view . . . Prioritizing civility facilitates effective communication, high-functioning teams, inclusive and productive communities, and civic engagement" (Kaslow & Watson, 2017, para. 1).
- "Incivility can be expressed in a variety of verbal and sometimes physical behaviours, including dismissing the views of others without explanation, repeatedly demeaning others who are subordinate to one's power, or patterns of disrespect based on minority status" (McCullough et al., 2023, para. 1).
- Occupational therapy practitioners have an ethical obligation to behave in a civil manner with colleagues, clients, and families, and in all professional communication.

Definitions

- *Implicit (or unconscious) bias*—Positive or negative "bias that occurs automatically and unconsciously, that nevertheless affects judgments, decisions, and behaviors" (National Institutes of Health, 2022, para. 2).
- *Microaggressions*—Subtle, often unintentional words or actions that convey some bias against people of a historically marginalized group (Limbong, 2020).
- *Lateral vs. vertical aggression*—Aggressive words or actions between colleagues or peers, vs. between colleagues at different power levels (Cascella, n.d.).
- *Prejudice*—"An irrational attitude of hostility directed against an individual, a group, a race or their supposed characteristics" (Merriam-Webster, n.d.).

Introduction

Civility includes many components. Ethical and social responsibility in a diverse world includes ethical decision making in collaboration with others. Communication includes the ability to communicate one's ideas while also respecting other people's opinions, even when they differ from one's own. Effective self-reflection, teamwork skills, and leadership abilities foster collaboration and serve to encourage others (Kaslow & Watson, 2017).

Incivility can take many forms, ranging from behavior that is annoying, disruptive, or intimidating; to behavior that is hateful, threatening, or violent. HR Search & Rescue (2021) defines *disruptive behavior in the workplace* as behavior that "prohibits others in the workplace from functioning normally" (para. 1). The Joint Commission (2021) defines *intimidating and disruptive behavior* as including "overt actions, such as verbal outbursts and physical threats, as well as passive activities such as refusing to perform assigned tasks or quietly exhibiting uncooperative attitudes during routine activities" (p. 1). Less aggressive behaviors, including facial expressions, eye rolling, avoidance, and demeaning comments are also disruptive (Rehder, 2020; Savrin, n.d.).

Workplace colleagues gossiping and spreading rumors, ignoring policies about dress code or lateness, or not completing their share of work; or clients and caregivers being late, not showing up for scheduled appointments, or not observing common hygiene practices can be annoying but typically do not severely impact a practitioner's mental health or ability to do their job. Behaviors such as telling offensive jokes, wearing clothing with certain slogans or symbols, or using derogatory or slang terms related to certain cultural groups can be annoying to some people but may be hateful and threatening to others. Verbal, written, and virtual exchanges between people that include offensive terminology or symbols based on characteristics such as race, ethnic origin, religion, gender identity, sexual orientation, political beliefs, ability status, socioeconomic status, or any other identity status can cause feelings of being belittled, marginalized, bullied, or attacked. These exchanges can derail collaboration and trust between the practitioners, clients, caregivers, colleagues, students, or other team members, and can lead to a variety of distressing emotions and affect the mental health of the persons involved. The effect on the reputation of the practitioners and employers or institutions can lead to financial repercussions if clients refuse further services, or if employees or students leave the facility or institution.

Vertical and Lateral Aggression

Vertical aggression between a supervisor and a subordinate can include bullying, name calling, and derogatory language (Cascella, n.d.). This behavior may be exhibited in the workplace by physicians, nurse managers, school principals, home health agency directors, rehabilitation managers, occupational therapy supervisors, deans or academic program directors, fieldwork educators, or other persons in leadership roles. The uncivil behavior may stem from unconscious bias about different populations and can be directed at a single practitioner, a group of people, or even the entire profession of occupational therapy.

Lateral aggression between peers can include interprofessional colleagues in the workplace. The phrase "eating their young" refers to the phenomenon of experienced practitioners not providing support to new practitioners, instead leaving them to learn on their own and make mistakes. This is often seen as a rite of passage, but it does not promote an atmosphere of teamwork (Alexis, 2021; Longo, 2010). This bullying behavior of ignoring questions, not returning phone calls or emails, or refusing to demonstrate a new technique can be further compounded if the supervisor or colleague also belittles or demeans the new practitioner for their mistakes.

Culture of Incivility

Brad Smith, Chief Science Officer of meQuilibrium, stated:

> Workplace incivility creates a toxic work environment that undermines team cohesion and collaboration, erodes trust between employees and their managers, and can ultimately damage the organization's reputation. . . . When employees are subjected to rude, disrespectful, or aggressive behavior in the workplace, it can lead to decreased job satisfaction, increased stress, and decreased productivity, which can result in higher rates of absenteeism, turnover, and decreased organizational performance. (Make a Difference, 2023, para. 2)

Allowing uncivil and unprofessional behavior to persist unchecked can create a company culture of toxicity. "In most organizations toxic workplace culture starts at the top. When leaders bring negative attitudes to work or treat employees poorly, it can have ripple effects throughout the organization" (Wasserman & Heston-Davis, 2023, para. 3). Toxic workplaces can flourish when employees do not report uncivil behavior because they are concerned about their job security, fear a lack of confidentiality, or there is a pattern of lack of follow-through by management (Longo, 2010). People subjected to incivility can experience fear, stress, sadness, moral distress, and humiliation; and may develop fatigue, headaches, or gastrointestinal issues, leading to increased absenteeism. This culture can result in decreased employee morale, job turnover, lower productivity, impaired interprofessional collaboration and teamwork, and increased employee absenteeism, and it can jeopardize the quality and safety of patient care (Cascella, n.d.; Deiratani, 2023; Longo, 2010; McCullough et al., 2023). Occupational therapy practitioners may be unable to remain employed at a position where they feel marginalized by their peers, colleagues, or supervisors; or they may be further traumatized by not being able to leave that position due to financial constraints. Clients and caregivers who feel demeaned or threatened by the words or actions of an occupational therapy practitioner may not participate in therapy, attend appointments, or follow recommendations. They may be unable to focus on recovery if they are dealing with emotional upheaval caused by disrespectful and uncivil behavior or actions. Students in occupational therapy or occupational therapy assistant programs may be unable to complete their didactic or fieldwork education if they feel offended or threatened by the words or actions of their classmates, faculty, or fieldwork educators, or if they are not supported by their faculty or educational institution.

Prejudiced Clients or Caregivers

Health care practitioners can be on the receiving end of uncivil behaviors by the clients and caregivers they serve. Karen Smith, PhD, director of ethics integration at the Henry Ford Hospital & Health System, said, "Everybody talks about patient rights, but we also need to talk about patient responsibilities. Caregivers work so selflessly . . . Patients absolutely have a duty to treat providers with respect and dignity" (Weiner, 2020, para. 11). It is not uncommon for health care practitioners of color to experience overtly racist behaviors by patients and clients. Sometimes it is reasonable to a patient to request a change in provider based on religious reasons, language barriers, or past trauma (e.g., sexual assault). However, the literature is growing regarding episodes of racial discrimination and the harm experienced by practitioners, and health care organizations must develop policies to determine how and when to respond to change requests (Garran & Rasmussen, 2019). The ethical challenges of providing support, care, and comfort to clients while being the recipient of repeated microaggressions or inappropriate and offensive behavior (e.g., touching a person's hair, flinching at their touch) affects not only the individual occupational therapy practitioner, but the entire field. Increased diversity in the workforce can lead to greater patient access to care, satisfaction, and outcomes (Institute of Medicine, 2004). However, when practitioners are belittled because of their race, religion, ethnic origin, gender identity, sexual orientation, or other characteristics, they may choose to switch jobs or leave the profession altogether.

Relation to the AOTA Code of Ethics

Many of the core values and ethical principles in the AOTA Code of Ethics (the Code) address the interaction between occupational therapy practitioners and their clients, colleagues, students, and others. These values and principles stress the need to treat others with respect and fairness. The values of *altruism* and *equality* and the ethical principle of *beneficence* guide occupational therapy practitioners to show concern for others and treat them fairly. The values of *equality* and *dignity* and the ethical principle of *autonomy* remind occupational therapy practitioners that other persons, groups, and populations may have different values, beliefs, and lifestyles; and that it is important to respect the uniqueness of others' cultural and social heritage, life experiences, and their choices and decisions. The value of *prudence* and the ethical principle of *fidelity* address the importance of discretion, moderation, intelligent reflection, and integrity in decision making and interaction with others. It can be difficult when an occupational therapy student or practitioner is faced with someone with disparate points of view, whether that be a client or caregiver, coworker or interprofessional colleague, faculty member, or employer. Similar to what is stated in the American Medical Association (AMA; n.d.) Code of Ethics, the relationship between health care providers and their clients is based on trust and should promote the clients' well-being and be nondiscriminatory, while also respecting the dignity and rights of the clients and the providers. Ethical behavior requires communication and actions that demonstrate cultural sensitivity and humility and encourages further communication that will not be harmful to either party. See Exhibit 34.1 for ethical standards from the Code related to professional civility.

EXHIBIT 34.1.
ETHICAL STANDARDS RELATED TO PROFESSIONAL CIVILITY

- Treat all stakeholders professionally and equitably through constructive engagement and dialogue that is inclusive, collaborative, and respectful of diversity of thought.
- Demonstrate courtesy, civility, value, and respect to persons, groups, organizations, and populations when engaging in personal, professional, or electronic communications, including all forms of social media or networking, especially when that discourse involves disagreement of opinion, disparate points of view, or differing values.
- Demonstrate a level of cultural humility, sensitivity, and agility within professional practice that promotes inclusivity and does not result in harmful actions or inactions with persons, groups, organizations, and populations from diverse backgrounds, including age, gender identity, sexual orientation, race, religion, origin, socioeconomic status, degree of ability, or any other status or attributes.
- Do not engage in actions that are uncivil, intimidating, or bullying or that contribute to violence.
- Conduct personal and professional communication with colleagues, including electronic communication and social media and networking, in a manner that is free from personal attacks, threats, and attempts to defame character and credibility directed toward an individual, group, organization, or population without basis or through manipulation of information.

Note. From the Standards of Conduct from the AOTA Code of Ethics.

Reference to Other AOTA Documents

Uncivil and unprofessional behavior may arise from implicit bias or not understanding the culture, values, and beliefs of others. The American Occupational Therapy Association's (AOTA's) Diversity, Equity, and Inclusion Learning Modules (AOTA, n.d.-a) and Resource Library (AOTA, n.d.-b) have many tools to help identify unconscious bias and learn how to better communicate with others. The resources include:

- case studies involving faculty, practitioners, and students
- research, scholarly articles, and practice examples from the *American Journal of Occupational Therapy, OT Practice, SIS Quarterly*, and others
- a Framework for Addressing Diversity, Equity, and Inclusion in Everyday Practice for Occupational Therapy
- AOTA's Guide to Addressing the Impact of Racial Discrimination, Stigma, and Implicit Bias on Provision of Services
- a Diversity, Equity, Inclusion, and Justice Vocabulary (Avarna Group, n.d.).

Reference to Other Standards

The Joint Commission recognized that intimidating and disruptive behaviors could foster medical errors, contribute to poor patient satisfaction and adverse outcomes, and cause qualified professionals to leave their fields for more professional environments. Recognizing that organizations that fail to address unprofessional behaviors are indirectly promoting it, in 2009 The Joint Commission developed Standard LD.03.01.01, which required that organizations develop a code of conduct defining acceptable and disruptive and inappropriate behaviors, and that leaders develop and implement a process for managing those behaviors. This standard was updated to include development of structures, policies, and procedures to address and prevent workplace violence (The Joint Commission, 2021).

Tips

- Self-reflect to determine unconscious biases. Consider taking a self-assessment such as those offered by Project Implicit at Harvard University (Project Implicit, 2011).
- Identify triggers that make you angry. It is not possible to control what other people say, but you can control your reaction to it. Think before speaking, and consider the impact your words or actions may have on other people.
- Do not seek out, respond to, or spread gossip. Do not contribute to the incivility of others.
- Speak up when you see or hear microaggressions. Behavior that is ignored and allowed to continue will not change. Provide specific examples of what was offensive or derogatory. Remember that unconscious bias starts in childhood with what we hear, see, and are taught by our parents, family, religious institution, and the media. Although the impact might be great, the intent may not have been to hurt.
- Do not assume you know the motive behind what someone else says. Ask questions and try to find the context for what they say or do before blaming them or retaliating. Listen more and show that you respect the opinions of others. Engage in dialogue, even if the end result is to agree to disagree (Lower, 2012).

CASE EXAMPLE 34.1. WHAT'S YOUR NAME?

An **occupational therapist** at City Rehabilitation Hospital gives nicknames to all the therapy staff. None of the nicknames is blatantly derogatory or bigoted, but some staff members are offended. Whenever someone complains about their own or someone else's nickname, the occupational therapist brushes it off and says they are overly sensitive. Three staff members nicknamed JLo, SenSei, and DruPaul file a complaint with the Human Resources department for verbal harassment.

Questions
1. Is this a case of vertical or lateral aggression?
2. Why might these nicknames be offensive?
3. What standards of conduct from the Code can the three practitioners cite in their complaint?

CASE EXAMPLE 34.2. NOT NOW, CASEY

Casey is an occupational therapy student on Level II fieldwork at an acute care hospital. Casey is appre-hensive about the acuity level of the patients, especially in the intensive care unit. Casey's Fieldwork Educator is **Morgan,** an occupational therapist with 10 years of experience in this setting. Morgan thinks Casey asks too many questions and resembles an unsuccessful fieldwork student Morgan su-pervised last year. Morgan sometimes leaves before their scheduled afternoon feedback meetings, and doesn't return Casey's calls or texts in a timely manner. Each Friday Morgan makes a list of all the ways Casey is not performing up to expected levels, but does not offer clarification or demonstration of what Casey is doing wrong. During review of the midterm evaluation, Casey begins to cry. "I'm not surprised, you're such a baby, Casey. That's typical for someone like you," says Morgan. Casey contacts the Academic Fieldwork Coordinator at school, and asks to be reassigned to another fieldwork place-ment, even if it delays graduation.

Questions
1. Is this a case of lateral or vertical aggression?
2. What standards of conduct from the Code do you think Morgan is violating?
3. If you were the Academic Fieldwork Coordinator, how would you respond to Casey's request?

Next Steps

To create a culture of civility in the work environment, it is necessary to have an organiza-tional commitment to change. Essential components to creating an environment of respect include the following:

- a code of conduct with a zero-tolerance policy that includes:
  - ○ a clear list of unacceptable behaviors that will trigger action, with specific examples to enhance clarity and understanding
  - ○ a process for reporting complaints and violations, which must include anonymous reporting
  - ○ an identified channel for communication between the reviewer and the person with the alleged uncivil behavior
  - ○ hierarchy of responses, including disciplinary action up to and including termination.
- organization-wide training on bullying, cultural humility, communication, and collaboration
- coaches and mentors available for feedback and monitoring
- available resources through Human Resources, Employee Assistance Programs, and mental health professionals
- review of policies and procedures, and assessment of efficacy (Cascella, n.d.; Longo, 2010).

Summary

Incivility in the workplace can affect occupational therapy practitioners, employers, colleagues, students, and clients and caregivers. Practitioners may be physically and emotionally unable to tolerate intimidating, derogatory, aggressive, or biased actions by administrators, supervisors, coworkers, or even the clients and caregivers. Employers may lose staff, and their reputation may be irreparably damaged. Clients and caregivers may not trust the providers, receive substandard care, or even decline care. The Code provides guidance for occupational therapy practitioners to conduct themselves in a civil manner. This conduct includes actions and behaviors, and all forms of written, electronic, verbal, and nonverbal communication. Practitioners can honor their own personal values while respectfully listening to others with whom they disagree. Professional civility facilitates successful interaction between occupational therapy practitioners and their students, clients and caregivers, employers, colleagues, and others with whom they engage in their work and professional spheres.

REFERENCES

Alexis. (2021). *Why nurses eat their young and how to stop this damaging practice.* American Association of Post-Acute Care Nursing. https://www.aapacn.org/article/why-nurses-eat-their-young-and-how-to-stop-this-damaging-practice/

American Medical Association. (n.d.). *AMA code of ethics opinion 1.2.2: Discrimination and disruptive behavior by patients.* https://code-medical-ethics.ama-assn.org/ethics-opinions/discrimination-disruptive-behavior-patients

American Occupational Therapy Association. (n.d.-a). *Diversity, equity, and inclusion learning modules.* https://www.aota.org/practice/practice-essentials/dei/diversity-equity--inclusion-toolkit-learning-modules

American Occupational Therapy Association. (n.d.-b). *Diversity, equity, and inclusion resource library.* https://www.aota.org/practice/practice-essentials/dei/diversity-equity--inclusion-toolkit-resource-library

Avarna Group. (n.d.). *Diversity, equity, inclusion, & justice vocabulary.* https://theavarnagroup.com/resources/equity-inclusion-diversity-vocabulary/

Cascella, L. M. (n.d.). *The corrosive effect of disruptive behaviors on staff morale and patient care.* MedPro Group. https://www.medpro.com/disruptive-behavior-staff-morale

Deiratani, A. (2023). *The ripple effect of disruptive behavior in the workplace.* https://www.teambonding.com/disruptive-behavior-at-work/

Garran, A. M., & Rasmussen, B. M. (2019). How should organizations respond to racism against health care workers? *AMA Journal of Ethics, 21,* 499–504. https://doi.org/10.1001/amajethics.2019.499

HR Search and Rescue. (2021). *What is considered disruptive behavior in the workplace?* https://hr-searchandrescue.com/what-is-considered-disruptive-behavior-in-the-workplace/

Institute of Medicine. (2004). *In the nation's compelling interest: Ensuring diversity in the health-care workforce.* The National Academies Press. https://doi.org/10.17226/10885

Kaslow, N. J., & Watson, N. N. (2017). *Civility: A core component of professionalism?* American Psychological Association's Psych Learning Curve. https://psychlearningcurve.org/civility/

Limbong, A. (2020). *Microaggressions are a big deal: How to talk them out and when to walk away.* NPR Life Kit. https://www.npr.org/2020/06/08/872371063/microaggressions-are-a-big-deal-how-to-talk-them-out-and-when-to-walk-away

Longo, J. (2010). Combating disruptive behaviors: Strategies to promote a healthy work environment. *Online Journal of Issues in Nursing, 15*(1). https://ojin.nursingworld.org/table-of-contents/volume-15-2010/number-1-january-2010/combating-disruptive-behaviors/

Lower, J. (2012). Civility starts with you. *American Nurse.* https://www.myamericannurse.com/civility-starts-with-you/

Make a Difference. (2023). *One in four workers experience workplace incivility, fueling toxic work environments.* https://makeadifference.media/culture/one-in-four-workers-experience-workplace-incivility-fueling-toxic-work-environments/

McCullough, L. B., Coverdale, J., & Chervenak, F. A. (2023). Professional virtue of civility and the responsibilities of medical educators and academic leaders. *Journal of Medical Ethics, 49,* 674–678. https://doi.org/10.1136/jme-2022-108735

Merriam-Webster. (n.d.). *Prejudice.* https://www.merriam-webster.com/dictionary/prejudice

National Institutes of Health. (2022). *Implicit bias.* https://diversity.nih.gov/sociocultural-factors/implicit-bias

Project Implicit. (2011). *Harvard Implicit Association Test.* https://implicit.harvard.edu/implicit/takeatest.html

Rehder, K. J. (2020). *Addressing disruptive behaviors in healthcare.* American Hospital Association Team Training. https://www.aha.org/system/files/media/file/2020/04/AHA_Team_Training_Webinar_Slides_April_2020.pdf

Savrin, R. (n.d.). *Incivility and disruptive behaviors in healthcare.* The Sullivan Group. https://blog.thesullivangroup.com/disruptive-behavior-in-healthcare

The Joint Commission. (2021). *The Joint Commission Sentinel Event Alert, 40.* https://www.jointcommission.org/-/media/tjc/documents/resources/patient-safety-topics/sentinel-event/sea-40-intimidating-disruptive-behaviors-final2.pdf

Wasserman, K., & Heston-Davis, R. (2023). *Toxic work environment: How to spot the signs and fix it* [Lyra Health Mental Health at Work Blog]. https://www.lyrahealth.com/blog/toxic-work-environment/

Weiner, S. (2020). Pushing back against patient bias. *AAMCNEWS.* https://www.aamc.org/news/pushing-back-against-patient-bias

The Ethics of Diversity, Equity, Inclusion, Justice, Access, and Belonging

ASHLEY WAGNER, OTD, OTR/L; SHANESE L. HIGGINS, DHSc, OTR/L, BCMH;
BRENDA KORNBLIT KENNELL, MA, OTR/L, FAOTA; RENA B. PUROHIT, JD, OTR/L;
NATALIE CHANG WRIGHT, MBA–HCM, COTA/L, ROH; and
BRENDA S. HOWARD, DHSc, OTR, FAOTA

Key Points

- Occupational therapy practitioners must not discriminate against clients, students, colleagues, or any other community members based on their age, gender identity, sexual orientation, race, religion, origin, socioeconomic status, degree of ability, or any other status or attributes.
- Occupational therapy practitioners are ethically obligated to provide the services they offer to all persons, groups, and populations.
- Diversity, equity, inclusion, justice, access, and belonging go beyond avoiding bias and include creating spaces of belonging for all persons.

Definitions

- *Diversity* means, "the representation of people of different races, ethnicities, genders, sexual orientations, ages, abilities, national origins, tribes, socioeconomic statuses, and religions" (National Board for Certification in Occupational Therapy [NBCOT®], 2023).
- *Equity* means, "providing equitable opportunities for everyone" (NBCOT, 2023).
- *Inclusion* means a community "where all members are and feel respected, have a sense of belonging, and are able to participate and achieve to their potential" (University of Iowa, n.d.).
- *Justice* means, "promoting fairness by eliminating the systems and structures that limit the opportunities for equity" (NBCOT, 2023).

- *Access* means, "participating in society, regardless of the internal or external factors that make every individual unique" (American Occupational Therapy Association [AOTA], 2020b, p. 1) and having the same opportunities and resources as others (AOTA, 2020b).
- *Belonging* means, "support[ing] the value of diversity. The idea of belonging allows individuals to show up as their authentic selves to work and school. Where inclusion, support, and acceptance are fostered in an organization, individuals have a sense of belonging" (AOTA, 2023a).
- *Intersectionality* is "a framework to describe how systems of power and oppression (for example, racism, sexism, heterosexism) interlock to shape people's lived experiences, health, and well-being, based on their multiple identities (for example, their race, gender, and sexual orientation, respectively)" (Michaels et al., 2023).

Introduction

It is the ethical responsibility of occupational therapy practitioners to value the diversity of our clients, colleagues, and other community members, and to enter therapeutic and professional relationships with cultural humility. Diversity, equity, and inclusion efforts of occupational therapy practitioners should go beyond nondiscrimination and avoiding bias; they should strive to create spaces where all individuals experience a sense of belonging. The American Occupational Therapy Association (AOTA) has adopted the acronym DEIJAB (diversity, equity, inclusion, justice, access, and belonging) to refer to these concepts as a whole. To address this ethical responsibility, practitioners must understand the nuances of harm, intersectionality, cultural humility, and belonging.

HARM

Discussions aligning ethics with concepts of DEIJAB must include an understanding of harm. *Harm,* in the context of diversity, equity, and inclusion, includes psycho-emotional harm, invalidation of one's personal identity, and undermining one's very right to exist (Beagan et al., 2022). Interpreting harm as only that which can result in physical risk or injury limits the discussion to only the most overt acts of discrimination. Doing so dilutes the true essence of the profession's call to nonmaleficence and overlooks the shared experiences of, and the mounting body of evidence on, the diffuse and varied types of harm sustained by members of oppressed communities (Beagan et al., 2022; Kung & Johansson, 2022). Therefore, an ethical occupational therapy practitioner must not only consider how their actions or the actions of those around them may inflict physical harm on clients, students, research participants, or colleagues, but must also consider the psycho-emotional or existential harm caused by bias, insensitivity, ignorance, and systemic re-traumatization (Beagan et al., 2022; Kung & Johansson, 2022; Subica & Link, 2022).

THE INTERSECTIONAL EXPERIENCE OF COLLEAGUES AND CLIENTS

To truly understand the potential depth of harm in relation to DEIJAB contexts and to fully practice cultural humility within the profession, occupational therapy practitioners must be aware of and accept that intersectionality results in a nuanced experience of and response to every situation (Jackson et al., 2016). Just as facets of DEIJAB are experienced and expressed distinctly and differently (e.g., diversity, equity, inclusion, accessibility, justice, belonging), the experience of intersectionality is also unique for each individual. By ensuring that one has an all-encompassing perspective of harm in all its forms, a practitioner can *begin* to recognize, acknowledge, and understand the totality of the experience of disparity for minoritized and oppressed communities (Michaels et al., 2023). This beginning step in understanding the disparity experience creates an opportunity for the practitioner to employ cultural humility and better ensures that their ethical decision-making framework is not limited by assumptions of harm based on their personal experiences and singular understanding of how a situation or interaction may affect another individual.

CULTURAL HUMILITY

Engaging in therapeutic and professional relationships with diverse populations requires an understanding of the practice of cultural humility. *Cultural humility* goes beyond focusing on cultural competence, which involves gaining knowledge about specific cultures and understanding cultural differences (Agner, 2020). It is important to consider the complexity of culture; diversity within cultural groups; and the unique, evolving cultural identities of individuals to avoid stereotyping and misunderstandings in our interactions with clients, colleagues, and others (Agner, 2020). Maintaining a cultural humility point of view emphasizes the process of continuous, lifelong learning when working with diverse populations; acknowledges assumptions and biases among practitioners; and recognizes power dynamics in health care (Agner, 2020; Foronda et al., 2016). The practice of cultural humility involves being open to interactions with diverse individuals, practicing self-awareness, and attempting to subdue one's own ego, while engaging in supporting interactions, self-reflection, and self-critique on an ongoing basis (Foronda et al., 2016). Practicing cultural humility can result in positive outcomes, including improved communication, empowerment, mutually respectful partnerships that are based on trust, improved care, and lifelong learning and self-reflection (Foronda et al., 2016). It is imperative that education and training be included within occupational therapy curricula and in the workplace to enhance the ability of practitioners to implement cultural humility concepts (AOTA, 2020a; Foronda et al., 2016).

BELONGING

Belonging is a fundamental human need and a core aspect of occupational therapy. It refers to the sense of connection, acceptance, and inclusion that individuals feel within their social and cultural contexts (Cornell University, 2023). Belonging goes beyond simply feeling included or accepted; it encompasses a deep sense of interpersonal connection, understanding, and acceptance within contexts and environments where persons engage in meaningful occupations. An occupational therapy practitioner can build a sense of belonging for colleagues and clients by analyzing how the space and systems around them account for a range of factors, including cultural identity, social support, and community participation of everyone involved. It is important to consider these factors in order to encourage and receive everyone's voices without the restrictions of barriers, or what some refer to as imposter syndrome (Glassdoor for Employers, 2021).

Belonging plays a vital role in occupational therapy practice, as it directly affects the well-being and overall success of clients, students, and practitioners. When individuals feel a sense of belonging, they are more likely to fully engage in meaningful activities and relationships, leading to better outcomes and increased satisfaction and well-being (Hammell, 2017). Belonging is also crucial for practitioners with diverse backgrounds and experiences, and by prioritizing DEIJAB within the profession, occupational therapy practitioners can ensure that all participants feel seen and heard (AOTA, 2019). An environment of belonging within the workplace goes a long way in supporting and enhancing the overall health and wellness of the practitioner.

Fostering belonging in occupational therapy practice requires a commitment to ethical principles such as diversity, equity, and inclusion; social justice; client autonomy; and empowerment. Prioritizing these values can create a safe and inclusive environment that promotes health, well-being, and a sense of connection and community for all who receive or deliver occupational therapy services (AOTA, 2020a, 2020b).

Relation to the AOTA Code of Ethics

The AOTA Code of Ethics (the Code) identifies core values and ethical principles of the occupational therapy profession. Core values relating to DEIJAB include equality, justice, and dignity; ethical principles include *beneficence, autonomy, justice,* and *fidelity*. The ethical principle of *justice* requires equitable treatment that is inclusive, collaborative, and respectful of diversity of thought. The ethical practitioner addresses *autonomy* by maintaining a collaborative relationship while respecting and honoring the wishes of service recipients, and demonstrates *beneficence* by providing evaluation and interventions specific to clients' needs. In upholding the principle of *fidelity*, an ethical occupational therapy practitioner must engage in cultural humility and professional civility when communicating with persons, groups, organizations, and populations from diverse backgrounds.

All occupational therapy practitioners should aspire to reflect these core values in their practice. The practitioner should also consider that equality is not the same as equity. "Equality means each individual or group of people is given the same resources or opportunities. Equity recognizes that each person has different circumstances and allocates the exact resources and opportunities needed to reach an equal outcome" (Milken Institute School of Public Health, 2020). Summarized in another way, "Equality is giving everyone a shoe. Equity is giving everyone a shoe that fits" (Anonymous). The Code itself does not define *equity* or *inclusion*, but it alludes to these principles in several standards of conduct related to therapeutic relationships, service delivery, communication, and professional civility. See Exhibit 35.1 for ethical standards from the Code related to diversity, equity, inclusion, justice, and belonging.

EXHIBIT 35.1.
ETHICAL STANDARDS RELATED TO DEIJAB

- Do not inflict harm or injury to recipients of occupational therapy services, students, research participants, or employees.
- Establish a collaborative relationship with recipients of service and relevant stakeholders to promote shared decision making.
- Provide appropriate evaluation and a plan of intervention for recipients of occupational therapy services specific to their needs.
- Provide information and resources to address barriers to access for persons in needs of occupational therapy services.
- Do not engage in communication that is discriminatory, derogatory, biased, intimidating, insensitive, disrespectful, or that unduly discourages others from participating in professional dialogue.
- Treat all stakeholders professionally and equitably through constructive engagement and dialogue that is inclusive, collaborative, and respectful of diversity of thought.
- Demonstrate a level of cultural humility, sensitivity, and agility within professional practice that promotes inclusivity and does not result in harmful actions or inactions with persons, groups, organizations, and populations from diverse backgrounds, including age, gender identity, sexual orientation, race, religion, origin, socioeconomic status, degree of ability, or any other status or attributes.
- Do not engage in actions that are uncivil, intimidating, bullying, or that contribute to violence.

Note. From the Standards of Conduct from the AOTA Code of Ethics.

Reference to Other AOTA Documents

The AOTA Diversity, Equity, and Inclusion toolkit (AOTA, 2023a) includes a learning center with a variety of resources, including

- case studies involving occupational therapy faculty, practitioners, and students;
- research and scholarly articles from the *American Journal of Occupational Therapy* (*AJOT*), *OT Practice*, *SIS Quarterly* articles, and others;
- a Framework for Addressing Diversity, Equity, and Inclusion in Everyday Practice for Occupational Therapy;
- AOTA's Guide to Addressing the Impact of Racial Discrimination, Stigma, and Implicit Bias on Provision of Services;

- learning modules;
- a DEI word bank (AOTA, 2023b); and
- a resource library, including handouts.

Reference to Other Standards

NBCOT (2023) states that "At NBCOT, justice, equity, diversity, and inclusion [JEDI] are woven into everything we do." To address these principles, NBCOT has provided several resources for certificants, including

- JEDI Reflection Points learning modules;
- resources on intersectionality, inequity, equality, equity, and justice; and
- access to implicit bias testing.

Tips

Occupational therapy practitioners have responsibilities as educators, practitioners, and colleagues to

- eliminate harassment, either intentional or perceived;
- protect self and students, clients, and colleagues from shame or loss of dignity;
- self-educate;
- address barriers to inclusion;
- conduct oneself in an ethical manner at all times (Kennell et al., 2022); and
- contribute to creating healthy environments.

There are many ways occupational therapy practitioners can help create a more diverse and inclusive environment and culture, including

- celebrating different backgrounds;
- encouraging collaboration and value contributions from diverse voices;
- providing resources and information regarding DEIJAB principles to colleagues and students;
- using inclusive language with clients, colleagues, and students;
- listening to understand;
- respecting differences;
- being an ally;
- speaking in an "I" voice;
- self-educating;
- leaning into discomfort;
- accepting critical feedback; and
- taking action to address concerns (Crawford, 2020; Denise, 2019; Reese, 2020; Simms, 2018).

CASE EXAMPLE 35.1. DEIJAB AND RESEARCH

An **occupational therapy researcher** evaluating the validity and reliability properties of their assessment tool recognizes that more than 90% of their sample population is made up of White, college-educated participants. They realize that this sample is not representative of their target population or of participant communities, but also recognize that this homogeneity is not uncommon when assessing the technical properties of an assessment tool. They have upheld their recruitment responsibilities according to the Internal Review Board overseeing the research, but still wonder if there is something more they should have done to improve the diversity and inclusion of their participants.

Questions

1. What are the ethical issues in this scenario?
2. What are the ethical principles and standards that apply?
3. Apply an ethical decision-making framework. What are the next steps the researcher should take?

CASE EXAMPLE 35.2. EQUALITY VS. EQUITY

Professor Taylor taught in an occupational therapy assistant program in a largely rural and economically depressed county. When the Program Director told Professor Taylor about the requirement to attend an upcoming DEI training, Professor Taylor said, "But I always try to make everything equal for all the students and not give extra help or advantages to anyone. Why do I need to go to DEI training?" The Program Director shared multiple student complaints with Professor Taylor, including the following:

- scheduling a required CarFit event on a Saturday afternoon, which conflicts with religious obligations for the Sabbath for Jewish and Adventist students
- requiring attendance for a synchronous discussion one evening at 7:30 pm, when several students were putting their school-age children to bed
- requiring all the students in the class to drink 3 oz of thickened liquid (to understand what it was like for clients), scheduled during Ramadan, when Muslim students were required to fast
- randomly assigning seats during an exam where a video was shown on the projected screen, which placed students with visual, hearing, or attention difficulties in non-optimal locations
- requiring the students to wear bathing suits while practicing simulated ADLs, which resulted in extreme distress for a transgender student.

Questions

1. How did Professor Taylor's actions affect the students? Does it matter that Professor Taylor had only good intentions?
2. Which standards from the Code were violated?
3. How could the distress and harm caused to the students have been avoided?
4. What should Professor Taylor do now to repair their relationship with the students?

CASE EXAMPLE 35.3. BELONGING

Yvette grew up in a low-income, spiritual family in a rural area where she spoke Spanish at home. She was the first in her family to go to college, and she chose to study occupational therapy because she was passionate about helping people with disabilities. After graduating from college with her Occupational Therapy Assistant degree, Yvette is hired in an inpatient rehabilitation hospital where she works with occupational and physical therapy practitioners. She is often sought out to translate or explain handouts to Spanish-speaking clients, but when she recommends creating Spanish versions of the handouts, she is told it is too much work for too few clients. After 3 years, Yvette is promoted to Rehabilitation Manager, as one co-worker put it, "because no one else wanted the job." Yvette is excited about the promotion but has some uncertainty due to experiencing marginalization and macroaggressions in a few ways.

As the only Afro-LatinX employee in her department, Yvette often feels like she is not being taken seriously by her coworkers, many of whom she is now supervising. Generally, she is busy and intricately involved in her work—treating clients and managing day-to-day operations—and she typically refrains from office politics and gossiping by staying in her office. She makes attempts to casually engage with her co-workers during normal clinical down time, but she notices these interactions are not typically initiated or reciprocated by her colleagues. She reflects that she is usually excluded from social events either at work or outside of working hours because in the past she has sometimes declined after expressing her commitment to family and spiritual activities. Over the years Yvette also faced difficulties accessing funding for education and training. After being promoted to Rehabilitation Manager, Yvette realized the inequity extended to wages. Despite receiving a minimal pay increase, she realizes that she earns less than her male colleagues at the same level of practice, even though she has the same or higher level of education, and more years of experience.

The marginalization that Yvette has experienced has had a significant impact on her sense of belonging. She has felt isolated and discriminated against, and she feels that she has had to work harder than her White colleagues to prove herself. This has led to feelings of burnout and frustration, and she is strongly considering leaving the profession.

Questions

1. What are the specific ways marginalization affect Yvette?
   a. In the profession of occupational therapy?
   b. In her career?
   c. Among her colleagues?
2. How might the intersectionality of Yvette's identities contribute to her nuanced experience of harm in this scenario?
3. What steps could Yvette take to feel a sense of belonging? What steps could her colleagues take?
4. What can be done to address and reduce marginalization of emerging majority or emerging minority practitioners in occupational therapy?

Next Steps

Promoting DEIJAB occupational therapy practice includes actively addressing and challenging biases and prejudices. Highlighting a person's autonomy and empowerment can also foster a sense of belonging (Hammell, 2017); this is important for both the practitioner and the client. Actively involving clients in their own care and decision-making processes can help them feel a sense of ownership and agency in their journey toward well-being. Valuing autonomy requires creating environments that respect choices and preferences; providing materials and resources; acknowledging various languages, cultures, and communication styles; utilizing assistive technology; incorporating various therapeutic, person-centered approaches that align with diverse cultural beliefs and values; and allowing individuals to feel competent and better suited to make informed decisions (Amodeo et al., 2020). Being aware of power dynamics within the therapeutic relationship and working to create collaborative and equal partnerships is also necessary (Agner, 2020).

Occupational therapy practitioners can continue to actively seek out opportunities to expand their knowledge and open themselves to learn from the diverse experiences of others. When individuals feel connected to others and their communities, they are more likely to experience a higher quality of life, improved well-being, and a greater sense of belonging (Hammell, 2017).

Summary

Ethical occupational therapy practice requires being firmly rooted in DEIJAB principles. Occupational therapy practitioners must address their own implicit biases, strive to reduce harm, and practice with cultural humility with all parties of interest including clients, students, and other professionals with whom they work. A true ethical emphasis on DEIJAB includes going beyond an absence of discrimination and addressing full belonging within therapeutic relationships, work teams and organizations, and the profession of occupational therapy. Only when belonging is addressed can occupational therapy practitioners begin to acknowledge and reduce the disparity experience for persons from minoritized groups.

REFERENCES

Agner, J. (2020). The issue is—Moving from cultural competence to cultural humility in occupational therapy: A paradigm shift. *American Journal of Occupational Therapy, 74*, 7404347010. https://doi .org/10.5014/ajot.2020.038067

American Occupational Therapy Association. (2019). AOTA board expands Vision 2025. *American Journal of Occupational Therapy, 73*, 7303420010p1. https://doi.org/10.5014/ajot.2019.733002

American Occupational Therapy Association. (2020a). Educator's guide for addressing cultural awareness, humility, and dexterity in occupational therapy curricula. *American Journal of Occupational Therapy, 74*(Suppl. 3), 7413420003p1–7413420003p19. https://doi.org/10.5014/ ajot.2020.74S3005

American Occupational Therapy Association. (2020b). Occupational therapy's commitment to diversity, equity, and inclusion. *American Journal of Occupational Therapy, 74*(Suppl. 3), 7413410030p1– 7413410030p6. https://doi.org/10.5014/ajot.2020.74S3002

American Occupational Therapy Association. (2023a). *Diversity, equity, and inclusion in OT.* https:// www.aota.org/practice/practice-essentials/dei

American Occupational Therapy Association. (2023b). *DEI toolkit: DEI word bank*. https://www .aota.org/practice/practice-essentials/dei/dei-toolkit-word-bank

Amodeo, A. L., Esposito, C., & Bacchini, D. (2020). Heterosexist microaggressions, student academic experience and perception of campus climate: Findings from an Italian higher education context. *PLoS One, 15*(4), e0231580. https://doi.org/10.1371/journal.pone.0231580

Beagan, B. L., Sibbald, K. R., Bizzeth, S. R., & Pride, T. M. (2022). Systemic racism in Canadian occupational therapy: A qualitative study with therapists. *Canadian Journal of Occupational Therapy, 89,* 51–61. https://doi.org/10.1177/00084174211066676

Cornell University. (2023). *Diversity and inclusion: Belonging at Cornell.* https://diversity.cornell.edu/ belonging

Crawford, C. (2020). *10 Ways to foster an inclusive workplace culture.* https://www.workingideal .com/10-ways-to-foster-an-inclusive-workplace-culture/

Denise, H. (2019). *3 ways to foster a diverse and inclusive company culture.* Give and Take Inc. https:// giveandtakeinc.com/blog/culture/3-ways-to-foster-a-diverse-and-inclusive-company-culture/

Foronda, C., Baptiste, D.-L., Reinholdt, M. M., & Ousman, K. (2016). Cultural humility: A concept analysis. *Journal of Transcultural Nursing, 27,* 210–217. https://doi.org/10.1177/1043659615592677

Glassdoor for Employers. (2021). *What is diversity, inclusion and belonging?* https://www.glassdoor .com/employers/blog/what-is-diversity-inclusion-and-belonging/

Hammell, K. W. (2017). Opportunities for well-being: The right to occupational engagement. *Canadian Journal of Occupational Therapy, 84,* 209–222. https://doi.org/10.1177/0008417417734831

Jackson, J. W., Williams, D. R., & VanderWeele, T. J. (2016). Disparities at the intersection of marginalized groups. *Social Psychiatry and Psychiatric Epidemiology, 51,* 1349–1359. https://doi .org/10.1007/s00127-016-1276-6

Kennell, B., Bennett, L., & Pavlovich S. (2022). *Infusing DEI and ethics into your curriculum and culture.* Innovation Summit for Health Professions Education.

Kung, W. W., & Johansson, S. (2022). Ethical mental health practice in diverse cultures and races. *Journal of Ethnic & Cultural Diversity in Social Work, 31,* 248–262. https://doi.org/10.1080/153132 04.2022.2070889

Michaels, E., Wesley, D. B., & O'Neil, S. (2023). *Intersectionality: Amplifying Impacts on health equity.* https://www.mathematica.org/blogs/intersectionality-amplifying-impacts-on-health-equity

Milken Institute School of Public Health. (2020). *Equity vs. equality: What's the difference?* https:// onlinepublichealth.gwu.edu/resources/equity-vs-equality/

National Board for Certification in Occupational Therapy. (2023). *An integral part of our mission and vision.* https://www.nbcot.org/jedi

Reese, A. J. (2020). An undergraduate elective course that introduces topics of diversity, equity, and inclusion into discussions of science. *Journal of Microbiology & Biology Education, 21*(1). https:// journals.asm.org/doi/10.1128/jmbe.v21i1.1947

Simms, C. (2018). *9 ways to foster diversity and inclusion at work.* https://www.helpscout.com/blog/ fostering-inclusivity/

Subica, A. M., & Link, B. G. (2022). Cultural trauma as a fundamental cause of health disparities. *Social Science & Medicine, 292,* 114574. https://doi.org/10.1016/j.socscimed.2021.114574

University of Iowa. (n.d.). *Defining diversity, equity, and inclusion at Iowa.* https://diversity.uiowa .edu/

When Ethics and Laws Conflict in Polarizing Political Times

BRENDA S. HOWARD, DHSc, OTR, FAOTA

Key Points

- Ethical conflicts occur when occupational therapy practitioners are legally bound to act in ways that differ from ethical standards.
- At times, practitioners may find their personal and professional values in conflict with those of colleagues and employer policies.
- Occupational therapy practitioners should carefully read laws and policies to acquire a thorough understanding of them, in order to clearly articulate how these may be in conflict with ethical care.
- Involvement in legal and political advocacy, taking an active role in organizational policy setting, documenting harm to clients, treating all clients with dignity, and resisting and challenging laws are some actions practitioners can choose to take.

Introduction

With increased polarization of social and political opinion in the United States, and changing laws regarding what is permissible in health care, occupational therapy practitioners are facing ethical challenges to the way they practice and interact in therapeutic relationships. The Dobbs vs. Jackson Women's Health (2022) decision and subsequent changes to laws in multiple states (Hensley & Washington, 2023), as well as laws prohibiting gender-affirming care for minors (Trans Legislation Tracker, 2023), are some examples of laws that are impacting the therapeutic relationship. Practitioners are asking themselves, "What can I discuss with my clients or their families? How will I document these conversations? How will I protect the autonomy and privacy of my clients and respect their right to care while observing laws in the jurisdiction where I practice?"

Previous issues have created similar ethical dilemmas for health care providers. These have included reporting abuse in contradiction to the client's wishes, rights of minors, and how to best support undocumented workers (Reamer, 2008). Although some have argued that all laws should be obeyed, "Blind obedience to the law can be shortsighted and harm clients, particularly when laws seem to be unjust" (Reamer, 2008, p. 1). Adjacent to the therapeutic relationship is addressing the concern of having healthy professional dialogue with colleagues who hold different perspectives. Educating oneself on the issues and the responses from professional organizations can help the practitioner engage in dialogue that is productive rather than emotionally charged. For example, both the American Medical Association (AMA; 2022) and the American College of Obstetricians and Gynecologists (ACOG; 2021) have published statements denouncing government intrusion on the physician–patient relationship, especially regarding patient care and reproductive health. In addition, the AMA, together with the Endocrine Society, passed a resolution to protect access to gender-affirming care and oppose criminal and legal penalties for those seeking care and those providing care (AMA, 2023). The American Psychological Association (APA; 2023b) also published a statement saying that scientific research is in direct opposition to the legislative bills that deny gender-affirming care to youth. The APA also denounced abortion bans, stating that abortion bans caused a disproportionate amount of harm to people of color and urging that psychologists keep patients' reproductive decisions confidential, despite laws mandating reporting (APA, 2023a). The American Occupational Therapy Association (AOTA; 2023) provides a number of documents, including societal statements, position statements, and policies, giving occupational therapy practitioners guidance on current issues.

At the heart of the discussion of law vs. ethics is the question of duty to the client and upholding the ethical principle of *beneficence* vs. upholding the law and the ethical principle of *justice*. This conflict is an example of a true ethical dilemma (Doherty & Purtilo, 2016). Some authors have argued that practitioners should be allowed to practice their convictions on either side of controversial issues (Eberl, 2021; Fox, 2021). Fox (2021) argued that if health care providers are allowed to refuse to provide legal care to honor their convictions, they should also be allowed to provide care that goes against the law in order to honor their convictions. In occupational therapy, this means that practitioners using their best reasoning skills for ethical decision making may come down on opposite sides of an issue. When this is the case, practitioners must use their best communication abilities to uphold professional civility and maintain their own beliefs while listening to and understanding opposing views (Kaslow & Watson, 2016). An ethical decision-making guide can help the practitioner take these difficult conversations out of the realm of the emotional and examine the issues with logic and thoughtful reflection (Doherty & Purtilo, 2016).

Relation to the AOTA Code of Ethics

The AOTA Code of Ethics states, "at times, conflicts between competing principles must be considered in order to make ethical decisions." When these conflicts occur, the occupational therapy practitioner must weigh professional values, their own beliefs, and laws and policies to determine a course of action. Consequently, it may be impossible to uphold all standards at the same time when laws and ethics are in conflict. The standards that apply in this situation are included in Exhibit 36.1.

EXHIBIT 36.1.
ETHICAL STANDARDS RELATED TO ETHICS AND LAWS CONFLICTING

- Comply with current federal and state laws, state scope of practice guidelines, and AOTA policies and official documents that apply to the profession of occupational therapy.
- Abide by policies, procedures, and protocols when serving or acting on behalf of a professional organization or employer to fully and accurately represent the organization's official and authorized positions.
- Inform employers, employees, colleagues, students, and researchers of applicable policies, laws, and Official Documents.
- Respect and honor the expressed wishes of recipients of service.
- Do not inflict harm or injury to recipients of occupational therapy services, students, research participants, or employees.
- Adhere to organizational policies when requesting an exemption from service to an individual or group because of self-identified conflict with personal, cultural, or religious values.
- Do not engage in actions or inactions that jeopardize the safety or well-being of others or team effectiveness.
- Provide information and resources to address barriers to access for persons in need of occupational therapy services.
- Report systems and policies that are discriminatory or unfairly limit or prevent access to occupational therapy.
- Maintain privacy and truthfulness in delivery of occupational therapy services, whether in person or virtually.
- Preserve, respect, and safeguard private information about employees, colleagues, and students unless otherwise mandated or permitted by relevant laws.
- Demonstrate a level of cultural humility, sensitivity, and agility within professional practice that promotes inclusivity and does not result in harmful actions or inactions with persons, groups, organizations, and populations from diverse backgrounds, including age, gender identity, sexual orientation, race, religion, origin, socioeconomic status, degree of ability, or any other status or attributes. practice that promotes inclusivity and does not result in harmful actions or inactions with persons, groups, organizations, and populations from diverse backgrounds, including age, gender identity, sexual orientation, race, religion, origin, socioeconomic status, degree of ability, or any other status or attributes.

Note. From the Standards of Conduct from the AOTA Code of Ethics.

Reference to Other AOTA Documents

AOTA has a number of official documents that may help occupational therapy practitioners understand the ethical conflicts involved when specific issues arise. Practitioners can rely on the *Occupational Therapy Practice Framework: Domain and Process (OTPF)* and Standards of Practice to provide information about occupational therapy's scope of practice. Societal statements from AOTA provide the Association's official stance on current issues. An example is

AOTA's societal statement denouncing conversion "therapy" (AOTA, 2022a). Policies provide professional guidelines for behavior (AOTA, n.d.). Examples include AOTA's policies on affirming sexual orientation (AOTA, 2022b) and affirming gender diversity and identity (AOTA, 2021). Lastly, AOTA's statement on diversity, equity, and inclusion provides support for reducing bias, supporting diverse communities, and protecting the rights of all people (AOTA, 2020).

Reference to Other Standards

Occupational therapy practitioners should carefully read their state, district, or territory licensure act. They should also carefully read any legislative acts, court decisions, or other documents that establish laws or rules that may conflict with providing ethical care. It may be helpful to consult legal representation for interpreting the law. Some laws criminalize actions or inactions that a practitioner may choose; other laws remove funding for organizations that do not follow rules. Practitioners should learn about rights given under law for both clients and providers (Reamer, 2008).

Tips

- Complete a careful reading of laws and policies to determine what is legal and permissible in one's location and organization when discussing and providing care to clients.
- Know what resources are available, including documents from professional associations, organizational policies, ethics committees, and ethics consultants who may be available through one's organization.

CASE EXAMPLE 36.1. CONFIDENTIALITY VS. MANDATORY REPORTING

An **occupational therapy practitioner** works with adolescents in a school system. A 15-year-old student with a cognitive disability reports she has been sexually active and has had a positive drugstore pregnancy test. The student states her mother is going to take her out of state at the end of the week for a medical abortion. The student lives in a state where there is a total ban on abortion, and school employees are mandated to report minors who have abortions to officials. Reporting the abortion could result in criminal charges for the student and her mother; not reporting the abortion could result in criminal charges against the practitioner.

Questions
1. Apply an ethical decision-making framework to this scenario. What are the ethical issues to consider?
2. What resources can the occupational therapy practitioner consult to help make a decision?
3. What options does the occupational therapy practitioner have? What are the potential consequences of each option?
4. Choose an option, and reflect on possible outcomes. Which ethical principle(s) would this option uphold?

CASE EXAMPLE 36.2. DISCRIMINATION AND BARRIERS TO ACCESS

A **38-year-old female client** was referred to an outpatient occupational therapy clinic for evaluation and treatment following removal of a brain tumor. The client is an undocumented worker from a Latin American country and does not have health insurance. She had previously been employed in a local factory, but was terminated when she had brain surgery. Deficits include hemiparesis, aphasia, and cognitive impairment. The outpatient supervisor tells the evaluating occupational therapist to limit services to evaluation and a home program, since the client does not have insurance, and states, "she doesn't speak English anyway, so therapy is not going to do her any good."

Questions

1. Apply an ethical decision-making framework to this scenario. What are the ethical issues to consider?
2. What are the issues regarding discrimination and bias in this case?
3. What resources can the occupational therapist access in order to make a determination for what to do in this case?
4. Choose an option, and reflect on possible outcomes. Which ethical principle(s) would this option uphold?

Next Steps

Occupational therapy practitioners can begin the process of ethical decision making when laws conflict with ethical care by recognizing their own implicit bias and educating themselves on current issues and the terms used to discuss the issues (Brous, 2019). Research has shown that even a small amount of continuing education can go a long way in increasing the practitioner's confidence for managing ethical issues (Bolding et al., 2022).

Upon encountering a conflict between the law and ethical care, the occupational therapy practitioner can begin the ethical decision-making process by thoroughly examining the law to determine what it requires of the practitioner, what is permissible or forbidden, and what exceptions are allowed. Furthermore, the consequences of not following the law should be reviewed. Penalties can range from loss of program or clinic funding to criminal charges brought against individuals or organizations. Next, it is helpful to clearly state how the laws conflict with ethical care. For example, ACOG (2021) pointed out specific instances when the law interfered with the relationship between physicians and patients and their ability to communicate confidentially and collaborate to determine the best, evidence-based course of care. By articulating the specific consequences, ACOG (2021) was able to advocate for changes to unjust laws. Similarly, it is important to detail how a law criminalizes differences (AMA, 2022).

After occupational therapy practitioners have articulated the issues in conflict between laws and ethical care, it is important to relate the conflicting issues to the occupational therapy scope of practice as outlined in the *OTPF* and analyze available resources and practice guidance documents to support professional reasoning (AOTA, n.d.). At times, organizational and employer policies may provide support for the practitioner's actions. As a critical part of the ethical decision-making process, the practitioner should remember that an ethical approach demands that the client be treated with dignity and respect (Walker et al., 2021).

Sometimes an occupational therapy practitioner reaches an impasse in which they are forced to either act against their own personal ethics or face legal consequences. "It is simply not possible for clinicians to do the right thing if ethical principles and legal requirements are in direct conflict" (Kusterbeck, 2019, para. 1). When this occurs, the occupational therapy practitioner may have very few options. When the law requires certain statements to be made to clients against the practitioner's own values, the practitioner may preface the statement with a phrase such as, "the state requires me to tell you. . ." (Kusterbeck, 2019). Even if the goal of acting within one's ethical values cannot be reached, it is important to keep the goal in mind and work toward the day when it can be achieved (Kusterbeck, 2019). If the situation becomes untenable, the practitioner may consider relocation and avoidance (Abreu et al., 2022) or engaging in civil disobedience when one believes the law is unjust and harmful, knowing that there may be legal consequences (Reamer, 2008). Challenging an unjust law in court may help to change it, especially when a practitioner or organization can band together with others in opposition to the law (Reamer, 2008).

Summary

Situations in which laws conflict with ethical care are extremely difficult to navigate. The occupational therapy practitioner must prepare to make hard choices. These decisions may entail choosing to follow a law that coincides with one's principles but creates professional controversy; following a law that goes against one's principles; advocating for changes to unjust laws; or resisting the law through civil disobedience. An ethical decision-making framework can assist the occupational therapy practitioner in examining the issue with logic and reflection, keeping the right thing to do in sight, even if an ideal solution is not always attainable.

REFERENCES

Abreu, R., Sostre, J., Gonzalez, K., Lockett, G., & Matsuno, E. (2022). "I am afraid for those kids who might find death preferable": Parental figures' reactions and coping strategies to bans on gender affirming care for transgender and gender diverse youth. *Psychology of Sexual Orientation and Gender Diversity, 9,* 500–510. https://doi.org/10.1037/sgd0000495

American College of Obstetricians and Gynecologists. (2021). *Legislative Interference with patient care, medical decisions, and the patient-physician relationship statement of policy.* https://www.acog.org/clinical-information/policy-and-position-statements/statements-of-policy/2019/legislative-interference-with-patient-care-medical-decisions-and-the-patient-physician-relationship

American Medical Association. (2022). *AMA announces new adopted policies related to reproductive health care.* https://www.ama-assn.org/press-center/press-releases/ama-announces-new-adopted-policies-related-reproductive-health-care

American Medical Association. (2023). *AMA strengthens its policy on protecting access to gender-affirming care.* https://www.endocrine.org/news-and-advocacy/news-room/2023/ama-gender-affirming-care#:~:text=In%20the%20resolution%2C%20the%20AMA,who%20provide%20gen-der%2Daffirming%20care

American Occupational Therapy Association. (n.d.). *Practice essentials: AOTA official documents.* https://www.aota.org/practice/practice-essentials/aota-official-documents

American Occupational Therapy Association. (2020). Occupational therapy's commitment to diversity, equity, and inclusion. *American Journal of Occupational Therapy, 74*(Suppl. 3), 7413410030. https://doi.org/10.5014/ajot.2020.74S3002

American Occupational Therapy Association. (2021). *Policy E.15: Affirming gender diversity and identity.* https://www.aota.org/-/media/corporate/files/aboutaota/officialdocs/policies/policy-e15-20211115.pdf

American Occupational Therapy Association. (2022a). AOTA's societal statement denouncing conversion "therapy." *American Journal of Occupational Therapy, 76*(Suppl. 3), 7613410320. https://doi.org/10.5014/ajot.2022.76S3010

American Occupational Therapy Association. (2022b). *Policy E.17: Affirming sexual orientation.* https://www.aota.org/-/media/corporate/files/aboutaota/officialdocs/policies/policy-e17-20220416.pdf

American Psychological Association. (2023a). *Abortion: Resources from APA.* https://www.apa.org/topics/abortion

American Psychological Association. (2023b). *Criminalizing gender affirmative care with minors: Suggested discussion points with resources to oppose transgender exclusion bills.* https://www.apa.org/topics/lgbtq/gender-affirmative-care

Bolding, D., Acosta, A., Butler, B., Chau, A., Craig, B., & Dunbar, F. (2022). Working with lesbian, gay, bisexual, and transgender clients: Occupational therapy practitioners' knowledge, skills, and attitudes. *American Journal of Occupational Therapy, 76,* 7603205130. https://doi.org/10.5014/ajot.2022.049065

Brous, E. (2019). Legal issues with sexual and gender minority patients in the emergency department. *Journal of Legal Nurse Consulting, 30*(2), 30–37.

Dobbs v. Jackson Women's Health Org., No. 19-1392, 2022 WL 2276808 (U.S. June 24, 2022) https://www.supremecourt.gov/opinions/21pdf/19-1392_6j37.pdf

Doherty, R. F., & Purtilo, R. B. (2016). *Ethical dimensions in the health professions* (6th ed.). Elsevier.

Eberl, J. (2021). What makes conscientious refusals concerning abortion different. *American Journal of Bioethics, 21*(8), 62–64. https://doi.org/10.1080/15265161.2021.1940372

Fox, D. (2021). Medical disobedience and the conscientious provision of prohibited care. *American Journal of Bioethics, 21*(8), 72–74. https://doi.org/10.1080/15265161.2021.1940361

Hensley, E., & Washington, J. (2023). *How major abortion laws compare, state by state.* The Fuller Project. https://fullerproject.org/story/how-major-abortion-laws-compare-state-by-state-map/

Kaslow, N. J., & Watson, N. N. (2017). Civility: A core component of professionalism? *Psychology Teacher Network, 26*(3). https://psychlearningcurve.org/civility/

Kusterbeck, S. (2019). Legal requirements may conflict with clinicians' ethical obligations. *Relias Media.* https://www.reliasmedia.com/articles/144497-legal-requirements-may-conflict-with-clinicians-ethical-obligations

Reamer, F. G. (2008). When ethics and the law collide. *Social Work Today, 8*(5). https://www.socialworktoday.com/archive/EoESepOct08.shtml#:~:text=Examples%20include%20statutes%20governing%20social,and%20the%20federal%20HIPAA%20laws

Trans Legislation Tracker. (2023). *2023 Anti-trans bills tracker.* https://translegislation.com/

Walker, K., McCune, K., & Kirby, A. V. (2021). Occupational therapy's role in gender-affirming surgeries. *OT Practice, 26*(10), 12–15.

Appendix A. Guidance for Case Questions and Discussion

This appendix provides additional resources for educators and practitioners to facilitate conversations using the questions at the end of each case example in chapters based on the ethics Advisory Opinions. Educators should use these case examples alongside an ethical decision-making framework. For practitioners, discussing ethical issues with peers and working through decision making with hypothetical cases can facilitate preparedness for facing ethical issues in practice.

Section 1. Professional Integrity, Responsibility, and Accountability

CHAPTER 10. ETHICAL GOVERNANCE

In Chapter 10, the authors offer questions for deep reflection in Table 10.1. Instructors can create learning activities using these questions. One learning activity could include dividing participants into groups and having them role-play various leadership roles in an organization such as the American Occupational Therapy Association (AOTA), including the Executive Director, Board President, Speaker of the Representative Assembly, Commission Chairperson, and so forth. Each group could then take one of the governance principles listed in Table 10.1 and consider the questions for that principle. They could then report the results of their discussion to the class. Another learning activity could be having participants interview a person serving in a leadership role in an occupational therapy organization and asking them how they live out each of these principles, using the questions included.

CHAPTER 11. ENGAGING IN BUSINESS TRANSACTIONS WITH CLIENTS: ETHICAL CONSIDERATIONS

CASE EXAMPLE 11.1. FINANCIAL TRANSPARENCY

1. *What are the ethical issues at stake in this scenario?*
   The occupational therapy practitioner has engaged in a conflict of interest in which they use their position as a practitioner for financial gain in their company. They have broken the principle of

(Continued)

CASE EXAMPLE 11.1. FINANCIAL TRANSPARENCY *(Cont.)*

fidelity to their client, and several standards in the Code regarding professional integrity, responsibility, and accountability regarding conflicts of interest. They were also not truthful, breaking the principle of veracity.

2. *What further information does the occupational therapy practitioner need to gather?*
The occupational therapy practitioner needs to gather information on the laws in their state regarding vending to clients, truth in advertising, and conflicts of interest. They also need to check into the policies of their employer to find out if sharing information on the sale of equipment through their separate company is a conflict of interest. Finally, they need to understand how selling to clients for personal gain could put a client, who is in a vulnerable position, at risk of harm.

3. *What actions could the occupational therapy practitioner take to salvage the therapeutic relationship and to avoid this situation in the future?*
The practitioner needs to talk with the client and apologize for the harm they have caused. They need to refund the client in full. At this stage, they may not be able to salvage the therapeutic relationship. If the client wants to switch to another practitioner, the practitioner needs to accommodate that request or make a referral to another facility to avoid abandoning the client. In the future, they must ensure that any advertisement they share with current clients discloses their ownership of the company. They also need to provide the client with multiple options for purchasing equipment instead of giving just one option from their own company.

CHAPTER 12. AVOIDING PLAGIARISM IN TODAY'S WORLD: A PROFESSIONAL RESPONSIBILITY

CASE EXAMPLE 12.1. REUSING FORMS AND HANDOUTS

1. *Apply an ethical decision-making framework to Tiffany's case. What standards of the Code were potentially violated by Tiffany's actions?*
Tiffany is passing off someone else's work as her own, which is the definition of plagiarism. When she copied someone else's handout and used websites without citing them, she plagiarized. The Code includes several standards on plagiarism, including those that state that occupational therapy practitioners must not participate in plagiarism, violate copyright laws, or illegally share resources. Standards also admonish practitioners to give credit and recognition when using the ideas and works of others.

    Participants can work through the decision-making framework to decide how they would gather information, what aspects of the Code are being violated, what options the practitioner has for resolving the ethical issue, what the desired resolution would be, and how each option would reflect the outcome.

2. *If a colleague of Tiffany at her new job found out about her actions, what steps should they take?*
The first thing the colleague should do is talk to Tiffany about the misuse of these materials and try to get her to secure permission for their use and properly cite the work of others. If that does not work, the colleague should talk with a supervisor and cite the Code and any facility policies on using materials created by other organizations. With the backing of official documents, the colleague will be able to make a stronger case to advocate for change.

(Continued)

CASE EXAMPLE 12.1. REUSING FORMS AND HANDOUTS *(Cont.)*

3. *What are several possible ways that Tiffany could rectify the situation to avoid violating the Code and plagiarism laws?*

   Tiffany could contact the Level II Fieldwork site and request to use their materials if she properly cites them. If they say no, Tiffany will need to develop new materials for the clinic. Tiffany could also edit her online article to contain proper citations for the information she provided. She should also remember to appropriately cite quotes with quotation marks and page or paragraph numbers.

CASE EXAMPLE 12.2. ACADEMIC COURSE CONTENT

1. *Does Bob need to cite sources when creating his academic PowerPoints for classroom use? Why or why not?*

   Bob should cite his sources when creating academic PowerPoints. First, he is legally and ethically bound to observe both copyright laws and the Code in regard to plagiarism. Second, he needs to set an example and expectations for students in the course.

2. *Do Bob's actions violate the Code and/or copyright laws? Why or why not?*

   Bob's actions do violate the Code. He is using outdated materials in his course, which is a violation of the Code, which requires practitioners to use evidence-based and current evaluation, planning, intervention techniques, assessments, and therapeutic equipment that are within the scope of occupational therapy practice. Additionally, works written by an organization are protected by copyright law even if the work (paper, website) is not officially copyrighted or trademarked. A person can be subject to fines for infringement of copyright laws.

3. *If Bob's supervisor finds out about Bob's actions, what should the supervisor do?*

   The first thing the supervisor should do is approach Bob and educate him on proper use of citations and references to avoid plagiarism and copyright infringement. The supervisor should also educate Bob on the need to use current, evidence-based materials. The supervisor should also let Bob know that just because something is well known, it does not mean that the information is in public domain. If the idea was not original to the speaker, then the speaker should cite a source for where the information can be found. Otherwise, Bob could be accused of stealing someone else's ideas and passing them off as his own, which is the definition of plagiarism.

CASE EXAMPLE 12.3. UNINTENTIONAL VS. INTENTIONAL PLAGIARISM

1. *Did both Isaac and Dina commit plagiarism? Why or why not?*

   Yes, both students committed plagiarism. Isaac committed unintentional plagiarism, because he appropriated the ideas of others and confused the thoughts of others with his own thoughts. Dina committed intentional plagiarism because she purchased a paper that she did not write and tried to pass it off as her own.

2. *What consequences should the students receive for their actions? Should these consequences be the same for both students? Why or why not?*

   Plagiarism constitutes academic dishonesty and should not be tolerated at any level in higher education. Although academic institutions may vary in their response, it is common for acts of unintentional plagiarism to be punished with lower grades and additional work, and for those who commit intentional plagiarism to be put on probation or dismissed from the academic program.

CASE EXAMPLE 12.4. IN-SERVICE PRESENTATION AND PLAGIARISM

1. *What are some ways in which Carlotta potentially violated copyright laws in this scenario?*
    Carlotta violated copyright laws by not citing works and then passing them off as her own, such as the PowerPoint slides and information copied and pasted from websites. Carlotta's work was careless and left her open to punishment for academic misconduct.
2. *Did Carlotta violate the Code? Why or why not?*
    Carlotta did violate the Code. Her actions violated copyright laws, which is expressly forbidden in the Code.
3. *What are some steps Carlotta could take to correct this situation?*
    If Carlotta is prone to omissions in her work, she could ask a friend to proofread her work. She also needs to obtain sources, use quotations for works used verbatim, and do her best to provide in-text citations and references to accurately show who owned the intellectual property she was using. She could refer to an online source for how to complete proper citations or use a citation management system.

Section 2. Therapeutic Relationships

CHAPTER 13. ESTABLISHING PROFESSIONAL BOUNDARIES: WHERE TO DRAW THE LINE

CASE EXAMPLE 13.1. SUPERVISOR AND STUDENT RELATIONSHIPS

1. *What are the ethical issues at stake in this scenario?*
    By maintaining dual relationships of both personal and professional natures, Sam's friendship with Camryn can compromise the occupational therapy practitioner's ability to provide supervision safely and competently. Additionally, there is a potential for exploiting the student because their relationship outside of work hours may conflict or interfere with Sam's professional judgment and objectivity, thus diminishing Camryn's opportunity for professional growth during fieldwork. Furthermore, occupational therapy practitioners and personnel must provide honest, fair, and accurate information on employee and student performance. Sam could face conflicts of interest, as well as difficulty maintaining professional boundaries and confidentiality and ensuring that their evaluation of Camryn is completely objective and unbiased.
2. *Who are the stakeholders who may be harmed in this scenario?*
    Stakeholders include Sam, Camryn, other team members and administrators at the hospital, the clients, Camryn's future clients, state licensing boards, and professional associations.
3. *What should Sam do to avoid a conflict of interest?*
    Sam should be supportive of Camryn in the work environment but refrain from spending social time with Camryn. Instead, Sam could connect Camryn with other students in the area or online affinity groups.
4. *What should Camryn do to advocate for themself?*
    Camryn could decline going out with Sam and, if needed, address the issue directly by requesting to meet with Sam to discuss the situation. While potentially difficult, the outcome of this conversation could result in a better supervisory experience for both Sam and Camryn.

CASE EXAMPLE 13.2. DATING AND ROMANTIC RELATIONSHIPS

1. *What are the ethical issues at stake in this scenario?*
   Taylor has shared many intimate moments with Aron during the course of their rehabilitation. As such, they would be entering into the relationship with far more information about Aron than they might naturally have In a normal dating relationship.
       This places Taylor in a situation in which they could potentially exploit the recipient of services physically, emotionally, or psychologically. Additionally, should the possibility of a sexual relationship arise, Taylor would find themselves breaching ethics standards from the Code that specifically state that practitioners, whether in paid or volunteer roles, must avoid dual relationships with those under their care (including family members); this includes sexual relationships.

2. *What further information does Taylor need to gather?*
   Taylor should gather information on company policy, state practice act requirements, the Code, and any other appropriate documents. It may also help Taylor to talk with a trusted colleague and consult ethics literature.

3. *What are the power dynamics in this situation, and how do they play into crossing ethical boundary lines?*
   By nature of the therapeutic relationship, clients are a vulnerable population. They depend on the occupational therapy practitioner for knowledge and skills that they need during a difficult time in their life. On this topic, groups could discuss the sense of closeness that may come from assisting with ADLs, the tendency for those in an unequal relationship to develop rescue fantasies or hero worship, the possibility of abuse when one person is vulnerable in a relationship, or any number of relationship issues that can result from unequal power dynamics.

4. *How can Taylor avoid unethical practice in this case?*
   The most appropriate response to Aron's request for a date is to let them know that the Code prohibits a relationship with them while they are a client. After Aron's discharge from the facility, Taylor should seriously consider the appropriateness of entering any type of relationship with Aron, as the relationship balance may be skewed because of their previous interactions as client and therapist. In addition, people who have been through a traumatic health event are vulnerable, and the professional burden is on the practitioner to set and maintain clear boundaries for the therapeutic relationship to protect their client. Taylor should also consult their state occupational therapy practice act and facility regulations for additional guidance.

CHAPTER 14. CULTURALLY RESPONSIVE CARE

CASE EXAMPLE 14.1. CULTURAL HUMILITY IN PEDIATRIC SERVICES

1. *What power dynamics might exist within this relationship between the practitioner and family?*
   There is an unequal distribution of power in this relationship, considering that the family is relying on the practitioner's knowledge and skills, and the practitioner is responsible for creating the interventions to help the child develop and thrive. Another aspect of power relates to the practitioner being in the family's home as a mandated reporter. The home is a personal space, and the family

(Continued)

CASE EXAMPLE 14.1. CULTURAL HUMILITY IN PEDIATRIC SERVICES *(Cont.)*

may be required to have the therapist within the home for the child's treatment. Other power dynamics may relate to the financial relationship between the practitioner and family, particularly if the family is paying for services; the education level of the practitioner as compared to the family; and the interactions among the multiple identities held by the practitioner and the family, such as gender, race, ethnicity, nationality, language, religion, socioeconomic status, and sexual orientation.

2. *Which standards of conduct from the Code are relevant to this scenario?*

Standards related to therapeutic relationships, service delivery, and professional civility are particularly relevant to this scenario. These include standards from the Code that require the practitioner to respect and honor the expressed wishes of service recipients; Susan must respect the family's wishes regarding food and toys that are brought within their home. The Code also states that the practitioner must establish a collaborative relationship with the child and family to promote shared decision making. This standard is helpful in providing guidance for Susan moving forward because collaboration appears to be lacking in terms of scheduling, planning sessions, and understanding beliefs and values. Additionally, Susan cannot abandon the service recipient, per the Code, and she must attempt to facilitate an appropriate transition. If Susan decides to request an exemption from providing services to this family because of a self-identified conflict with personal, cultural, or religious values, then the Code requires that Susan follow organizational policies and appropriate procedures to find a provider for the family. Susan is required by the Code to plan interventions that are specific to this family's needs. Susan should ask questions and acknowledge and incorporate their cultural and religious needs into her intervention plan. Susan must conduct herself in a civil manner by respecting different points of view and demonstrating cultural humility in her interactions with the family.

3. *What would it look like if Susan practiced cultural humility in this situation? And how does this look different from cultural competence?*

By practicing cultural humility, Susan would be comfortable with not knowing everything about the family's culture, self-aware, supportive when interacting with the family, and open to learning and engaging in self-reflection on an ongoing basis. Susan would engage in identifying her biases and recognize and attempt to minimize the impact of power imbalances in the relationship with the family. Cultural competence would have Susan already knowledgeable about the culture of the family, including their cultural and religious needs, preferred types of foods and toys, and view of independence. Attempting to be fully knowledgeable does not consider the complexity of culture, or the multiple intersecting identities of family members, and can lead Susan to make false assumptions when working with the family.

4. *What course of action do you recommend for Susan?*

Susan must not abandon this child and leave the family without an occupational therapy practitioner. By practicing cultural humility and collaborating with the family, Susan has the opportunity to change her perspective and learn about this family's life experience in a nonjudgmental way. Through introspection, she may recognize that as an occupational therapy practitioner, she values independence, but certain cultures place great importance on caring for family members as opposed to encouraging them to do for themselves. After each therapy session, it may be helpful to reflect on what went well and what could improve. Susan can reassess the situation after a reasonable amount of time is given to develop the therapeutic relationship.

CASE EXAMPLE 14.2. CULTURALLY RESPONSIVE THERAPEUTIC USE OF SELF

1. *What is the difference between ethnocentrism and cultural humility?*
   Ethnocentrism means that one believes that their own group, ethnicity, or nationality is superior to others. *Cultural humility* means that a person understands their own biases and privileges, manages power imbalances, and maintains openness to others in relation to aspects of their cultural identity. In terms of practical application, cultural humility allows the occupational therapy practitioner to recognize that although their own cultural values and beliefs are important to them and guide their daily occupational engagement and performance, they need to be flexible and allow that same freedom for their clients to let their personal cultural values and beliefs to guide their occupational engagement and performance.

2. *How can occupational therapy practitioners move from cultural awareness to cultural humility?*
   Being aware of what culture is and that there are various cultures and various cultural beliefs across populations, communities, groups, and individuals is just the foundational basis for a journey toward cultural sensitivity and humility. To truly reflect cultural humility, one must commit to the understanding that they will never fully reach competency. Instead, practitioners must work daily to be intentional about acknowledging personal cultural values, beliefs, and preferences for engaging in occupation, acknowledging the uniqueness of each individual client. Practitioners must recognize how multiple perspectives affect the therapeutic relationship, including those of the profession of occupational therapy and the institution where services are provided.

3. *What did Sasha need to do differently to employ the best evidence-based practice and culturally responsive and humble care with Kendra?*
   Sasha needed to acknowledge their own ethnocentrism and cultural awareness and beliefs. Then Sasha needs to acknowledge that even if they perceive similarity and affinity with a client, they need to complete a client profile and gain insight into the client's unique perspective and preferences for treatment, goals, and relevant tasks with guidance on current evidence and trends for best practice.

4. *What is the next step of the occupational therapy process for Sasha and Kendra?*
   To repair lost trust and rapport, Sasha should move to the re-valuation phase of the occupational therapy process. They should reassess current progress towards goals and make any necessary updates to the current plan of care based on current progress and Kendra's feedback before proceeding with the intervention plan.

CASE EXAMPLE 14.3. RESPECTING CULTURAL TRADITIONS IN HEALTH CARE

1. *In what ways did Terry disrespect Mr. Guillermo and his culture?*
   Terry disrespected Mr. Guillermo immediately upon entering the home by not starting with introductions or engaging in brief small talk. Terry mispronounced his name and did not ask how he would like to be addressed or how to pronounce his name. Instead of asking questions, Terry badgered Mr. Guillermo with questions and accusations based on stereotypes of Latino culture, such as assuming he was drinking tequila, was lazy and uncooperative, and was not following doctor's orders. Terry also referred to Mr. Guillermo and his other care providers as Mexican when they were from a different country.

(Continued)

CASE EXAMPLE 14.3. RESPECTING CULTURAL TRADITIONS IN HEALTH CARE *(Cont.)*

2. *What standards of conduct from the Code did Terry violate?*
   Terry violated the ethical principles of autonomy, justice, and fidelity by not respecting Mr. Guillermo's choices or treating him with fairness and respect. Standards that were violated include:
   - *Respect and honor the expressed wishes of recipients of service:* Terry made no effort to determine what Mr. Guillermo's concerns were or what he wanted to do.
   - *Establish a collaborative relationship with recipients of service and relevant stakeholders to promote shared decision making:* Terry asked no questions about the other care providers and what they did or whether they could meet.
   - *Do not engage in communication that is discriminatory, derogatory, biased, intimidating, insensitive, or disrespectful or that unduly discourages others from participating in professional dialogue:* Terry was disrespectful to Mr. Guillermo and spoke about him in derogatory terms to the agency director.
   - *Engage in collaborative actions and communication as a member of interprofessional teams to facilitate quality care and safety for clients:* Terry made no effort to learn about the other care providers or to work with them.
   - *Demonstrate professional civility:* Terry was uncivil to Mr. Guillermo and was not respectful of diversity of thought. Terry did not demonstrate courtesy nor cultural humility.

3. *What could Terry do to learn more about Latino cultures in general, and Mr. Guillermo's cultural priorities specifically?*
   Terry could learn more about Mr. Guillermo's culture by first recognizing Mr. Guillermo's country of origin and culture, and not assuming all LatinX people are Mexican. He could ask Mr. Guillermo about his homeland, his preferences, his favorite foods, and so forth. Terry could also do research on Salvadoran culture or attend conferences or seminars about culture and health care. There may be an International Center where Terry lives, which could provide a lot of information.

4. *How can an occupational therapy practitioner work collaboratively with a* yerbero *(herbalist),* sobandero *(similar to a massage therapist), and other healers?*
   Terry could reach out to the *yerbero* and the *sobandero* and learn about their practices. Terry could request a meeting where they learn about each other's professions and determine how to collaborate. The *yerbero's* suggestions could be incorporated into occupational therapy sessions on meal preparation. They might want to schedule OT after sessions with the *sobandero*, when Mr. Guillermo will be more relaxed. They might be able to collaborate on a home program that incorporates recommendations from all of them.

CHAPTER 15. SOCIAL JUSTICE, OCCUPATIONAL JUSTICE, AND ETHICAL PRACTICE

CASE EXAMPLE 15.1. SERVICES FOR PEOPLE WITH LIMITED RESOURCES

1. *What are the ethical principles and standards in question in this scenario?*
   The principles of *justice* and *fidelity* apply. Other principles and standards from the Code apply as well and can be discussed as a group.

2. *Apply an ethical decision-making framework to this case. What steps should the occupational therapy practitioner take to address Jackie's needs?*

(Continued)

CASE EXAMPLE 15.1. SERVICES FOR PEOPLE WITH LIMITED RESOURCES *(Cont.)*

Participants can work through the decision-making framework to decide how they would gather information, what aspects of the Code are being violated, what options the practitioner has for resolving the ethical issue, what the desired resolution would be, and how each option would reflect the outcome.

3. *Choose one possible solution to this ethical problem. What would be the possible outcomes? What issues would remain outstanding?*
   Participants may provide various responses to this scenario, including creative solutions for pro bono care or referral to other sources. Participants should consider outcomes and outstanding needs as a way of reflecting on their solution to this scenario.

CASE EXAMPLE 15.2. CENTER FOR UNSTABLY HOUSED PEOPLE

1. *What are the occupational justice and social justice issues in this scenario?*
   Participants might discuss how a lack of resources affects occupational engagement and what role the occupational therapy practitioner may have in advocating for more resources or finding creative ways to meet needs when the principle of justice is at stake.
2. *What are some possible solutions to sustainably source the supplies needed?*
   Finding sustainable solutions in under-resourced environments can be quite challenging. The student has a limited amount of time in this setting to come up with a solution. They could do anything from a one-time drive to finding community groups to "adopt a month" and ensure the center has the personal products needed. Discussions may produce other options.
3. *How would these solutions reflect ethical practice and the principles of occupational and social justice?*
   Participants can come up with many creative solutions and reflect on how these solutions relate to the Code. They can also discuss the realistic effectiveness of the outcomes for this population.

CASE EXAMPLE 15.3. FACILITY POLICIES VS. SOCIAL JUSTICE

1. *What ethical principles and standards in the Code are at stake in this scenario?*
   In this scenario, the practitioner is encountering a true ethical dilemma between the principles of *justice* and *fidelity*.
2. *Apply an ethical decision-making framework. What options does the occupational therapy practitioner have?*
   Although it is necessary to have money to "keep the lights on" and pay the bills, the clinic could explore creative solutions to manage attendance, transportation, and other challenges for people with insufficient resources. Participants can use the ethical decision-making framework to brainstorm options, discuss the merits of each option, and reflect on possible outcomes for creating just opportunities for underserved clients.
3. *Which of these options would bring about the greatest result for social and occupational justice for clients?*
   To advocate for occupational justice, the occupational therapy practitioner could collaborate with colleagues in the setting to present the director with creative solutions to the attendance problem. A sustainable solution with the most support from practitioners and management would bring about the most desirable outcomes.

CHAPTER 16. BALANCING CLIENT RIGHTS AND PRACTITIONER VALUES

CASE EXAMPLE 16.1. CONFLICT OF VALUES AND UNSAFE ENVIRONMENT

1. *How might Keisha balance Rafaella's right to autonomy and client-centered, collaborative care against Keisha's personal values regarding relational health and safety for her client?*
   Keisha's first step is to evaluate whether she is at risk of physical harm or significant moral injury. At the beginning of the case, Keisha does not seem to feel physically unsafe or that her mental health is threatened. If either became a concern, Keisha would need to reflect on whether she held any biases or misconceptions influencing that concern. She may consider seeking advice from a trusted supervisor or reading relevant literature from a reputable source to inform her reflection. Would supporting Rafaella's goals for independence and wellness, while knowing that Rafaella engages in situations that contradict Keisha's own standards for wellness and safety, cause Keisha significant mental health strain to the extent that she may experience symptoms of depression, trauma and stress-related disorders, or other moral injury? If Keisha can continue seeing Rafaella without personal or moral injury, she should provide Rafaella with collaborative, client-centered care. Keisha's moral objection to Rafaella's ongoing abuse is not a reason to undermine Rafaella's right to autonomy, beneficence, and best-practice occupational therapy. However, at the end of the case Keisha does feel unsafe. She now must consider the potential danger to herself and Rafaella. Note that Keisha has an ethical obligation to report the abuse if she lives in a state, territory, or region where Rafaella's abuse falls under mandatory reporting laws.

2. *What aspects of this case should Keisha document in her initial assessment?*
   Keisha should document the reports of abuse and continue to document what she observes.

3. *Is Keisha ethically obligated to stay in the home with Rafaella in this scenario?*
   Occupational therapy practitioners are never ethically obligated to put themselves in danger to deliver client care or fulfill professional responsibilities. If Keisha feels that continuing to treat Rafaella in her home puts Keisha at risk of physical harm, she is not obligated to continue seeing Rafaella in that context. However, Keisha is obligated to seek alternative options to maintain the therapeutic relationship with Rafaella, if possible. Following the procedures and policies of her employer and all relevant legislation, Keisha should attempt to continue the therapeutic relationship while collaborating with Rafaella to find a safe alternative to in-home treatment. If collaboration fails to avail Keisha of an acceptably safe way to provide Rafaella with care, then Keisha can ethically step away from the therapeutic relationship in a way that limits Rafaella's risk of harm or perception of abandonment.

4. *Is Keisha ethically obligated to continue working with Rafaella in her home once the situation described in the scenario is resolved?*
   Keisha is obligated by the Code not to abandon the client. However, if she is traumatized by the scenario and fearful of reentering the home, she can fulfill her obligation to Rafaella by transferring care to another occupational therapy practitioner or another site of care.

CASE EXAMPLE 16.2. TRIGGERING SYMBOL

1. *Does the occupational therapy assistant have an ethical obligation to treat the client? Why or why not?*

   The Code states that an occupational therapy practitioner is not to abandon the service recipient, but it goes on to say that the practitioner may facilitate appropriate transitions when unable to provide services. It also states that the practitioner should adhere to organizational policies when requesting an exemption from service. Such an exemption may be requested when the practitioner self-identifies a conflict due to personal, cultural, or religious values.

2. *Is it ethical for the supervisor to require the occupational therapy assistant to treat this client? Why or why not?*

   In this scenario, we do not know what the organizational policies are regarding an exemption for service. It is possible that the supervisor is following policy. Participants may wish to discuss whether such a policy would be ethical. A caring response would be for the supervisor to find another practitioner to provide treatment to avoid causing trauma to the occupational therapy assistant.

Section 3. Documentation, Reimbursement, and Financial Matters

CHAPTER 17. ETHICAL CONSIDERATIONS FOR PRODUCTIVITY, BILLING, AND REIMBURSEMENT

CASE EXAMPLE 17.1. BILLING GROUP TREATMENT AT THE HIGHER INDIVIDUAL RATE

1. *What is the proper procedure for billing services done simultaneously?*

   Blake can find out the proper procedure for billing by gathering the facts pertaining to the case. What information do they know, and what additional information might they need? Blake must first be certain about how Parker's treatment sessions are being billed, which could include checking charge sheets, if available. It is of paramount importance that Blake know the specific rules and regulations that pertain to Parker's billing practices before proceeding further. Does the health care organization where Blake is employed have a reimbursement compliance program or compliance officer? If so, Blake could seek further clarification by referring to the health care payer organization's reimbursement policies and procedures. They could make a fact-finding appointment with the compliance officer to discuss the situation. There would be no need to disclose the name of the practitioner at this point, and the discussion could occur as a "hypothetical situation."

2. *What standards from the Code did Parker violate?*

   The principle of *veracity* indicates that occupational therapy practitioners should be truthful and accurate in billing and documentation. Likewise, the principle of *justice* directs practitioners to be aware of laws, policies, and official documents that apply to practice; this includes billing and coding for services. Blake also has the obligation to report to the appropriate authorities any illegal practice actions or any breaches of the Code.

(Continued)

CASE EXAMPLE 17.1. BILLING GROUP TREATMENT AT THE HIGHER INDIVIDUAL RATE *(Cont.)*

3. *What is Blake's best course of action, not knowing whether the clinic supports Parker's billing practices?*

Blake should continue to gather information and try to work within the organization to address this error before reporting the potential fraud. If it is determined that the billing practice was not permissible, Blake would have an obligation to act. In this scenario, the compliance officer checked the payer policies and procedures and determined that billing for four individual *CPT* codes while providing the treatment in a group setting was not permissible. The plan of care and all documentation and billing records that were obtained did not accurately reflect the services provided and were not in alignment. After the facts were determined, several options were open to Blake. He could speak directly to Parker, notify his supervisor, report Parker to the compliance officer, or report the situation directly to the payer. To resolve the ethical problem internally, Blake decided to speak directly to Parker first as a potential opportunity to educate them and observe the ethical principle of *fidelity*. Blake first sought to determine Parker's knowledge of reimbursement and coding regulations. Parker told Blake that they had recently attended a conference during which several other occupational therapy practitioners were discussing billing practices for group treatment as individual sessions. They thought the logic of billing at the higher individual rate seemed to be sound and were unaware that it was against payer guidelines. Parker thanked Blake for informing them of the rules and said they would stop this practice immediately.

Both agreed that the overpayment should be returned to the payer. Blake, Parker, and the supervisor met, and the supervisor notified the compliance officer, who notified the payer and returned the funds. Although the reimbursement issue was documented in Parker's personnel file, no disciplinary action was taken. Parker was provided with training to help ensure that they would not make any further inaccurate claim requests and would have the knowledge necessary to use appropriate resources and information to enable compliance.

If the issue was not addressed internally within the organizational structure, Blake might have had additional options. Blake might have decided not to work in an environment in which unethical and illegal practices were not addressed. Blake also could have decided to report to external entities, such as the payer organization's fraud and abuse hotline or state or federal agencies. Doing so might have been the only option they had left to disentangle themselves from unethical and illegal activity.

Blake also could have done nothing. However, doing nothing could have resulted in moral distress and would not have met ethical obligations. If Blake had gone along with fraudulent billing practices, Blake could have been subject to fines, loss of license, loss of employment, and even criminal conviction and incarceration.

CASE EXAMPLE 17.2. UNREALISTIC PRODUCTIVITY EXPECTATIONS

1. *What standards were violated by the skilled nursing facility company and the Rehab Manager?*
   Unrealistic productivity expectations violate the principles of *justice* and *fidelity* regarding employees because it is unjust to expect employees to work off-the-clock to complete documentation and other non-billable tasks.
2. *What avenues of recourse are available to Jing?*
   Jing chose to resign from this position, but other options may be available. One of the best ways to address unjust actions from an employer is to band together as employees and address the employer as a group. The group can present the employer with laws and professional standards for productivity to seek a fair solution.
3. *What would you do if you were asked to maintain an unrealistic productivity standard?*
   Participants may share a variety of possible solutions.

CHAPTER 18. ORGANIZATIONAL ETHICS

CASE EXAMPLE 18.1. ORGANIZATIONAL LOYALTY VS. CLIENT AUTONOMY

1. *What ethical issues are in conflict for this occupational therapist?*
   The occupational therapist wants to respect the client's autonomy, yet they feel a responsibility to maintain a positive working relationship with the physician. Although the practitioner–client relationship is typically the theoretical focus for conflict resolution, the practitioner also must maintain other relationships to ensure safe, effective, and ethical delivery of occupational therapy services, as reflected in the ethical principle of fidelity.
2. *What may be some of the organizational consequences for failing to follow this physician's order? Conversely, what are some of the ethical consequences for following the order?*
   A physician's order that is contrary to the ethical principle of *autonomy* would make it difficult for the occupational therapist to know how to proceed. If the therapist chooses the autonomy of the client over fidelity to the organization and physician, they could risk losing the physician as a referral source. If the organization values the relationship with the physician over the judgment of the occupational therapist, the consequences for the therapist could be severe. If, however, the organization supports the therapist, there could be several options for resolution to this scenario.

   If the therapist is to violate the trust of the client by forcing them to participate in therapy against their will, it could lead to many adverse outcomes, including a decline in trust between client and practitioner; the potential harm—both psychological and physical—imposed on the client; the lack of benefit incurred when a client is treated against their will (which is also a legal issue, because it can be construed as assault and battery); and, ultimately, a decline in trust among occupational therapy practitioners, organizations, and the individuals served. Continuing to treat a client who is refusing services and has decision-making capacity is not ethically justifiable.
3. *Apply an ethical decision-making framework to this scenario. What options does the occupational therapist have?*
   One option is for the occupational therapist to ask their supervisor to help them communicate with the physician. If a supervisor is not available, a medical director or administrator may be able

(Continued)

CASE EXAMPLE 18.1. ORGANIZATIONAL LOYALTY VS. CLIENT AUTONOMY *(Cont.)*

to facilitate communication with the physician. Often, organizational management can communicate with physicians in a way that minimizes power imbalances. In addition, a supervisor or administrator should be familiar with and able to locate clients' rights policies that objectively identify client and practitioner roles and can assist the employee in the identification of other organizational resources. The hospital ethics committee or consultation services may help resolve conflict between practitioners within the confines of the organization. In addition, organizational structures, such as incident reporting systems or safety hotlines, can be used to influence the behavior of practitioners to protect client rights while keeping the reporting source anonymous to avoid strained relationships among team members. The occupational therapist walks a difficult line in balancing these team relationships with their responsibilities to the client. The therapist should approach the physician again, ideally, with rational and objective support based on conversation with a supervisor, administrator, and/or ethics consultant.

4. *Choose an option and reflect on the potential outcome. What positive and negative outcomes would be produced by the selected option?*

The occupational therapist should pursue opportunities for communication with the physician. However, if the physician continues to rebuff their attempts at dialogue, the therapist should pursue another avenue for communication involving the administration. Depending on the organization's understanding of its role in fostering relationships between practitioners and clients, the therapist may or may not encounter a supportive advocate for resolution of the ethical dilemma. If this option does not resolve the conflict, they may ultimately decide to transfer the client's care to another practitioner; refuse to treat the client, which may result in termination of employment; or continue treating the client. The therapist should consider the legal implications of each option as well. It is important to actively advocate for the client, but this should be done in a respectful manner that is least damaging to the relationship between physician and therapist. Although client trust is essential, one must also work to maintain trust among colleagues and team members.

Section 4. Service Delivery

CHAPTER 19. ETHICAL CONSIDERATIONS RELEVANT TO EMERGING TECHNOLOGY-BASED INTERVENTIONS

CASE EXAMPLE 19.1. PARENT OF PEDIATRIC CLIENT AND 3D PRINTING

1. *What are the ethical issues at stake in this scenario?*

The occupational therapy practitioner must weigh the evidence regarding risks and benefits, effectiveness, and safety of this device before agreeing to educate the client in its use. These factors correspond with the ethical principles of *beneficence* and *nonmaleficence*.

2. *What additional information does the occupational therapy practitioner need to gather?*

The practitioner needs to gather more information on what the literature is saying about the efficacy of this device and safety of its use.

(Continued)

CASE EXAMPLE 19.1. PARENT OF PEDIATRIC CLIENT AND 3D PRINTING *(Cont.)*

3. *What actions could the occupational therapy practitioner take?*

   After researching the device, the practitioner needs to inform the parent of what they learned about its efficacy, safety, and benefits versus the device's cost and difficulty of use. If there is no research available on the device, the practitioner should caution the parent that potential benefits are not verified. If the practitioner cannot recommend the device, then they should consider what other options they might offer the parent and child. If the practitioner finds that the device is well-researched and would benefit the child, then they should consider becoming educated in the use of the device so that they can train the parent in its use.

CASE EXAMPLE 19.2. PRODUCT PROMOTION

1. *What are the ethical issues at stake in this scenario?*

   There are several ethical issues at stake in this scenario. One major ethical concern is the potential conflict of interest. Accepting free robotic gloves from the developer may create a financial interest in promoting and using the product, which could compromise the objectivity and best interests of the clients. The practitioner might feel pressure to use the gloves even when they may not be the most suitable intervention for a particular client. Informed consent is also an ethical issue in this scenario. Introducing a new technology, like the robotic glove, without obtaining informed consent from clients could infringe on their autonomy. Clients have the right to make informed decisions about their treatment options, and this includes being informed about the use of new technologies. The practitioner should also consider the evidence supporting the robotic glove's effectiveness in stroke rehabilitation. Ethical concerns arise if the practitioner is pressured to use the gloves without clear evidence of their benefit, or if they compromise evidence-based practice. Finally, there may be concerns about equity in health care access. If the robotic gloves are offered for free, disparities in access to rehabilitation services could occur because not all clients may receive the same benefits or opportunities.

2. *What additional information does the occupational therapy practitioner need to gather?*

   Before making a decision, the occupational therapy practitioner should gather more information. They should investigate the scientific evidence supporting the efficacy of the robotic glove in stroke rehabilitation and whether it is a proven and effective intervention. They should discuss the potential use of the robotic glove with clients, considering their preferences, goals, and individual needs, and understand whether they are open to using this technology. They should also consider who will cover the costs of maintenance, repair, and ongoing support for the robotic gloves and assess the long-term sustainability of using this technology. They may wish to consult with colleagues, professional organizations, and legal experts to understand the ethical and legal implications of accepting the developer's offer. Finally, they should explore alternative rehabilitation interventions that may be more appropriate for specific clients and assess the potential impact on client outcomes.

(Continued)

CASE EXAMPLE 19.2. PRODUCT PROMOTION *(Cont.)*

3. *What actions could the occupational therapy practitioner take?*
The practitioner should consult the ethical guidelines and standards of practice established by their professional organization (e.g., AOTA) to ensure compliance with ethical principles. They should engage in shared decision making with clients, explaining the pros and cons of using the robotic glove and obtaining informed consent. They need to be transparent with clients about the nature of the offer from the developer, potential conflicts of interest, and the source of the equipment. They should consider the appropriateness of using this glove on a case-by-case basis and in line with evidence-based practice. It would be important to continuously monitor and document the outcomes of using the robotic gloves to ensure that they are beneficial for clients and used in accordance with ethical principles. Finally, the practitioner should consult with legal and ethical experts to ensure that the decision aligns with professional and legal standards. Ultimately, the occupational therapy practitioner should prioritize the best interests of their clients and maintain their professional integrity while carefully considering the offer from the product developer.

CHAPTER 20. ETHICAL CONSIDERATIONS IN TELEHEALTH

CASE EXAMPLE 20.1. TELEHEALTH AND INFORMED CONSENT

1. *Despite having followed all anticipated issues during telehealth, situations may arise that change the outcome and cause a dilemma related to ethics. What ethical standards were met or not met during this session?*
   * *Informed consent:* The informed consent standard was not fully met. Although Serena explained the teleconferencing session to Becky and her mother, the request for Becky to undress partially during the session may not have been adequately explained in advance. Informed consent should include clear communication about what will happen during the session, and consent should be obtained for each specific action or intervention.
   * *Privacy and dignity:* The request for Becky to undress in front of a video camera without her prior understanding or consent may have violated her privacy and dignity. Protecting the client's dignity and privacy is a fundamental ethical principle, and this situation appears to have compromised both.
   * *Competence and scope of practice:* Both Serena and Nell followed the standards of their profession by confirming their state licensure and consulting with the caregiver and client to ensure the appropriateness of the telehealth consultation. However, Nell's request to assess pelvic mobility through videoconferencing may have raised questions about the scope of practice and competence in this specific context.
   * *Beneficence and nonmaleficence:* The practitioners' intentions to improve Becky's seating system were driven by the principle of *beneficence,* aiming to enhance her functioning and comfort. However, the request to undress Becky caused distress and emotional harm to the client, thus conflicting with the principle of nonmaleficence.

(Continued)

CASE EXAMPLE 20.1. TELEHEALTH AND INFORMED CONSENT *(Cont.)*

2. *How could this telehealth session have been better planned so a successful outcome would have been obtained?*

   To ensure a successful telehealth session while upholding ethical standards, several steps could have been taken:

   - *Observe all applicable laws and policies:* Sammy and Casey both checked to be sure they were compliant with their individual state's licensure and reviewed payor sources prior to the visit.
   - *Obtain enhanced informed consent:* Prior to the session, Serena and Nell should have provided a detailed explanation of what to expect during the consultation, including the possibility of physical assessments, and obtained explicit informed consent from Becky and her mother for each step. Sammy explained the process and expected outcomes for the telehealth visit and obtained consent from both. Sammy and Casey might have avoided the problem if they had more fully explained what to expect during the session. Sammy did respect Becky's right to refuse by ending the session when she started to cry.
   - *Address privacy and modesty:* Consider alternative ways to assess pelvic mobility without compromising the client's privacy and modesty. This could include using adaptive clothing or instructing the caregiver on how to assist without undressing Becky during the video session. Sammy or Casey might have asked Becky to wear something more form fitting to allow visualization of the anatomical areas of concern for mobility and positioning.
   - *Use secure platforms:* Ensure the use of a secure, HIPAA-compliant video conferencing platform to protect client data and privacy.
   - *Set boundaries:* Both practitioners should establish clear boundaries and limitations for the telehealth session, including what is and isn't feasible in a remote assessment.
   - *Be culturally sensitive:* Consider the client's cultural background and preferences when planning the session. Some clients may have cultural or religious sensitivities to certain requests.
   - *Have a contingency plan:* Develop a contingency plan in case a situation arises where an action like the one Nell requested might cause distress to the client. This plan could include alternatives for assessing pelvic mobility, rescheduling, or involving a local health care provider if necessary.
   - *Provide regular communication:* Regularly check in with the client and caregiver to ensure their comfort and understanding during the session. Encourage them to speak up if they have concerns or feel uncomfortable at any point.

   By taking these steps, the occupational therapy practitioners could better plan and conduct a telehealth session that respects the client's rights, privacy, and dignity while still providing valuable assessments and recommendations for care.

CASE EXAMPLE 20.2. SUPERVISION AND TELEHEALTH

1. *According to the Code, what ethical issues were created in the above scenario?*
   During their weekly virtual meetings, Jamie had been helping Chris develop competency for providing intervention through telehealth. During the first session, Jamie did obtain consent for the session but did not fully explain the purpose of the session. Jamie did provide supervision and education necessary for Chris to complete the telehealth sessions, however, when Jamie left unexpectedly Chris continued with the telehealth sessions with no supervision. Finally, Jamie's participation during the telehealth sessions did not allow for the client's expected privacy.

2. *Apply an ethical decision-making framework. How could the ethical issues in this scenario have been avoided?*
   Participants can work through the decision-making framework to decide how they would gather information, what aspects of the Code are being violated, what the options are, what the desired resolution would be, and how they would reflect on the outcome. To avoid some of the issues experienced by Jamie and Chris, the client could have been told what to expect during the telehealth sessions, including that Jamie would be attending some of the sessions for supervision purposes and observations of client's progress. When Jamie left on medical leave unexpectedly, Chris could have postponed treatment until another occupational therapist could assume supervision.

CASE EXAMPLE 20.3. SAFETY IN TELEHEALTH

1. *What are some of the ethical concerns identified in this scenario?*
   Terry did not follow the organization's policies and procedures related to obtaining contact information prior to the session or requesting informed consent.

2. *What could Terry have done differently prior to this telehealth evaluation?*
   In anticipation of the evaluation process, Terry should have inquired about the veteran's functional mobility and balance and explored the need for a family member or care extender (e.g., friend, neighbor) to be present during portions of the evaluation if balance was a concern.

3. *What could Terry have done differently during this telehealth evaluation?*
   Terry demonstrated concern for and did not abandon the veteran by contacting the appropriate emergency number and remaining online with both parties until the veteran was safe. However, Terry may have been able to avoid this situation altogether by addressing safety and explaining the need for a counter, chair, or other stabilizing surface for the veteran to grab in the event he lost balance.

CHAPTER 21. ETHICAL CONSIDERATIONS IN PRIVATE PRACTICE

CASE EXAMPLE 21.1. MULTIPLE REFERRALS WITHIN THE SAME FAMILY UNIT REQUIRING PROFESSIONAL COLLABORATION

1. *What are the ethical issues in this scenario?*
   The following ethical issues are at stake:
   - *Veracity*: Two of the three children qualify for services, and the practitioner is considering "creating" deficits to allow for qualification of the third.
   - *Beneficence*: An occupational therapy practitioner is considering treating out of their scope and training based on reimbursement rates.
   - *Justice*: Discovery of the reimbursement rate is driving the therapy process instead of evaluation data and standards of care.

2. *What are the ethical principles and standards that apply?*
   Several principles and standards apply, including the following:
   - *Veracity*: The practitioner is held to honesty and truthfulness.
   - *Nonmaleficence*: The practitioner must refrain from causing harm, injury, or wrongdoing to the client.
   - The practitioner must ethically report outcomes to payers and referring entities as well as to relevant local, regional, and national databases and registries, when appropriate.
   - The practitioner must provide services within their own level of competence.
   - The practitioner must refer clients to appropriate resources when the needs of the client can best be served by the expertise of other professionals.
   - The practitioner should not provide false and misleading information to qualify the third child for services.

3. *Apply an ethical decision-making framework. What are the next steps the practitioner should take?*
   Participants can work through the decision-making framework to decide how they would gather information, what aspects of the Code are being violated, what the options are, what the desired resolution would be, and how they would reflect on the outcome. The third child who did not qualify for occupational therapy should not be seen based solely on reimbursement and the parent request. The qualification and direct need for services should be based on deficits. Deficits were not present in the initial evaluation. The practitioner who is considering treating out of their scope of practice should be held to the ethical standard to appropriately refer to another clinician trained in feeding. This may include collaboration with a provider trained in swallowing, while the original provider manages other aspects of the feeding therapy needed, including sensory and motor needs. The family should be informed of the ethical standard to practice within one's scope and training and the need for therapy services; they cannot justify services on a monetary basis.

CASE EXAMPLE 21.2. HIPAA VIOLATION WITH ONLINE PAYMENT SERVICE

1. *What are the ethical issues in this scenario?*
   There are several ethical issues in this scenario:
   - *Confidentiality and privacy:* The parent's inadvertent disclosure of their child's evaluation payment on a publicly visible online payment platform compromised the confidentiality and privacy of the child's health care information. The occupational therapy practitioner has an obligation to use a secure billing platform to ensure the client's confidentiality is protected on both the payment and receipt sides of the billing transaction.
   - *Informed consent:* The child's information was shared without the informed consent of the child or their legal guardian. The parent may not have realized the potential consequences of making the payment publicly visible, but because the occupational therapy practitioner is responsible for protecting the client's information, they have an obligation to make sure the information is secure.
   - *Professional boundaries:* The business owner, who is an occupational therapy practitioner, may face a dilemma related to professional boundaries when their personal relationship with the parent is tested by the friend's inquiry about the child's evaluation.
   - *Transparency and honesty:* The business owner must balance the need to maintain transparency and honesty with the ethical obligation to protect the child's privacy and confidential information.
   - *Beneficence:* The clinic owner should ensure they are competent to evaluate the needs of the child.

2. *What are the ethical principles and standards that apply?*
   - *Autonomy:*
     - *Confidentiality:* Occupational therapy practitioners have a duty to protect the confidentiality and privacy of the information obtained during evaluations and treatments.
     - *Informed consent:* Informed consent is a fundamental ethical principle, and individuals (or their legal guardians) must be informed and give consent for any disclosure of their health information.
   - *Nonmaleficence:* Practitioners must maintain professional boundaries, which may be challenged when a personal relationship with a client's family is involved.
   - *Veracity:* Practitioners should be transparent and honest with clients about the use and disclosure of their health information.

3. *Apply an ethical decision-making framework. What are the next steps a practitioner should take?*
   To address this situation, the practitioner should consider the following steps:
   - The practitioner should first evaluate the extent of the privacy breach and its potential consequences for the child and their family.
   - The primary responsibility is to protect the child's and family's confidentiality. The practitioner should ensure that the online payment transaction is immediately made private to prevent further disclosure of sensitive information. The practitioner should inform the parent about the unintended disclosure and advise them to adjust their privacy settings to avoid future breaches. The practitioner should also educate the parent about the importance of maintaining privacy settings for online transactions involving sensitive health care information.

(Continued)

CASE EXAMPLE 21.2. HIPAA VIOLATION WITH ONLINE PAYMENT SERVICE *(Cont.)*

- The practitioner should acknowledge the inquiry from the mutual friend but refrain from sharing any specific details about the child's evaluation. Instead, they can express a commitment to respecting the child's privacy and the importance of confidentiality in health care.
- The practitioner should implement procedures within the clinic to ensure that online payment transactions for health care services are kept confidential, and staff should be educated about the potential privacy risks associated with online payment platforms.
- The practitioner should document the incident, the actions taken to address it, and any future preventive measures implemented.
- The practitioner should reflect on the incident and review the clinic's policies and procedures to further safeguard client privacy and confidentiality.

CHAPTER 22. THE ROLE OF THE OCCUPATIONAL THERAPY PRACTITIONER AS AN EXPERT WITNESS

CASE EXAMPLE 22.1. ACTING AS AN EXPERT WITNESS

1. *At different times, Tonya violated various standards of the Code. Which standards were violated and when?*
   - *Nonmaleficence:* Tonya may have violated the principle of nonmaleficence by failing to disclose critical information regarding Charley's competence and the potential harm caused by outdated techniques used. This violation occurred when Tonya did not mention these issues to Parent B's attorney or during her deposition.
   - *Veracity:* Tonya violated the principle of veracity by failing to provide a complete and accurate report about Charley's competence. She withheld information about the outdated techniques and potential harm, which was relevant to the case.
   - *Fidelity:* Tonya may have violated the principle of fidelity by not acting in the best interests of both parents and the child. She failed to provide critical information that could have affected the outcome of the case.
   - *Justice:* Tonya's failure to disclose relevant information about Charley's practices and her knowledge of the potential harm may have undermined the pursuit of justice in the case, because it could have affected the legal proceedings and fairness of the trial.
2. *It appears that Tonya recognized some issues when reviewing the medical records. What should she have done at that point?*
   When Tonya recognized the issues in Charley's documentation and the potential harm associated with the outdated techniques, she should have taken the following steps:
   - Tonya should have reported her concerns to Parent B's attorney as soon as she identified them. It was her ethical duty to provide all relevant information to the attorney, even if it could potentially harm Charley's case.
   - Tonya should have amended her expert witness report to include the information about the potential harm of outdated techniques. This would have ensured that all parties had access to complete and accurate information.

(Continued)

CASE EXAMPLE 22.1. ACTING AS AN EXPERT WITNESS *(Cont.)*

- As an occupational therapist and an expert witness, Tonya had a professional obligation to prioritize client safety, the best interests of the child, and ethical standards over her personal interests or her desire to help Charley. This means providing complete and accurate information to legal authorities, regardless of the potential consequences.

By failing to report her concerns and withholding relevant information, Tonya not only compromised her professional ethics but also negatively affected the case's outcome and the welfare of the child involved.

3. *After the Ethics Commission receives the complaint, what should the next steps be?*

The Ethics Commission will follow the steps in the Enforcement Procedures to ensure that the complaint is duly considered regarding whether Tonya committed a violation of the Code. Those steps include:

- *Complaint submission:* The process begins when a complaint is submitted to the AOTA Ethics Commission. Complaints can be submitted by AOTA members or non-members.
- *Initial review:* The Ethics Commission conducts an initial review of the complaint to determine if it falls within the scope of the Code and Standards of Practice for Occupational Therapy.
- *Response from the practitioner:* If the complaint is accepted for further review, the practitioner against whom the complaint was filed is notified and provided with an opportunity to respond to the complaint.
- *Investigation:* The Ethics Commission may conduct an investigation to gather information and evidence related to the complaint. This may involve contacting the parties involved and requesting documentation.
- *Review and decision:* After the investigation, the Ethics Commission reviews the complaint, any responses from the practitioner, and the gathered evidence. The Commission then deliberates and makes a decision regarding the complaint.
- *Resolution options:* The Ethics Commission may decide to resolve the complaint in several ways, which can include:
  - *Dismissal:* If the complaint is not substantiated or does not fall within the scope of the Code or Standards of Practice for Occupational Therapy, it may be dismissed.
  - *Resolution through education:* The practitioner may be provided with education on ethical considerations or standards.
  - *Censure:* The Commission may issue a formal censure if they determine that the practitioner's actions warrant it.
  - *Sanction:* In more serious cases, the Ethics Commission may impose sanctions, such as probation, suspension, or revocation of AOTA membership.
  - *Notification of authorities:* In cases where the complaint involves potential violations of the law, the Ethics Commission may notify the appropriate authorities.
- *Notification:* The practitioner and the complainant are notified of the Ethics Commission's decision, and they are informed of any actions that will be taken as a result of the decision.
- *Appeal:* Practitioners who are subject to sanctions have the right to appeal the decision within the AOTA's established appeal process.
- *Publication:* Sanctions or censures may be published in AOTA publications, as deemed appropriate.

CHAPTER 23. CLIENT ABANDONMENT

CASE EXAMPLE 23.1. LEAVING IN THE MIDDLE OF THE SCHOOL YEAR

1. *Does leaving a school district in the middle of a school year constitute client abandonment?*
The practitioner has found themself in one of the appropriate and unavoidable instances where they will be stepping away from clients who still need occupational therapy services. Although it sounds like their supervisor would like them to feel guilt for this situation, the practitioner has no reason, at this point, to worry about having crossed an ethical line. They informed their supervisor with enough time for the supervisor to accommodate the departure. They even went above and beyond by offering to assist in finding and training a replacement.

2. *What steps can the practitioner take to address the ethical uncertainty they are experiencing?*
The practitioner has an obligation to minimize the potential harm to clients by giving them (and their families and teachers) notice of the upcoming transition, collaborating with them on how to transition care, and completing all paperwork to support incoming service providers.

CASE EXAMPLE 23.2. RESEARCH IN A RURAL COMMUNITY

1. *Knowing that some clients will need services beyond what is offered during the research intervention, what ethical responsibilities must the researcher fulfill to avoid client abandonment?*
The researchers know even before establishing a plan of care and a therapeutic relationship that there may be a need to terminate services before the client has fully met all goals on the treatment plan. Recognizing the need to employ a strategy to avoid client abandonment is a good first step for the researchers in preventing an ethical breach. There are multiple avenues for them to address the potential for client abandonment because of their proactive consideration of the possibility. Regardless of which specific solution they employ, if the researchers follow ethical guidelines in mitigating harm to the client when services are terminated, they will have handled the situation ethically. They should clearly communicate expectations for the duration of the relationship from the onset. They should collaborate with clients on the transition of care at the termination of the relationship. They should also provide the client with any documentation, resources, or recommendations at the end of the study to support the clients in continuing to get their therapeutic needs met.

CHAPTER 24. RESPONDING TO PUBLIC HEALTH CRISES

CASE EXAMPLE 24.1. COMMUNITY-BASED SETTING DURING A PANDEMIC

1. *What are the competing ethical issues Brianna must decide among?*
The case example of Briana highlights ethical issues of duty to provide care vs. duty to self and family, resource allocation, and scope of practice.

2. *How might Brianna use a framework for ethical decision making to help her decide what to do?*
Following a framework for ethical decision making, Brianna first identified the ethical problem: the competing duties to her employer (fidelity) and to herself and family (justice). Second, she

(Continued)

CASE EXAMPLE 24.1. COMMUNITY-BASED SETTING DURING A PANDEMIC *(Cont.)*

considered all those involved, including clients, coworkers, supervisors, family members, and self. Next, she sought more information through discussing the issue with her employer. Next, she learned all she could about options and resources, as well as consequences of those options. Finally, she decided to discuss the issue again with her employer to seek out a compromise, creating a new option. Reflecting on the outcome could help Brianna and her colleagues set new standards and come up with creative care solutions as they continued to provide care to their clients during the pandemic.

3. *What resources could Brianna use to help guide her ethical decision making?*
   Brianna sought guidance from the Code. She understood this situation required careful consideration of ethical obligations as they related to the ethical principles of *beneficence, nonmaleficence,* and *fidelity.* Brianna used an ethical decision-making framework to contemplate options and the likely consequences of each. She also relied on other sources of information, such as the Centers for Disease Control and Prevention (CDC) and her local public health agency, each of which relayed that the virus could be spread by persons who were asymptomatic and strongly discouraged gathering in groups.

   Brianna requested a follow-up discussion with the early intervention program director regarding her concerns. Based on the discussion, they reached a compromise in which they agreed that a group limited to three staff members would gather to assemble the materials. The trio worked at separate workstations, following CDC guidelines related to social distancing, wearing masks and gloves, proper handwashing techniques, and appropriately disinfecting surfaces. Brianna was satisfied with her contribution to the project and believed she successfully participated while taking appropriate precautions.

CASE EXAMPLE 24.2. ACUTE CARE SETTING DURING A PANDEMIC

1. *Who could Lee turn to for assistance in clarifying options in this situation?*
   Lee decided to meet with his supervisor to outline his concerns and sources of moral distress. Other options could have been to discuss the situation with an ethicist, consult the literature, or email the AOTA Ethics Program.

2. *What are at least three other options Lee could choose besides not going to work?*
   Lee and his supervisor could review current personal protective equipment (PPE) guidelines, consult with infection control administrators, and set up additional training for all the occupational therapy practitioners in the department to practice donning and doffing PPE. These options may help reassure Lee that he could stay as safe as possible and protect his family while fulfilling his duty to clients. Perhaps they could consider having the occupational therapy team rotate care of COVID-positive clients to provide respite from the challenges of working with this population. Lee could also seek counseling and self-care to protect his mental health to reduce the moral distress and self-doubt he felt in light of his role and the negative comment made by the physician.

(Continued)

CASE EXAMPLE 24.2. ACUTE CARE SETTING DURING A PANDEMIC *(Cont.)*

3. *What ethical principles could Lee use to help select a course of action?*

   This case highlights beneficence versus risk to self in an acute care setting. Lee is experiencing moral distress, because his employer is unable to provide PPE and guidelines for its use to assure safety for the health care team and clients, yet he has a duty to care for the clients. He is also contemplating the ethical dilemma of fidelity to his colleagues weighed against the risk of personal harm and harm to others through transmission of COVID-19. Together, Lee and his supervisor could review the Code to understand their ethical obligations to clients during a pandemic. Lee could then realize that the principles of *fidelity* and *beneficence* could help guide his decision, but that he would still have to do his own personal risk assessment.

4. *To whom could Lee talk to communicate his decision?*

   Lee would want to complete his ethical decision-making process by discussing the outcome of his decision with his supervisor.

CHAPTER 25. OUTDATED AND OBSOLETE ASSESSMENT TOOLS

CASE EXAMPLE 25.1. USING STANDARDIZED ASSESSMENTS

1. *What are areas of concern regarding this occupational therapist's assessment?*

   Pat submitted an evaluation report based on a speech-language pathology assessment tool, an outdated version of an occupational therapy tool, and a simulated version of another occupational therapy tool with made-up norms because the tool was validated for a different age group.

2. *What standards in the Code have been violated?*

   The evaluation that Pat submitted was not accepted by New City Clinic. This could cause the staff at New City Clinic, and probably Taylor's parents, to have reduced trust in occupational therapy, violating the standard not to reduce the public's trust in occupational therapy. One of the assessment tools was not appropriate for Taylor's age, violating the standard for use of assessment tools appropriate to the specific client. Pat also used an assessment tool that is for speech-language pathologists, not occupational therapy practitioners, so it was outside of the scope of practice. Another assessment tool was outdated and thus did not meet the standard to be current. By making up norms, Pat did not record and report accurate evaluation data.

3. *How would you proceed if you were the clinic director?*

   If Pat is retained on the job, the director needs to be sure that Pat attends relevant continuing education regarding assessment. The clinic might voluntarily report a revocation of the charges to Taylor's insurance company because the evaluation was not competent or accurate. If this happens, Pat might be required to pay back the clinic or return wages for that evaluation. If Taylor's family reports this situation to the state regulatory board and/or the insurance company, the clinic and/or Pat might incur significantly more severe penalties.

CASE EXAMPLE 25.2. USING UPDATED ASSESSMENTS

1. *What are areas of concern regarding this occupational therapist's assessment?*
    Ken misrepresented his occupational therapy assessment as complete and appropriate for his client.
2. *What standards in the Code could have been violated by submitting these results?*
    Ken chose an assessment tool that would have been appropriate for his client if the assessment tool was complete. By using an incomplete tool and presenting it as a complete assessment, Ken's report was not accurate, violated the Code, and could affect the public's trust in occupational therapy and his competence.

CHAPTER 26. INFORMED CONSENT

CASE EXAMPLE 26.1. INFORMED CONSENT IN PRACTICE: WHOOPS!

1. *What informed consent procedures did Alex omit?*
    Alex omitted several important informed consent procedures:
    *   *Failure to verify client identity:* Alex did not properly verify the identity of the client before initiating the intervention. This is a crucial step in ensuring that the right client receives the right care.
    *   *Failure to communicate treatment plan:* Alex did not adequately communicate the treatment plan or seek consent from the client before initiating the activity. Informed consent involves explaining the nature and purpose of the intervention and its potential risks, and obtaining the client's agreement.
2. *How could have Alex prevented this from happening?*
    To prevent such incidents, Alex could have taken the following steps:
    *   Double-check client identification: Always verify the client's identity using at least two identifiers (e.g., name, date of birth) before initiating any intervention.
    *   *Review client information:* Review the client's medical chart or electronic health record to confirm the correct client, diagnosis, room number, and any specific precautions or contraindications.
3. *What should Alex do after this happened?*
    After realizing the mistake, Alex should take the following steps:
    *   *Apologize and communicate:* Apologize to the client (Alice) for the error and any discomfort caused.
    *   *Report the incident:* Report the incident to the appropriate supervisor or manager and follow the hospital's established procedures for adverse events.
    *   *Learn from the mistake:* Use the incident as an opportunity for self-reflection and continuous improvement. Identify factors that contributed to the mistake and implement strategies to prevent similar errors in the future.

CASE EXAMPLE 26.2. INFORMED CONSENT IN RESEARCH: VULNERABLE POPULATION

1. *Was Charlie correct that they did not have to inform parents or go through an IRB?*
   Charlie's understanding of the need to inform parents and seek Institutional Review Board (IRB) approval is not accurate in this case. In educational research involving human subjects and a vulnerable population, it is required to obtain informed consent from the parents or guardians of the students, especially when there are changes in the students' educational environment. Even if Charlie believes that the study does not involve direct physical interaction with the students, changes to the learning environment can still affect students' experiences and falls under the definition of human subjects research. Therefore, IRB approval is necessary.

2. *What consequences would Charlie face if they proceed with this research?*
   If Charlie proceeds with the research without obtaining informed consent from parents and without securing IRB approval, there could be serious consequences. This may include ethical violations, potential harm to participants, and legal implications.

3. *What procedures would Charlie need to follow to adhere to informed consent processes?*
   Charlie should develop a clear and comprehensive informed consent form that explains the nature of the research, the purpose of the study, the study's potential risks and benefits, and the right to withdraw from the study at any time. The consent form should also include information about how data will be handled, stored, and reported. Charlie should submit the research proposal to the school's IRB or an external IRB for review and approval before initiating the study.

Section 5. Professional Competence, Education, Supervision, and Training

CHAPTER 27. STATE LICENSURE AND ETHICS

CASE EXAMPLE 27.1. PRACTICING WITHOUT A LICENSE

1. *What are the ethical implications of this scenario?*
   Regardless of personal situations, each occupational therapy practitioner is responsible for ensuring that their license is active before providing occupational therapy services in every instance. The occupational therapy practitioner should consider the relevant ethical standards of the Code that were in violation as well as pertinent regulations of the state and other governing agencies, such as the National Board for Certification in Occupational Therapy (NBCOT®). The practitioner violated the principle of *beneficence,* including standards of the Code that require complying with applicable laws, accurately representing credentials, and demonstrating they have maintained competence. Practitioners who practice without a license may face legal or disciplinary action, including loss of licensure, resulting in the inability to work. The unlicensed practice of occupational therapy in a state may be reported by a consumer, employers, colleagues, organizations, individuals, or the occupational therapy practitioner themself.

2. *What actions should the practitioner take?*
   In this case, the occupational therapy practitioner should be honest with their employer, immediately stop providing occupational therapy services, and contact their state or territory regulatory board. State and territory licensure and regulation protect the safety of consumers by ensuring that only qualified individuals can provide occupational therapy services.

CASE EXAMPLE 27.2. CONTINUING EDUCATION AND LICENSE RENEWAL

1. *What are the ethical implications of this scenario?*
   Occupational therapy practitioners must be knowledgeable about the requirements for continuing competence or education necessary for renewal of state licensure to ensure timely completion. The occupational therapy practitioner should consider the relevant ethical standards of the Code that were violated as well as pertinent state regulations and regulations of other governing agencies such as NBCOT. If they are unable to comply with the continuing education requirements of their state license, they risk violating the ethical principles of *beneficence* and *justice,* and standards requiring compliance with the law and maintaining competence.
2. *What actions should the occupational therapy practitioner take?*
   In this case, the occupational therapy practitioner should contact their state regulatory board and/or state occupational therapy association for advice and direction related to options for completing continuing education. Practitioners who fail to complete required continuing education and continue to practice may be subject to fines, disciplinary action, or contingencies until the requirements for licensure renewal are fulfilled. Falsification of continuing education hours is unlawful and unethical and may subject the practitioner to legal ramifications, and/or disciplinary action from the state regulatory board as well as other governing agencies such as the AOTA Ethics Commission and NBCOT. Creating a professional development plan, pursuing meaningful professional development activities, and maintaining a record of those activities is highly encouraged not only to qualify for and meet criteria for renewal of state licensure but also to advance one's continuing competence.

CHAPTER 28. PROMOTING ETHICALLY SOUND PRACTICES IN OCCUPATIONAL THERAPY FIELDWORK EDUCATION

CASE EXAMPLE 28.1. THE ABSENT FIELDWORK EDUCATOR

1. *What ethical standards of the Code have been violated?*
   The following standards were violated:
   - Ensure that documentation for reimbursement purposes is done in accordance with applicable laws, guidelines, and regulations.
   - Do not follow arbitrary directives that compromise the rights or well-being of others, including unrealistic productivity expectations, fabrication, falsification, plagiarism of documentation, or inaccurate coding.
   - Provide appropriate supervision in accordance with AOTA official documents and relevant laws, regulations, policies, procedures, standards, and guidelines.
2. *What should Sam do next?*
   Sam needs to contact their academic fieldwork coordinator (AFWC) regarding their concerns. The AFWC can provide support to students while out on fieldwork rotations, especially when there are ethical concerns. Sam should not document treatments they did not complete.
3. *What are the appropriate actions to take at this point in the fieldwork rotation?*
   The AFWC should schedule a meeting with Alex and Sam first thing Monday morning to discuss these concerns. In this way, all interested parties can work together to create a corrective course of action for the remainder of Sam's fieldwork experience that includes ethically sound practices. Adequate supervision is the main issue that must be addressed for both the benefit of Sam and the safety of all clients and family members.

CASE EXAMPLE 28.2. CURRENT AREAS OF ETHICAL CONCERN

1. *For each of the identified ethical issues, what sections of the Code of Ethics have been violated?*
   With the numerous ethical issues the AFWC found, potentially every section of the standards of the Code has been violated. Examples include:
   - Accessing medical records of family, friends, or others not on caseload—this violates the principle of *autonomy* and the standards for communication and maintaining confidentiality and privacy.
   - Social media posting of pictures or identifying client information—this violates the principle of *autonomy* and the standards for communication and maintaining confidentiality and privacy.
   - Fieldwork educators not thoroughly vetting the competency of a student prior to the start of hands-on care—this violates the principle of *beneficence* and standards of the Code for providing appropriate supervision and ensuring competence.
   - Crossing professional boundaries of relationships with students, clients, and fieldwork educators (FWEs), including having inappropriate sexual relationships—this violates the principle of *nonmaleficence* and standards for avoiding dual relationships and maintaining professional boundaries.
   - Student failing to disclose any conflict of interest prior to the start of fieldwork—this violates the principles of *nonmaleficence* and *fidelity* and standards for not engaging in conflicts of interest.
   - Dishonesty in documentation and billing practices—this violates principles of *justice* and *veracity* and standards for billing and documenting in accordance with laws, guidelines, and regulations.
   - Failure to maintain confidentiality and privacy of student and client information—this violates the principles of *fidelity* and *autonomy* and the standards for communication and maintaining confidentiality and privacy.
   - Failure to provide adequate supervision—this violates the principle of *beneficence* and standards of the Code for providing appropriate supervision and ensuring competence.
   - Impaired practice—this violates the principles of *fidelity* and *beneficence* and standards of the Code for not engaging in actions or inactions that jeopardize the safety or well-being of others or taking action to resolve impaired practice.
   - Incompetent practice—this violates the principles of *fidelity* and *nonmaleficence* and standards of the Code that require practitioners not to engage in actions or inactions that jeopardize the safety or well-being of others; and taking action to resolve incompetent practice.
   - Inappropriately accepting gifts from clients and others—this violates the principle of *justice* and the standard of the Code that states that one should not accept gifts that would unduly influence the therapeutic relationship.
   - Professional incivility, including bullying in the workplace—this violates principles of *justice* and *fidelity* and standards of the Code relating to professional civility.

2. *What potential laws may have been broken?*
   One law that may have been broken is The Health Insurance Portability and Accountability Act (HIPAA) of 1996.

3. *Using an ethical decision-making framework, what is one course of action the AFWC could take?*
   Using the ethical decision-making framework, the AFWC would need to gather all the facts that are known and unknown. These facts would include knowledge that several ethical standards have

(Continued)

CASE EXAMPLE 28.2. CURRENT AREAS OF ETHICAL CONCERN *(Cont.)*

been violated. Students, FWEs, and other occupational therapy practitioners are crossing professional boundaries, breaking confidentiality laws, and not acting in a civil and professional manner. It is important for the AFWC to assess what is going on and then determine the best course of action. In this case, it is necessary to address these concerns within the fieldwork curriculum at the school before students are placed on fieldwork. However, the AFWC needs to address concerns with the organizations they currently use for fieldwork. The AFWC could provide an in-service presentation or offer to host an Academic Fieldwork Educator Certificate Program for FWEs. This is a systemic problem and requires intervention at multiple levels.

CHAPTER 29. SUPERVISION AND COLLABORATION BETWEEN OCCUPATIONAL THERAPISTS AND OCCUPATIONAL THERAPY ASSISTANTS

CASE EXAMPLE 29.1. OCCUPATIONAL THERAPY ASSISTANT AS MANAGER

1. *Which ethics standards of the Code are relevant in this case?*
   - Kelly reminds the occupational therapy practitioners to provide evaluation and intervention that is specific to the needs of the service recipient in compliance with standards in the Code.
   - Kelly is proactively addressing workplace conflict so that it does not affect professional relationships and the provision of services.
   - The occupational therapist is violating the standards of professional civility in the Code by engaging in derogatory and disrespectful communication.
   - The occupational therapist violated the Code by disparaging and disrespecting occupational therapy assistants.
2. *How should the practitioners proceed?*
   The situation involves ethical and professional issues as well as potential workplace misconduct. For Kelly (occupational therapy assistant and Rehab Manager):
   - *Documentation:* Document all relevant incidents, including the occupational therapist's comments during the staff meeting and the social media post. This documentation will be essential for the disciplinary meeting.
   - *Disciplinary meeting:* Conduct a formal disciplinary meeting with the occupational therapist. During the meeting, Kelly should address the inappropriate behavior, emphasizing that such behavior is unprofessional, unethical, and unacceptable in the workplace. She should clearly communicate any consequences for the behavior as determined by the organization and any expectations moving forward.
   - *Review policies:* Review the facility's policies and procedures regarding workplace conduct, social media usage, and professional behavior, and ensure that the occupational therapist is aware of these policies.
   - *Conflict resolution:* Encourage open and respectful communication among team members. If there are underlying issues causing tension, explore ways to address these conflicts constructively.

(Continued)

CASE EXAMPLE 29.1. OCCUPATIONAL THERAPY ASSISTANT AS MANAGER *(Cont.)*

- *Client-centered care:* Reinforce the importance of client-centered care and ethical practice in the facility. Emphasize the need to prioritize individualized treatment plans based on clients' needs rather than revenue generation.
- *Professional development:* Encourage ongoing professional development and respect for all team members' contributions, regardless of their titles or educational backgrounds.
- *Follow up:* After the disciplinary meeting, Kelly should monitor the occupational therapist's behavior and ensure compliance with facility policies and ethical standards.
- *Supervisory role:* Kelly should continue to supervise and ensure ethical practice and client-centered care within the department. She should maintain an open line of communication with her team.

For the occupational therapist:

- *Acknowledgment:* Acknowledge the inappropriate behavior and comments made during the staff meeting and on social media.
- *Apology:* Issue a sincere and professional apology to Kelly, other staff members, and anyone else who may have been affected by the social media post. This apology should be made in person and in writing, and it should express remorse for the unprofessional behavior.
- *Commitment to ethical practice:* Commit to adhering to ethical standards, client-centered care, and professional behavior in the workplace.
- *Social media removal:* Promptly remove the inappropriate social media post and refrain from making further derogatory comments about colleagues.
- *Participation in resolution:* Actively participate in any efforts to resolve underlying conflicts within the team.
- *Self-reflection:* Reflect on the behavior and strive to improve their interpersonal skills, professionalism, and teamwork.

For both practitioners:

- *Team building and conflict resolution:* Consider organizing team-building activities and conflict resolution training for the entire occupational therapy department to promote better collaboration and understanding among team members.
- *Professional boundaries:* All team members should respect each other's roles and expertise and maintain professional boundaries in the workplace.
- *Continual improvement:* The facility should support ongoing education and professional development for all staff members to enhance their skills and knowledge.
- *Policy review:* The facility should periodically review and update its policies related to professional behavior, social media usage, and ethical standards to prevent future incidents.

Resolving this situation requires clear communication, adherence to ethical standards, and a commitment to improving workplace relationships and professionalism. For resolution to be successful, Kelly will need support from the facility's administration. The goal is to create a more respectful, collaborative, and client-centered environment within the occupational therapy department.

CASE EXAMPLE 29.2. OCCUPATIONAL THERAPIST–OCCUPATIONAL THERAPY ASSISTANT CLINICAL SUPERVISION

1. *Which ethics standards of the Code are relevant in this case?*
   By reassigning the child to a different practitioner, Casey is upholding the Code, which states that we must ensure that all duties delegated to other occupational therapy personnel are congruent with their competencies.
2. *How should the practitioners proceed?*
   Casey and the occupational therapy assistant can work together to create a professional development plan and goals that are beneficial to the occupational therapy assistant and the clinic.

CASE EXAMPLE 29.3. OCCUPATIONAL THERAPIST–OCCUPATIONAL THERAPY ASSISTANT COLLABORATIVE PARTNERSHIP

1. *Which ethics standards of the Code are relevant in this case?*
   - To uphold the standard for collaborative decision making, Avery and the occupational therapy assistant need to establish a collaborative relationship.
   - Avery and the occupational therapy assistant should uphold the Code by proactively addressing their workplace conflict.
   - The occupational therapy assistant felt that the original assessment tool was a better choice to determine whether goals are being achieved because it was used for the initial evaluations. It would be the best tool to determine whether intervention plans should be revised. Using an appropriate assessment tool upholds service delivery standards from the Code.
2. *How should the practitioners proceed?*
   - Since this assessment tool was relevant to this setting, Avery should achieve and maintain competence in its use. Then Avery would be able to provide appropriate supervision. Both these actions uphold the standards of the Code.
   - Avery and the occupational therapy assistant need to collaborate and communicate to facilitate quality care and safety for clients per the Code.

CHAPTER 30. ETHICAL CONSIDERATIONS FOR STUDENTS AND PRACTITIONERS WITH DISABILITIES

CASE EXAMPLE 30.1. STUDENT DISCLOSURE OF DISABILITY

1. *What would you do if you were the AFWC?*
   This is a complicated but common scenario that involves many ethical considerations. Participants in this discussion may have multiple responses as to what they would do in this situation.
2. *What standards of conduct do you think apply to this situation?*
   There are many parts of the Code that apply. First, the AFWC must maintain the confidentiality of all communication, including verbal, written, electronic, augmentative, and nonverbal communications. The AFWC must also consider the principle of justice and the standard of the Code that requires occupational therapy practitioners to be familiar and comply with institutional rules and federal laws.

(Continued)

CASE EXAMPLE 30.1. STUDENT DISCLOSURE OF DISABILITY *(Cont.)*

Additionally, the ethical principle of *autonomy* applies to Tanisha having the right whether to disclose. This prevents the AFWC from forcing Tanisha to disclose, and legally and ethically prohibits directly answering Jeremy's question about whether Tanisha has a disability. By providing Tanisha with access to accurate information regarding the educational requirements and academic policies and procedures of fieldwork and this site, the AFWC is fulfilling their ethical obligation outlined in the Code.

Taking a step back and looking at the whole scenario, the principle of *justice* applies to all faculty involved in this case. Faculty have an ethical responsibility to be aware of and follow practice guidelines, policies, and procedures that are relevant to educating students with disabilities in higher education. Although it might seem harmless to give a student regular extended time on tests and deadlines, best practice is to have students go through the formal accommodation application process to ensure their civil rights are being met. Faculty and clinical educators are under no obligation to approve or make any accommodations that have not been formally approved by the Office of Disability Services of the educational program. The ethical standard in the Code that requires practitioners to inform others of applicable policies, laws, and official documents also applies. It is important that Tanisha be made aware of her options as a student and then for faculty to follow formal policies and procedures for implementing reasonable accommodations.

3. *What laws apply to this scenario?*
   Americans with Disabilities Act (ADA), HIPAA, and the Family Educational Rights and Privacy Act (FERPA) laws apply.
4. *What are the ethical obligations of the fieldwork coordinator?*
   The only thing the AFWC can legally do is let Tanisha know what resources are available to her and discuss the pros and cons of disclosing, and then simply let Jeremy know that Tanisha does not have any accommodations. As an autonomous person with freedom to exercise choice and self-direction with all the information she has been given, Tanisha must make the final decision as to whether to disclose or apply for accommodation. Autonomous people can and do take risks. Tanisha may be risking failure of her first Level II Fieldwork by not applying for accommodations, but taking the risk is her choice.
5. *How would you navigate this challenging conversation with Tanisha?*
   Given that Tanisha has been struggling at fieldwork, it would be natural for Jeremy, the fieldwork educator, to feel an ethical tension between his obligation to allow her to have autonomy and their obligation to ensure occupational therapy recipients (in this case, recipients of her care) do not get harmed. As it relates to this specific case, Jeremy has a greater obligation to avoid breaching confidentiality with Tanisha, because there is no evidence at this point that Tanisha's behavior is putting clients at risk. It is imperative that Jeremy follow the standard in the Code that requires him to be honest, fair, accurate, respectful, and timely in gathering and reporting fact-based information about Tanisha's student performance. If there was information to indicate that clients were at risk, Jeremy would have a greater obligation to protect the clients and to focus on Tanisha's lack of competence in client safety. It might be hard to do this in a way that would not break Tanisha's right to privacy, but students must be proficient in adhering to the Code, adhering to safety regulations, and ensuring the safety of self and others during fieldwork. In this specific case, Tanisha's struggles due to her disability are not protected because she did not formally apply for and have reasonable accommodations approved. Although she did ask Jeremy for additional time on her notes, this reasonable accommodation request needed to go through her university's Office of Disability Services and be formally approved.

(Continued)

CASE EXAMPLE 30.1. STUDENT DISCLOSURE OF DISABILITY *(Cont.)*

Tanisha was made aware of her right to accommodation and given information on how to request them. As a result, the ethical obligations of the occupational therapy educational program, university, and site were met. Tanisha ultimately chose not to follow the processes outlined to her and was therefore not legally protected and not discriminated against for having a disability.

6. *To whom would you reach out for additional support and knowledge about this scenario?*
Jeremy could reach out to other practitioners at his site who have been fieldwork educators or to the AFWC. He could also use professional documents from AOTA to find out more about how to manage this situation.
Tanisha could reach out to her university's Office of Disability Services and to the AFWC.

CASE EXAMPLE 30.2. ESSENTIAL JOB FUNCTIONS

1. *What would you do if you were the AFWC?*
As occupational therapy practitioners and educators, it can be hard to separate the two different lenses through which one views teaching and supporting students with disabilities. Occupational therapy practitioners are naturally skilled and trained to help people adapt their environment to achieve their desired outcome. However, educators must remain objective and practice the principle of *fidelity* and maintain their role first and foremost as educators to set students up for success, not just during an occupational therapy educational program, but, more importantly, afterward. Ultimately, students desire to be successful practitioners, not just successful students. It might be difficult and uncomfortable to speak to Adam about how his limitations might prevent him from being employed in an inpatient setting; however, being honest about how many sites declined his accommodation (with legally appropriate reasons) shows the principles of *beneficence* and *veracity*. This discussion with Adam will objectively and honestly make him aware of very realistic future challenges in this setting and demonstrate concern for his success after graduation, without making assumptions about the range of his abilities.

2. *What standards of conduct do you think apply to this situation?*
As counterintuitive as it might sound, this information is constructive and promotes inclusivity by helping Adam navigate the professional world and learn where and how his disability will not limit his success as a practitioner. Additionally, this discussion will make Adam aware of the principle of *nonmaleficence* and the standard in the Code to not inflict harm or injury to recipients of occupational therapy services. Although Adam will not have to transfer during fieldwork, he admits he would not be able to keep a client safe if they were to start to lose their balance or need immediate physical support. Adam is ethically responsible for providing occupational therapy services that are within his competence and scope of practice, as outlined by the Code.

3. *What laws apply to this scenario?*
The Americans with Disabilities Act (ADA) applies to this scenario.

4. *What are your ethical obligations as a fieldwork coordinator?*
By guiding Adam through this conversation, as painful and challenging as it might be, the AFWC fulfills the ethical responsibility for recognizing and taking appropriate action to remedy occupation

(Continued)

CASE EXAMPLE 30.2. ESSENTIAL JOB FUNCTIONS *(Cont.)*

therapy personnel's personal problems and limitations that might cause harm to recipients of service. Although Adam has an accommodation not to have to transfer clients, he still must ensure their safety as well as his own, including when clients are not being transferred. By talking to Adam about the pros and cons of doing his Level II Fieldwork in this setting, what is required for him to pass the Fieldwork Performance Evaluation, and what accommodations will likely be or not be reasonable as an employee, the AFWC is meeting their ethical obligations of providing him with the information he needs to make a decision for his educational setting. This is critical information he might not have known about before considering this setting for fieldwork, and he is now empowered to make decisions about his educational experience (i.e., principle of *autonomy*).

5. *How would you navigate this challenging conversation with Adam?*
   Participants in this discussion may have varying responses.

CASE EXAMPLE 30.3. REASONABLE ACCOMMODATIONS

1. *Are the accommodations that Alex applied for reasonable? Why or why not (what information is needed to determine if they are reasonable)?*
   This case encompasses two very real scenarios: Practitioners who develop a disability after they have become established practitioners, and practitioners who have depression and anxiety. Alex is an autonomous person with freedom to exercise choice and self-direction and ultimately has the right to decide whether to disclose or apply for accommodations, even if choosing not to have an accommodation could lead to probation or termination at work. People discussing this case may have a variety of responses to Adam's requests for flexible scheduling, proofreaders for documentation, and immunity from previous safety incidents. Organizational policies and local laws may need to be consulted to determine whether these accommodations are reasonable. Human resources (HR) could be a great help in determining Alex's rights to accommodation.

2. *What standards of conduct do you think apply to this situation?*
   Alex's employer must maintain the confidentiality of all verbal, written, electronic, augmentative, and nonverbal communications to comply with the Code and applicable laws, including HIPAA. Alex's boss must also consider the principle of *justice* and the standard in the Code that requires occupational therapy practitioners to be familiar and comply with institutional rules and federal laws, which in this case is ADA. Additionally, the ethical principle of *autonomy* applies to Alex having the right whether to disclose. Alex's boss must therefore refrain from forcing Alex to disclose and must provide reasonable accommodations. The only thing the employer can do is remind Alex how to apply for reasonable accommodation. By providing Alex with access to policies and procedures of the site, the employer is fulfilling their ethical obligation outlined in the Code by informing employers, employees, colleagues, students, and researchers of applicable policies, laws, and official documents. Given that Alex's performance has resulted in safety issues, it is imperative that Sam follow the standard in the Code that requires them to gather information in an honest,

(Continued)

CASE EXAMPLE 30.3. REASONABLE ACCOMMODATIONS *(Cont.)*

fair, accurate, respectful, and timely way about Alex's performance. Because Alex's disabilities are resulting in safety issues, there are indicators that clients are at risk, and therefore Sam has an obligation to protect the clients as outlined in the Code and avoid inflicting harm or injury to recipients of occupational therapy services. Although it is natural for Sam to be empathetic to Alex's situation, it is more important for Sam to follow the ethical obligations outlined by the Code.

3. *What federal laws apply to this scenario?*
   - *Family and Medical Leave Act (FMLA):* FMLA allows eligible employees to take up to 12 weeks of unpaid, job-protected leave in a 12-month period for specific family and medical reasons, including the employee's own serious health condition or the serious health condition of a family member. In this case, Alex used FMLA for personal reasons. FMLA protects the employee's job during the leave period.
   - *ADA:* ADA prohibits discrimination on the basis of disability and requires employers to provide reasonable accommodations to qualified employees with disabilities. In this scenario, when Alex disclosed the diagnosis of depression and anxiety, it triggered ADA protections.

4. *Did the workplace meet its ethical obligations to support Alex's disability leading up to this point?* When Alex first returns to work, Sam is understandably compassionate and recognizes that Alex might be having a hard time returning to work. The Code comes into play when that empathy ultimately starts to put clients in harm's way. In this specific case, since Alex never applied for any reasonable accommodations, Alex remained on probation. The HR office let Alex know that previously having a disability without accommodations was not enough to prevent probationary action but that Alex was welcome to apply for other accommodations at this time. After working with HR through the interactive process, Alex recognizes that the presence of depression and anxiety now required more time for documentation and additional support with scheduling. Together, Alex, Sam, and HR came up with accommodations that supported Alex's needs, were reasonable for the site, and did not result in an undue burden on coworkers.

Section 6. Communication

CHAPTER 31. ETHICAL COMMUNICATION

CASE EXAMPLE 31.1 CLIENT INTERACTION

1. *How did Janelle's paraverbal and nonverbal communication impact her interaction with the child's mother?*
   - *Paraverbal communication:* Janelle's tone of voice and speaking slowly and enunciating every syllable when addressing the mother indicated condescension and impatience. Her tone and manner of speaking conveyed a lack of respect for the mother's ability to understand and communicate effectively in English.

(Continued)

CASE EXAMPLE 31.1 CLIENT INTERACTION *(Cont.)*

- *Nonverbal communication:* Janelle's nonverbal cues, such as rolling her eyes, using offensive gestures (like pointing to herself and the child), and her body language (sitting on the floor without consent) all contributed to the mother's perception of disrespect and insensitivity.

2. *What standards of conduct from the Code did Janelle violate?*
   - *Demonstrate a level of cultural humility, sensitivity, and agility:* Janelle failed to respect the mother's cultural background by not seeking permission before entering the house and starting to interact with the child. She also did not consider how her actions and gestures might be perceived based on the mother's cultural background and life experiences.
   - *Provide services that are culturally sensitive; provide evaluation and intervention specific to their needs:* Janelle displayed a lack of respect for the mother by speaking to her condescendingly, using offensive gestures, and assuming a lack of English proficiency. These actions violated the core value of dignity and the ethical principle of *autonomy* by not respecting the parent's right to make informed choices about their child's care.
   - *Respect and honor the expressed wishes of recipients of service:* Janelle's communication style and use of sarcastic language violated honoring the mother's wishes. She failed to establish a rapport with the mother, which is crucial in providing early intervention services.
   - *Respect the client's autonomy and establish a collaborative relationship with them:* Janelle must learn to work with clients and family members to create therapeutic, collaborative relationships.

3. *What action(s) do you think Janelle and the supervisor should take to avoid situations like this in the future?*
   Participants may discuss several outcomes. Some possibilities include:
   - *Self-reflection and awareness:* Janelle should reflect on her own biases and assumptions and work on increasing her cultural sensitivity and awareness. She needs to recognize the importance of respecting cultural differences and understanding the impact of her paraverbal and nonverbal cues.
   - *Cultural sensitivity training:* Janelle should undergo training in cultural sensitivity to better understand and interact with individuals from diverse cultural backgrounds. This training can help her develop the skills necessary to build rapport and trust with families from different cultural backgrounds.
   - *Effective communication training:* Janelle should participate in training for effective communication, emphasizing the importance of empathy, active listening, and respectful language. This training should focus on building positive relationships with the families she serves.
   - *Apologize and rebuild trust:* Janelle should reach out to the mother to apologize for her behavior and express her commitment to improving her approach. Rebuilding trust may take time, but acknowledging her mistakes is a crucial first step.
   - *Supervisory guidance:* The supervisor should provide ongoing guidance and support to Janelle, monitoring her interactions with families, and helping her improve her cultural sensitivity and communication skills.
   - *Assigning cases based on cultural sensitivity:* The supervisor should consider assigning cases to practitioners who have demonstrated cultural sensitivity and the ability to work effectively with families from diverse backgrounds.

CASE EXAMPLE 31.2. PROFESSIONAL COMMUNICATION

1. *How did Dr. Avery's verbal, paraverbal, and nonverbal communication affect the professional–student relationship?*
   - *Verbal communication:* Dr. Avery's use of incorrect gender pronouns when referring to Shea demonstrated a lack of respect for their gender identity, which is unprofessional and disrespectful. Additionally, Dr. Avery's comments about Ling's quiz performance conveyed microaggression, and his negative comments about Marcus and Carson's work were not constructive and could have been phrased more diplomatically.
   - *Paraverbal communication:* Dr. Avery's fast and loud speech, along with his use of acronyms that the students hadn't learned, created a challenging and intimidating environment for the students. This paraverbal style made it difficult for the students to engage effectively in the conversation.
   - *Nonverbal communication:* Dr. Avery's nonverbal cues, such as standing and walking around, crossing his arms, and making a thumbs-down gesture, conveyed a sense of dominance and judgment. These behaviors can be perceived as hostile and unapproachable.
2. *What standards of conduct from the Code did Dr. Avery violate?*
   - *Dignity and autonomy:* Dr. Avery's critical and judgmental comments toward Ling, Marcus, and Carson did not respect the dignity and autonomy of the students, because it undermined their self-esteem and their agency as students.
   - *Diversity and promoting inclusivity:* Dr. Avery failed to respect Shea's gender identity by misgendering them, which is not in alignment with this standard. Dr. Avery made assumptions about Ling based on cultural stereotypes.
   - *Autonomy and privacy:* Dr. Avery failed to respect the students' privacy by talking about academic performance in front of the other students.
3. *Using an ethical decision-making framework, what course of action do you think the program director should take with the students and with Dr. Avery?*
   - *Gather:* The program director should meet with the students to learn more about the situation. The program director should also consult institutional policies, the Code, and other relevant professional documents. They may consider consulting with the Title IX office at the university.
   - *Identify:* The program director should document specifically how Dr. Avery violated policies and the Code.
   - *Prioritize:* The program director must consider the possible courses of action, the targeted outcome of any action, and the most likely course of action that would lead to the desired outcome.
   - *Implement:* Possible actions may include meeting with Dr. Avery to discuss the concerns raised by the students and provide feedback on his behavior during the meeting. Dr. Avery should be made aware of the specific instances where his behavior was inappropriate and the impact it had on the students. The program director should offer Dr. Avery training and support to improve his communication and interpersonal skills. This could include sensitivity training, diversity and inclusion training, and effective communication workshops to help him interact more professionally and respectfully with students. Dr. Avery should apologize to Shea for the misgendering, and offer a sincere apology to Ling, Marcus, and Carson for his critical comments.

(Continued)

CASE EXAMPLE 31.2. PROFESSIONAL COMMUNICATION *(Cont.)*

Making amends could involve providing additional support, such as additional tutoring or resources, to help them improve their performance.

- *Feedback:* The program director should monitor and document Dr. Avery's progress and interactions with students to ensure that he is making efforts to change his behavior and communication style. This may involve a performance improvement plan and regular feedback. After reflection, the program director may also want to explore further actions to create a supportive and inclusive environment for all students, ensuring that they feel safe and respected.

CHAPTER 32. ETHICS AND SOCIAL MEDIA

CASE EXAMPLE 32.1. SHARING CLIENT INFORMATION

1. *What standards of conduct may have been violated?*
   The principle of *autonomy* and standards for maintaining privacy were violated. Posting pictures of clients, even if they are smiling and having a good time, on a public platform like Instagram without obtaining proper consent violates the clients' right to autonomy, confidentiality, and privacy. Additionally, Janine's Instagram post is well-intentioned but blurs the line between her personal and professional life and could be seen as a violation of the standard admonishing practitioners not to engage in dual relationships. Janine may have damaged public trust in occupational therapy as a profession, violating the standard for not engaging in damaging actions.

2. *What do you think is the appropriate course of action?*
   For the families who requested to be moved to another practitioner, Janine should apologize to the affected families, acknowledge her mistake in posting pictures without proper consent, and assure them that she values their trust and privacy. She should also work with the clinic to facilitate the transfer of these families to another practitioner. For the families transferring to another clinic, Janine should also apologize and express understanding for their decision to transfer. It is essential to maintain professionalism and goodwill, as these families may encounter other practitioners in the future.

3. *Which type(s) of dilemmas do you think were illustrated?*
   An integrity dilemma surfaced when privacy and confidentiality laws were violated by posting photos of clients without written consent. This ethical dilemma focuses on autonomy and justice. These principles conflicted with Janine's exuberance and attempt to show fidelity to her new colleagues and clients.

CASE EXAMPLE 32.2. BLURRING WORK AND PERSONAL LIFE

1. *What standards of conduct may have been violated?*
   The coworkers' participation in a protest with anti-LGBTQ+ signs and hateful messages goes against the core value of respecting diversity and justice, a principle that requires occupational therapy practitioners to provide a safe and inclusive environment for all clients. Professional civility standards for creating inclusive and respectful dialogue and for demonstrating cultural humility were not observed. Participating in such a protest while wearing their company's insignia on their polo shirts blurs the line between personal activities and professional conduct, violating the standard for maintaining professional boundaries. There is also the potential for reducing the public's trust in the employer and the profession of occupational therapy.

2. *What do you think is the appropriate course of action for each scenario?*
   Roger and his friend who discovered the Instagram post should express their concerns and feelings to their coworkers if they are comfortable doing so. They can communicate their discomfort with the coworkers' actions and have an open dialogue to understand their perspective. Depending on the outcome of this conversation, they can decide whether they want to continue working with them. The coworkers who were terminated should reflect on their actions and their impact on their professional reputation and the clients' trust. If they genuinely regret their participation in the protest and are willing to learn from this mistake, they may consider apologizing to their former employer and coworkers. They should also take this opportunity to educate themselves about the importance of respect for diversity and maintaining professional boundaries. The company should respect the clients' choices and assign them to other health care professionals who do not have a history of participation in such protests. It is crucial to ensure that the clients' comfort and well-being are prioritized.

3. *Which type(s) of dilemmas do you think were illustrated?*
   A speech dilemma emerged when two employees were captured in a social media post that exposed behavior that was not aligned with civility. The coworkers' participation in a protest with hate messages created an ethical dilemma, because it involved the conflict between their personal beliefs and their professional responsibilities to respect diversity and provide quality care to all clients.

CASE EXAMPLE 32.3. SHARING WORKPLACE FRUSTRATIONS

1. *What standards of conduct may have been violated?*
   Sara's TikTok post, in which she used derogatory language and danced suggestively while mentioning her supervisor and a resident by name, clearly violated the standard in the Code not to engage in communication that is derogatory or insensitive. These actions were disrespectful and unbecoming of a health care professional. By mentioning a resident's name in a negative context in a public video, Sara violated the principle of *autonomy,* including confidentiality. This action breaches the trust between health care providers and clients, violating the standard admonishing practitioners to refrain from actions that reduce the public's trust in occupational therapy. Sara's actions showed a lack of ethical behavior by ridiculing her supervisor and a resident. It is unethical

(Continued)

CASE EXAMPLE 32.3. SHARING WORKPLACE FRUSTRATIONS *(Cont.)*

to make disparaging comments about colleagues and clients in a public forum. Sara's impatience and frustration with residents during the day demonstrated a lack of respect for their dignity (core value) and autonomy (ethical principle).

2. *What do you think is the appropriate course of action?*

Belinda, as Sara's supervisor, should address the issue immediately. She should discuss the inappropriate TikTok video and confront Sara about her unprofessional behavior and attitude at work. This conversation should be constructive and aimed at helping Sara understand the seriousness of her actions. Belinda should review the professional conduct and ethical expectations of occupational therapists and the facility's policies with Sara. She should emphasize the importance of confidentiality, respect for dignity, and professionalism. Sara should consider making a public apology for her unprofessional TikTok video and remove it from her account. This will help mitigate some of the damage done to the facility's reputation. Sara should be required to undergo additional training and education to improve her understanding of professional conduct, ethics, and therapeutic relationships. This may help her learn from her mistakes and become a more responsible practitioner. The facility and the AFWC from Sara's educational program may need to take disciplinary action against Sara for her unprofessional behavior and violation of standards of conduct. This could include a formal warning, additional training, or even termination from her Level II Fieldwork placement.

3. *Which type(s) of dilemmas do you think were illustrated?*

A tempo dilemma appeared when an occupational therapy student posted content with the click of a button and without thought to professionalism. She now must grapple with the consequences of her unethical behavior carried out in the heat of the moment.

CHAPTER 33. OCCUPATIONAL THERAPY ETHICS ROUNDS IN PRACTICE

CASE EXAMPLE 33.1. SMOKING AS AN OCCUPATION

1. *How do you react to John's goal? Do you think it has the potential to cause ethical tension in the interprofessional team? Why or why not?*

A variety of answers are possible in response to this scenario, ranging from strong opposition to John's smoking to believing that if John wants to smoke, he should not be forced to quit against his will and the occupational therapy practitioner should help him achieve his goal. Because of this variety of reactions, this scenario could indeed lead to ethical tension in the interprofessional team.

2. *What ethical principles or standards from the Code are relevant to this case? Do any of the principles or standards conflict with each other?*

Principles from the Code that may be in conflict include the client's *autonomy* and right to make his own decisions about his life, and *beneficence,* or what is truly the best and most caring course of action in this situation. Multiple answers may apply.

(Continued)

CASE EXAMPLE 33.1. SMOKING AS AN OCCUPATION *(Cont.)*

3. *What is the role of interprofessional care in this case?*
   The team should discuss a plan so that they are unified in their approach to John's desire to smoke. They should include John and his family in the decision-making process, because they are also part of the interprofessional team.
4. *What resources exist to assist the occupational therapy practitioner in confronting this ethical dilemma?*
   Codes of ethics and facility policies on smoking may help with decision making. There may be a facility ethicist who can help mediate discussions with John and his family.
5. *What are the practitioner's potential next steps?*
   Discuss John's case with the person who can bring forward John's case at the next ethics rounds or team meeting. Provide a clear summary of the issues at hand and the questions John's case brings forward. Clarify that the team's actions in this case may inform the team approach in similar cases in the future.

CASE EXAMPLE 33.2. PRODUCTIVITY

1. *What challenges exist to meeting productivity standards in practice?*
   Discussions may bring up a variety of issues, since productivity standards vary from setting to setting.
2. *What other resources should the team seek to provide data and support for challenging existing productivity standards?*
   Resources may vary depending on the setting and may include investigating Medicare and private insurance guidelines and their impact on productivity, guidance documents provided by professional organizations on workload, *AOTA's Salary and Workforce Survey*, staff turnover in the setting, and other data showing the cost versus benefit of high productivity requirements in the setting.
3. *Using an ethical decision-making framework, what additional steps should the team take in addressing productivity standards?*
   The team should gather more information on why productivity is an issue in order to state the issue in factual terms; name ethical principles and standards as well as policies, procedures, guidance documents, and licensure laws that have a say in productivity standards; determine the team's goals for addressing this issue (reduce productivity requirements? request overtime pay? hire more help?); make a decision on a plan to act on the team's decision and carry out the plan; and reflect on the outcome and determine if the team's goal was achieved.
4. *How does the Code apply to the topic of productivity?*
   The Code addresses productivity and billing in several standards, including: bill and collect fees justly and legally in a manner that is fair, reasonable, and commensurate with services delivered; Ensure that documentation for reimbursement purposes is done in accordance with applicable laws, guidelines, and regulations; and do not follow arbitrary directives that compromise the rights or well-being of others, including unrealistic productivity expectations, fabrication, falsification, plagiarism of documentation, or inaccurate coding.
5. *What are the team's potential next steps? What strategies could the team employ to take their concerns to management?*
   A variety of answers may be discussed.

CASE EXAMPLE 33.3. PEDIATRIC TEAM AND FAMILY WISHES

1. *What are the ethical principles in conflict between the interprofessional team and the child's parents?*

   The team may be considering the principle of *nonmaleficence* in that they do not want to cause the child undue suffering, and *beneficence* to provide the most caring action they can for the child. The parents may also be focusing on beneficence because they want their child to live and have not yet been able to accept that their child will not survive their disease. They also want the right to make choices for their child (i.e., principle of *autonomy*).

2. *What resources might the team use in their ethical decision-making process?*

   This scenario would be an excellent situation in which to employ a medical ethicist to facilitate hard conversations between members of the health care team and between the health care team and the family. First, the health care team needs to discuss what would be the most caring response for this child; the physician may have given in to pressure from the parents to order therapies even though they do not believe rehabilitation is possible. Therapists could discuss their role in palliative care with the health care team and discuss what appropriate therapeutic intervention could look like for this child. In mediation with the family, the health care team could explain that they would re-evaluate the plan of care at every step in the process, and if the child's condition changes, they would certainly provide the most appropriate care needed in light of those changes. The family may also benefit from referral to social services and/or pastoral care.

3. *What additional information does the team need to achieve a plan of action with the child's parents?*

   This could include gathering more information from the parents regarding any religious or cultural needs; finding out what other team members are thinking and reaching team consensus; reading literature on palliative care; and involving other team members, such as chaplains and social workers.

Section 7. Professional Civility

CHAPTER 34. PROFESSIONAL CIVILITY

CASE EXAMPLE 34.1. WHAT'S YOUR NAME?

1. *Is this a case of vertical or lateral aggression?*

   This is a case of lateral aggression in which a peer bullies, demeans, or fails to provide support to colleagues.

2. *Why might these nicknames be offensive?*

   These nicknames appear to be related to the staff members' racial, ethnic, or gender identity characteristics.

3. *What standards of conduct from the Code can the three practitioners cite in their complaint?*

   The practitioners can cite the core values of equality and dignity, and the ethical principle of *fidelity,* all of which relate to treating all persons without bias, acting with cultural sensitivity and humility, and treating others with respect and integrity. Relevant standards of conduct include demonstrating courtesy, respect, cultural humility, and civility to persons, groups, and populations from diverse backgrounds.

CASE EXAMPLE 34.2. NOT NOW, CASEY

1. *Is this a case of lateral or vertical aggression?*
   This is a case of vertical aggression since Morgan is Casey's fieldwork educator and acting in a supervisory capacity.
2. *What standards from the Code do you think Morgan is violating?*
   This scenario reflects violation of the core values of altruism and dignity, as well as the ethical principle of *fidelity*, because Morgan was not concerned with Casey's welfare, did not value Casey's inherent worth, and did not treat Casey with respect or integrity. Standards of conduct that were violated include those related to providing appropriate supervision to Casey, ensuring that Casey was competent to provide services to clients of high acuity, and being accurate in evaluating Casey's performance. Instead, Morgan's feedback was vague and provided no clarification. Morgan addressed Casey in a manner that was intimidating, bullying, and perceived as a microaggression about one or more of Casey's characteristics (e.g., racial or ethnic origin; "you of all people").
3. *If you were the AFWC, how would you respond to Casey's request?*
   Participants' answers may vary. After meeting with Casey to discuss the issue, possible responses include meeting with Morgan and Casey together, meeting with Morgan alone, or meeting with Morgan and the director of the occupational therapy department at the hospital. If Casey and the AFWC felt that continuing at the facility could be detrimental to Casey's emotional health and not conducive to learning, the AFWC may choose to relocate Casey to another facility, despite the possible delay in graduation. Depending on the response from Morgan and the occupational therapy director, the AFWC may also choose not to place any further students with Morgan or at that facility.

CHAPTER 35. THE ETHICS OF DIVERSITY, EQUITY, INCLUSION, JUSTICE, ACCESS, AND BELONGING

CASE EXAMPLE 35.1. DEIJAB AND RESEARCH

1. *What are the ethical issues in this scenario?*
   The researcher's sample population is not representative of the target population, indicating a lack of diversity. This can lead to biased results and limit the generalizability of the assessment tool. The core value of equality requires that occupational therapy practitioners avoid bias. Additionally, the researcher has an ethical responsibility to conduct research that respects the dignity, autonomy, and needs of all potential participants, not just those from the majority group. The lack of diversity raises concerns about inclusivity and equity in research and practice. It may perpetuate disparities and contribute to the exclusion of underrepresented groups from the research process.
2. *What are the ethical principles and standards that apply?*
   Core values of equality, justice, and dignity apply. Principles of *autonomy* and *justice* apply. Standards related to inclusion and cultural sensitivity apply.
3. *Apply an ethical decision-making framework. What are the next steps the practitioner should take?*
   - *Gather:* Seek guidance and input from colleagues, experts, or community leaders who can provide insights on how to make the study more inclusive. Engage in a dialogue with the

(Continued)

CASE EXAMPLE 35.1. DEIJAB AND RESEARCH *(Cont.)*

Institutional Review Board (IRB) overseeing the research to discuss strategies for improving diversity and inclusion. The IRB may have recommendations or requirements to address these concerns.

- *Identify:* Determine the nature of the problem and the ethical issues at stake, including autonomy, justice, inclusion, and cultural sensitivity.
- *Prioritize:* Determine the desired outcome of the ethical decision-making process, which in this case would involve ensuring the validation of the assessment tool included addressing diverse populations.
- *Implement:* The researcher should review their recruitment strategies and try to diversify the sample population. This may involve reaching out to underrepresented communities and collaborating with community organizations to enhance recruitment efforts. They should also seek guidance and input from colleagues, experts, or community leaders who can provide insights on how to make the study more inclusive and appealing to a broader range of participants. They could consider collaborating with researchers who have expertise in recruiting underrepresented populations to ensure a more diverse and inclusive sample. They could modify the research plan to address the lack of diversity, which may include extending the recruitment period, targeting specific demographic groups, or adjusting the inclusion criteria. If these courses of action are not possible at this late stage in the research process, the researcher should be transparent about the limitations of the current sample and provide a clear description of the recruitment process, acknowledging the lack of diversity.
- *Feedback:* The researcher should consider this incident and make a commitment to ongoing efforts to enhance diversity and inclusion in future research endeavors and acknowledge the importance of representative samples in research validity and generalizability.

CASE EXAMPLE 35.2. EQUALITY VS. EQUITY

1. *How did Professor Taylor's actions affect the students? Does it matter that Professor Taylor had only good intentions?*
   Professor Taylor's actions had a negative impact on the students, regardless of their good intentions. By scheduling events that conflicted with the religious obligations of Jewish and Adventist students, Professor Taylor created an environment that was not inclusive or accommodating, making affected students feel excluded and disrespected. Requiring synchronous discussions late in the evening can be challenging for students with child care responsibilities, making it difficult for them to balance their academic and family responsibilities. This places an undue burden on these students and may affect their academic performance and well-being. Requiring students to drink thickened liquid during Ramadan, when Muslim students are fasting, is highly insensitive and can be distressing for those students. It demonstrates a lack of cultural sensitivity and understanding of diverse religious practices. Randomly assigning seats during an exam without considering the needs of students with visual, hearing, or attention difficulties shows a lack of consideration for their individual needs and potential academic disadvantages. Requiring students to wear bathing suits

(Continued)

CASE EXAMPLE 35.2. EQUALITY VS. EQUITY *(Cont.)*

without considering the feelings and distress it may cause to a transgender student is a violation of their dignity and autonomy. It creates an unwelcoming and insensitive learning environment.

2. *Which standards from the Code were violated?*
   - *Beneficence:* Professor Taylor failed to consider the well-being and best interests of the students in these situations.
   - *Justice:* There were issues of fairness, inclusivity, and cultural sensitivity in Professor Taylor's actions, indicating a violation of the principle of justice.
   - *Autonomy:* Several scenarios demonstrated a lack of respect for the dignity and autonomy of students, including those with religious beliefs, family responsibilities, disabilities, and gender identities.
   - *Maintaining competence:* Professor Taylor's actions showed a lack of competence in understanding and accommodating the diverse needs of students.
   - *Treating students professionally and equitably:* Professor Taylor did not provide an inclusive learning environment for students with disabilities, students from marginalized groups, and for students with varying socioeconomic backgrounds.

3. *How could the distress and harm caused to the students have been avoided?*
   The distress and harm caused to the students could have been avoided by practicing flexibility, considering individual needs, and taking an inclusive and sensitive approach. Professor Taylor could have provided alternative scheduling options for students with religious obligations, family responsibilities, or fasting requirements, so they could participate without conflicts. They could tailor teaching and assessment methods to accommodate the individual needs of students with disabilities, such as providing appropriate seating arrangements and alternatives to video-based exams. They could also demonstrate sensitivity to the experiences and feelings of all students, including those with diverse gender identities, and avoid activities that may cause distress. In the case of the lab with bathing suits, Professor Taylor could find other ways to simulate ADLs, such as having students wear form-fitting clothing or asking for a few volunteers to play the role of the clients.

4. *What should Professor Taylor do now to repair their relationship with the students?*
   Professor Taylor should apologize to the affected students for the insensitivity and harm caused by the previous actions and acknowledge that the intention was not enough to justify the impact on the students. They should encourage open dialogue with students to understand their concerns and needs better, and actively involve them in finding solutions for future events and coursework. Professor Taylor should fulfill the requirement to attend diversity, equity, and inclusion training to gain a better understanding of inclusivity, cultural sensitivity, and diversity in education and health care. Finally, Professor Taylor should ensure that future activities and requirements consider the diverse needs of all students and are more inclusive and accommodating and take proactive steps to create a learning environment that values diversity, respects individual needs, and fosters inclusion and equity.

CASE EXAMPLE 35.3. BELONGING

1. *What are the specific ways marginalization impacts Yvette?*
    a. In the profession of occupational therapy?
    b. In her career?
    c. Among her colleagues?

    Yvette experienced marginalization through barriers related to language and cultural differences, including lack of recognition and appreciation for unique attributes such as her culture and linguistic skill set; lack of recognition of her academic accomplishment as having both a Bachelor of Science and the credential of an occupational therapy assistant; lack of recognition as evident through minimal financial compensation; and perhaps discrimination due to her identity as Afro-LatinX woman. Lack of belonging creates a sense of isolation caused by marginalization within the workplace.

2. *How might the intersectionality of Yvette's identities contribute to her nuanced experience of harm in this scenario?*

    Yvette's diverse intersectionality as an Afro-LatinX, Spanish-speaking woman from a low-income background creates layers of challenges that contribute to her experiences of harmful exclusion. Diversity should be celebrated, not criticized, because consumers of occupational therapy services benefit from an inclusive and diverse mix of practitioners. By embracing diversity of culture, language, and spirituality, these experiences will be minimized and will benefit the profession.

3. *What steps could Yvette take to feel a sense of belonging? What steps could her colleagues take?*

    To create a sense of belonging, Yvette and the organization could:
    *   Encourage open conversations about experiences and concerns with colleagues and supervisors/administrators.
    *   Create inclusive policies and procedures within the department and organization.
    *   Recruit diverse staff, students, and volunteers
    *   Promote understanding of various cultures through culturally focused activities, discussions, seminars
    *   Identify safe and supportive groups that can provide mentorship, counseling, validation, and DEIJAB advocacy efforts.
    *   Engage in mindful habits, such as meditating or praying, breathing exercises, stretching or yoga, using time off, taking mental health breaks, or reciting positive affirmations for self-promotion and protection.

4. *What can be done to address and reduce marginalization of emerging majority or emerging minority practitioners in occupational therapy?*

    Methods to address and reduce marginalization take a combination of effort between those marginalized and those creating the marginalization as evidenced by micro and macro aggressions. Various steps include equitable and fair compensation, professional development, diverse and inclusive policies at a departmental and organizational level to eliminate various forms of discrimination and systemic racism, and creation of safe spaces and opportunities to report discrimination or biases without reprisal. These are just a few strategies that can be adopted in the profession to foster employment and education spaces that will help create more diverse, equitable, and inclusive environments and communities. A population shift is taking place in which the White population will become minor to Black, Indigenous, and people of color (BIPOC) populations. These populations include, but are not limited to, Black, Hispanic/Latin, Asian, and other diverse cultures. Being aware of these cultural shifts in one's geographic region may help occupational therapy practitioners remain culturally sensitive.

CHAPTER 36. WHEN ETHICS AND LAWS CONFLICT IN POLARIZING POLITICAL TIMES

CASE EXAMPLE 36.1. CONFIDENTIALITY VS. MANDATORY REPORTING

1. *Apply an ethical decision-making framework to this scenario. What are the ethical issues to consider?*
   Once a practitioner has identified an ethical problem or dilemma, a decision-making framework can facilitate their analysis of the situation. The process should involve gathering the relevant facts, considering additional information and resources, determining alternatives for action, choosing the best course of action, and evaluating the results of the action or outcome. The practitioner in this scenario is caught between the law, or justice, and upholding autonomy and confidentiality for the client. Examining this issue from the perspective of an ethical decision-making framework may help the practitioner make a rational decision rather than an emotional one.

2. *What resources can the occupational therapy practitioner consult to help make a decision?*
   The practitioner should check organizational policies and association documents, and they should thoroughly read state and local law.

3. *What options does the occupational therapy practitioner have? What are the potential consequences of each option?*
   Options could include stay silent and risk personal jeopardy, discuss the law with the student and her mother, report the abortion and risk criminalization of the mother and student, and read the law carefully for any provisions for confidentiality and try to find another option.

4. *Choose an option and reflect on possible outcomes. Which ethical principle(s) would this option uphold?*
   Many possible responses may be included. A practitioner could personally believe abortion is wrong but still not want to criminalize the student. The practitioner could choose to uphold the principles of *autonomy* and *beneficence,* at risk of personal consequences. A careful reading of the law may indicate that the consequences would entail fines. The practitioner should seek an attorney and be prepared to challenge the law in court. If the school system is willing to support the practitioner, this could help the practitioner in challenging the law.

CASE EXAMPLE 36.2. DISCRIMINATION AND BARRIERS TO ACCESS

1. *Apply an ethical decision-making framework to this scenario. What are the ethical issues to consider?*
   The ethical principles of *beneficence,* providing due care, and *justice,* following the letter of the law, are in conflict. Further, the standards for addressing barriers to services, reporting discriminatory systems, and addressing systems that limit access to services are in jeopardy.

2. *What are the issues regarding discrimination and bias in this case?*
   The client is being discriminated against because of their ethnic and socioeconomic status. This discrimination goes against the core values of the profession, including altruism and justice, and against the ethical principle of *beneficence.* Other values, principles, and standards may also apply.

3. *What resources can the occupational therapist access to make a determination for what to do in this case?*
   The occupational therapist may check with institutional policies and resources, including possible funds from a foundation for persons unable to pay for services. They might also check with community resources or the client's past employer for potential resources to assist them in their care.

4. *Choose an option and reflect on possible outcomes. Which ethical principle(s) would this option uphold?*
   Many possible responses may be included.

Index

Note. Page numbers in *italic* indicate exhibits, figures, and tables.

A

abandonment. *See* client abandonment

abortion, 351, 352, 354, 406

ACA (Affordable Care Act, 2010), health disparities, 101

academic course content, plagiarism, 133, 361

academic fieldwork coordinators (AFWCs), 273–280

  AOTA Code of Ethics, 277, *277*

  billing and reimbursement, 275

  case example, 279, 387–388

  current areas of concern, 279, 387–388

  disabilities, 295–297, 390–393

  other AOTA documents, 278

  responsibilities, 273–274

  student responsibilities, 275–277

  tips, 278

academic rules and resources, plagiarism, 132

access

  defined, 342

  discrimination and barriers, 355, 406

accessibility

  disabilities, 290–291, 297, 393–394

  justice, 157, 158

  organizational ethics, 185

  private practice, 220–221

accommodations

  fieldwork education, 276–277

  reasonable, 290–291, 297, 393–394

accountability

  organizations, 185

  private practice, 219

Accreditation Council for Occupational Therapy Education (ACOTE) standards, 273–274

ACE (Aid to Capacity Evaluation), *62*

ACLS–5 (Allen Cognitive Level Screen), 80

ACOG (American College of Obstetricians and Gynecologists), physician-patient relationship, 352

acronyms, 307

action, ethical reasoning, 34

active learning strategies, 5–6

activities of daily living (ADLs), cognitive impairment, 55, 57

acute care setting, public health crises, 248, 382–383

AD (Alzheimer's disease), capacity assessment, 65

ADA. *See* Americans with Disabilities Act (ADA, 1990)

administrative supervision

  AOTA Code of Ethics, 282–284, *283*

  case example, 285, 388–389

  defined, 281, 282

  other AOTA documents, 284

  other standards, 284

  tips, 284–285

advance directives, 60, 61, 66

Advisory Opinions, 4, 5

advocacy

  governance, 113, *119*

  school setting, 47

  social justice, 158

affinity bias, 147

Affordable Care Act (ACA, 2010), health disparities, 101

AFWCs. *See* academic fieldwork coordinators (AFWCs)

AGB (Association of Governing Boards of Universities and Colleges), 112

aggression

  see also incivility

  vertical and lateral, 331, 332–333, 336–337, 401–402

AI (artificial intelligence), 131, 197

AIDET acronym, 262

Aid to Capacity Evaluation (ACE), *62*

Allen Cognitive Level Screen (ACLS–5), 80

altruism

  AOTA Code of Ethics, 9, 31, *75*

  civility, 334

  health care crises, 244–245

Alzheimer's disease (AD), capacity assessment, 65

ambassadorship, governance, 113, *119*

mandatory reporting, *vs.* confidentiality, 354, 406

marginalization, 343–344, 348, 405

MCI (Mild cognitive impairment), 65

media sharing, 311

Medicaid, health disparities, 102–103

medical records, accessing, 387

mental health diagnoses, as metaphors, 307

Mental Health Parity and Addiction Equity Act (MHPAEA, 2008), health disparities, 101

microaggressions, 147, 304–305, 331

Mild cognitive impairment (MCI), 65

Mini-Mental State Examination (MMSE), 64

mission, governance, 116, *119*

Montreal Cognitive Assessment (MoCA), 64, 65

moral agent, 19–20

moral code, 74

moral courage, 21–22

moral distress, 19–24

  background, 19–20

  case example, 24

  categories, 20–21

  communication, 22–23

  contributing factors, 20–21

  defined, 19, 20, 319

  educational strategies, 22

  ethical decision making, 15

  ethical leadership, 23

  ethics rounds, 23, 319–320

  healthy work environment, 23

  implications, 21

  learning activity, 24

  occupational therapy ethics rounds, 23

  organizational ethics, 186–187

  practical applications, 21–23

  public health crises, 242

  recognizing, 22

  research, 20, 22

moral injury, 165, 166

moral norms, 74

moral objection, 166

morality, defined, 3, 27

multiple perspectives, ethical decision-making framework, 17–18

N

name calling, vertical aggression, 332

National Board for Certification in Occupational Therapy (NBCOT)

  ethics outcomes and enforcement, 31–32

  ethics rounds, 322

  justice, equity, diversity, and inclusion (JEDI), 307–308, 346

  resources on communication, 305

  state licensure, 270, 385, 386

  technology-based interventions, 201

National Healthcare Quality and Disparities Report (Agency for Healthcare Research and Quality), 98

neuropsychological assessments, 64

nicknames, 336, 401

nonmaleficence

  cognitive impairment, 51, 52, 53, 57, 61, 68

  defined, 11, 81

  evaluation, *77*, 81–84

  governance, 116

  health care system, 28

  health disparities, 99

  informed consent, 260

  moral distress, 19

  private practice, 219

  related standards of conduct, 82

  school setting, *41*

nonverbal communication, 304, 395, 396

Nuremberg Code, 259

O

obsolete assessment tools. *See* outdated and obsolete assessment tools

occupational justice, 155–162

  AOTA Code of Ethics, 100, 158

  as core value, 10

  bringing about, 157–158

  case examples, 160–161

  defined, 156

  injustice issues, 156–157

  next steps, 161–162

  other AOTA documents, 159

  overview, 156

  tips, 160

  WFOT standards, 156, 159–160

occupational possibilities, 100

occupational therapy

  ethics, 30–32

  public health crises, 243–244

  regulating bodies, 178

occupational therapy assistants

  as occupational therapy managers. *See* administrative supervision

  collaboration, 282–287, *283*, 388–390

  supervision. *See* clinical supervision